PREFACE

Oncology is a fast-evolving field. The last decade had witnessed enormous, complex discoveries in cancer biology, genetics, mutations, diagnostics and new targeted biological therapies. The team of expert contributors to this book tried to present these major aspects including, cancer traits, exogenous factors of cancer, the biology of cancer, growth factors of cancer, signaling pathways of cancer and epigenetic factors of cancer, in a simple but, at the same time, using up to date information. The book will be a great resource for medical students, scientists, physicians and other healthcare professionals involved in cancer care and cancer research.

Faris Q.B. Alenzi
Professor of Immunology
College of Applied Medical Sciences
Prince Sattam Bin Abdulaziz University
Saudi Arabia

DEDICATION

I dedicate this book to those who lost their lives because of this disease. May Allah bless them all!

To,

Fatema S. Albady Alanazi

Talal H. Almosaieed Alanazi

Saeed A. Baqader

Abdulla S. Alsiary

Moqaeem A. Alanazi

Nadda F. Alhassainan

Shaikha A. Alhabrdi

Hawazn W. Alnaam

Halah F. Alnaam

Hanan G. Alanazi

Eida S. Alhussani

Fryah A.M. Alshammari

Abdulrahman Zekri

Ghaytha Alshammari

List of Contributors

Abdulaziz Bin Saeedan	College of Pharmacy, Prince Sattam Bin Abdulaziz University, Alkharj, Saudi Arabia
Abeer A. Alsofyani	King Abdullah International Medical Research Center, King Saud bin Abdulaziz University for Health Sciences, Jeddah, Saudi Arabia
Afaf Ahmed Aldahish	College of Pharmacy, King Khalid University, Abha, 62529, Asir, Saudi Arabia
Aisha Al Anazi	Department of Paediatrics, Division of Endocrine and Diabetes, Prince Sultan Military Medical City, Riyadh, Saudi Arabia
Amal Almohisen	King Saud University, Riyadh, Saudi Arabia
Baraa T. Alhajhussein	King Saud Bin Abdulaziz University for Health Sciences (KSAUHS), Jeddah, Saudi Arabia
Fahad Nasser Alonazi	Saudi Public Health Authority, Riyadh, Saudi Arabia
Hajir A. Al-Saihati	Department of Clinical Laboratory Sciences, College of Applied Medical Sciences, University of Hafr Al-batin, Hafr Al-batin, Saudi Arabia
Hanadi A. Katouah	Chemistry Department, Faculty of Applied Sciences, Umm Al-Qura University, 21955, Makkah, Saudi Arabia
Hanaa I. Sharaf	Chairperson of Molecular Pathology at King Saud Medical City, Riyadh, Saudi Arabia
Hesham Hamdy Amin	Hotat Bani Tamim General Hospital, Riyadh, Saudi Arabia
Hiba S. Al-Amodi	Department of Biochemistry, Faculty of Medicine, Umm Al-Qura University, P.O. Box 715, Makkah 21955, Saudi Arabia
Khalid A. Asseri	College of Pharmacy, King Khalid University, Abha 62529, Asir, Saudi Arabia
Kate Shearston	UWA Dental School, The University of Western Australia, Nedlands, 6009 WA, Australia
Majed H. Wakid	Department of Medical Laboratories Technology, Faculty of Applied Medical Sciences, King Abdulaziz University, Jeddah, Saudi Arabia
Mashael Al-Toub	Department of Clinical Laboratory Sciences, College of Applied Medical Sciences King Saud University, Riyadh, Saudi Arabia
Manjari Singh	Department of Pharmaceutical Sciences, College of Pharmacy, Assam University, Silchar (Assam), India
Mohd Nazam Ansari	College of Pharmacy, Prince Sattam Bin Abdulaziz University, Alkharj, Saudi Arabia
Najwa Mohamad Alsawi	Alhabib Hospital Group, Riyadh, Saudi Arabia
Omar Kujan	UWA Dental School, The University of Western Australia, Nedlands, 6009 WA, Australia
Rawiah A. Alsiary	King Abdullah International Medical Research Center (KAIMRC), WR King Saud Bin Abdulaziz University for Health Sciences (KSAU-HS), P.O. Box 9515, Jeddah, Saudi Arabia

Ravi Teja Chitturi Suryaprakash	UWA Dental School, The University of Western Australia, Nedlands, 6009 WA, Australia
Talat Abdullah Albukhari	Faculty of Medicine, Um Al Qura University, Makkah, Saudi Arabia
Waheed A. Filimban	Pathology Department, Faculty of Medicine, Um Al Qura University, Makkah, Saudi Arabia
Yazan Samih Said	King Fahad Specialist Hospital, Dammam, Saudi Arabia

CHAPTER 1

Introduction

Abdulaziz Bin Saeedan[1,*], Mohd. Nazam Ansari[1] and **Amal Almohisen[2]**

[1] *College of Pharmacy, Prince Sattam Bin Abdulaziz University, AlKharj, Saudi Arabia*

[2] *King Saud University, Riyadh, Saudi Arabia*

Abstract: Cancer is a complex family of diseases that usually begins with carcinogenesis, in which abnormal cells divide or develop wildly by not following the regular path of cell division and likewise can invade nearby tissues. Cancer cells demonstrate transformations in metabolism, which is frequently more anaerobic than normal and probably can tolerate hypoxic surroundings. The remarkable variability of the disease, at all levels, is the major challenge for cancer medicine. Six biological abilities gained during the multi-stage advances of human tumors are the maintenance of proliferative signaling, the prevention of growth suppressors, cell death resistance, replicative immortality allowance, angiogenesis induction, invasion, and metastasis activation. In this chapter, we discuss the features of cancer cells and the epidemiology of cancer for better understanding.

Keywords: Cancer, Characteristics, Definition, Epidemiology, Features.

INTRODUCTION

The biological revolution of the 20th century completely redesigned all fields of biomedical knowledge, including cancer research. The revolution partially produced by Watson and Crick's finding of the DNA double helix, which began in the mid-century, and continues to this day [1]. Furthermore, understanding its true significance and its long-standing ramifications is still in process. The stream of molecular biology, derived from this finding, provided answers to the most insightful problem of 20th-century biology and described how the genetic structure of a cell or organism determines its outlook and function [2].

Like many other biological disciplines, modern cancer research would have remained a theoretical science if this molecular foundation did not exist. By exploiting the evolution in the sciences of molecular biology and genetics, many

* **Corresponding author Abdulaziz Bin Saeedan:** College of Pharmacy, Prince Sattam Bin Abdulaziz University, AlKharj, Saudi Arabia; E-mail: a.binsaeedan@psau.edu.sa

diverse biological phenomena, including cancer, currently have been partially explained. Surprisingly, it is also seen that most of the perceptions of the origins of malignant disease are out of the laboratory benches of cancer researchers. As a substitute, significant knowledge that drives the need to achieve rapid development in cancer research is delivered from the study of diverse organisms, ranging from yeast to worms to flies [3].

Definition

Cancer is a disease in which an assembly of abnormal cells divides or develops wildly by not following the regular path of cell division and likewise can invade nearby tissues. Persistent subjection of the normal cells to signals that control whether the cell should rest, divide into another cell or die. A degree of autonomy from these signals could result in uncontrolled growth and proliferation develops cancer cells. This could become lethal if this development continues and expands, leading to a major cause of cancer-related deaths owing to the spreading of tumors, and a procedure termed metastasis [4].

The concepts of modern cancer biology are based upon unpretentious principles. Fundamentally, all mammalian cells share analogous molecular networks that control cell proliferation, differentiation, and cell death. Ordinary cells are malformed into cancers as an effect of alterations in these networks at several levels, including the molecular, biochemical, and cellular ones. Such mechanisms for these changes are limited and can be determined.

In the past decade, phenomenal research developments in cancer have given us a perception of how cancer cells progress this autonomy. The present definition of cancer is that it is a disease that involves alterations or mutations in the cell genome. These alterations (DNA mutations) yield proteins that spoil the delicate cellular stability between cell division and quiescence, causing cells that keep multiplying to form cancers [5].

Characteristics of Cancer

Cancer is a complex family of diseases that usually begins with a process called carcinogenesis. Such a complex process involves converting an ordinary cell into a cancer cell in the body. The cancer cells display cellular and nuclear pleomorphic, then lose normal arrangement of cells, therefore developing alterations in the cell membranes and organelles, and hence exhibit abnormal mitoses and chromosomal abnormalities [6].

Intervallic cellular adhesiveness (for the solid surface) and contact inhibition (amid cells) may be the consequences of alterations in the cell surface glycoproteins and the underdeveloped tight junctions and desmosomes in malignant cells. Fluctuations in motility, adhesiveness, and contact inhibition possibly will promote invasion and the consequent formation of secondary malignant development metastasis.

Compared to a normal cell, cancer cells demonstrate transformations in metabolism. This metabolism of malignant cells is frequently more anaerobic than compared to normal hastily separating cells and is immensely speeded. Malignant cells can probably tolerate hypoxic surroundings. Glucose and amino acid uptake might be greater than before. These cells have extraordinary levels of hexokinase accumulation in their glucose consumption. In this scenario, the cancer cells lose the ability to synthesize specialized proteins distinct from segregated cells. Tumor growth is based on enzymes and other proteins produced by cancer cells [6].

The Hallmarks of Cancer

The remarkable variability of the disease at all levels, is the major challenge for cancer medicine. In the fall of 1999, Robert A. Weinberg and Hanahan depicted there were no credible organizational rules for the biological characteristics of tumors. In January 2000, they published an article "The Hallmarks of Cancer" to summarize these rules. The hallmarks of cancer constitute a fundamental belief that may deliver a rational basis for refining this complexity to better understand the mechanisms of the disease in its various manifestations [7].

For rationalizing the dynamics of neoplastic disorder, the hallmarks represent an organizing concept. Six biological abilities gained during the multi-stage advances of human tumors are the hallmarks of cancer. They comprise the maintenance of proliferative signaling, the prevention of growth suppressors, cell death resistance, replicative immortality allowance, angiogenesis induction, invasion, and metastasis activation. Underlying these hallmarks is genome instability, which produces the genetic variation which fast-tracks their acquisition, and inflammation, which nurtures several hallmark roles. Former era, conceptual advancement has added two emerging hallmarks of future generality to this list: energy metabolism reprogramming and evading immune destruction [7]. Apart from cancer, cell tumors demonstrate another measurement of complexity: they include a repertoire of engaged, ostensibly normal cells that contribute to the acquisition of hallmark characteristics by creating the "tumor microenvironment". Increasingly, awareness of the extensive application of these ideas will inspire the creation of innovative ways of treating human cancer.

The conceptualization includes eight acquired abilities-cancer hallmarks, and two generic neoplastic disease characteristics that promote their acquisition during the multi-stage neoplastic growth and malignant progression phase. Numerous cell types inhabiting the tumor microenvironment, including heterogeneous populations of cancer cells, especially cancer stem cells, and three prominent groups of stromal support cells, are part of integrating these hallmark competencies into the symptomatic disease. One assumption is that cancer hallmarks are a valuable heuristic method for determining the mechanistic basis and interrelationships between various types of human cancer with future cancer therapy applications [8].

Features of Cancer Cell

Cancers or Malignant neoplasms have numerous unique characteristics that facilitate the experimental cancer biologist or pathologist to distinguish them as not normal. Epithelium (The External or internal surfaces covering cells of the body) is the origin of the most common types of human neoplasms [9]. The sympathetic stroma of blood vessels and connective tissue are available in these cells. Malignant neoplasms may look similar to normal tissues in growth and development in the early stages. Neoplastic cells can grow in any body tissue that comprises cells with the capacity for cell division. Their cultivation rate is frequently based on the surrounding normal tissue and may cultivate fast or slowly. Though this is not a static feature, the degree of cell renewal in several normal tissues (such as hair follicles, bone marrow, and gastrointestinal tract epithelium) is as swift as that of a fast-developing tumor. Neoplasm means "novel growth", and is frequently mentioned and renamed with the word "tumor" to indicate a cancerous growth, to be more specific. Tumors can be classified into basic categories of two types: benign and malignant. The capability of classifying benign and malignant tumors is essential for providing appropriate treatment and prognosis for the patient with a tumor. The characteristics which differentiate a malignant tumor from that a benign tumor are as follows [10-12]:

1. Malignant tumors have the capability to invade and destroy neighboring normal tissue, whereas benign tumors develop by spreading out, do not attack surrounding tissue and are usually encapsulated. Benign tumors could become highly dangerous in certain cases. One of which is if the benign tumors press on nearby nerves or important blood vessels (might push aside normal tissue), or amend normal homeostatic mechanisms by releasing different biologically active elements, such as hormones.

2. Malignant tumors spread to other sites in the body using blood circulation or the lymphatic system and metastasize whereas, benign tumors remain localized and do not spread to other sites in the body.

3. Malignant tumor cells are likely to be "anaplastic", or scarcely distinguished from normal cells of the tissue in which they originate. Benign tumors typically

look like normal tissue when compared to malignant tumors. A few malignant neoplastic cells resemble the normal tissue at first structurally and functionally in which they originate. As the malignant neoplasm evolves in the course of time, it enters neighboring tissues, and metastasizes, and the malignant cells could look different from the original cell. The growth of a least distinguished malignant cell in a population of differentiated normal cells in some cases is called dedifferentiation. This word is possibly inaccurate for the procedure, due to the implication that a differentiated cell goes backward in its evolving procedure after carcinogenic abuse. The anaplastic malignant cell type is more likely to emerge from the posterity of a "stem cell" tissue (the one that continues to show renewal potential and cannot be completely differentiated) that has been choked or redirected in its course to form a fully differentiated cell. Examples of neoplasms that retain a differentiation modicum include pancreatic islet cell tumors that still make insulin, gland-forming colonic adenocarcinoma cells, such as epithelial structures and secrete mucin, and breast carcinomas that make abortive attempts to shape structures that imitate ducts of the mammary gland.

Conversely, the response controls handling normal tissue development or negative physiologic response handling hormonal secretion do not respond to Hormone producing tumors. For instance, in the face of severe hypoglycemia, and lung carcinoma-producing ectopic adrenocorticotropic hormone (ACTH), an islet cell tumor may continue to secrete insulin and possibly will continue to harvest ACTH while circulating levels of adrenocortical steroids are adequate to induce Cushing's syndrome. Many malignant neoplasms, predominantly the aggressively developing and invasive ones, only imprecisely look like their regular counterpart tissue structurally and functionally. Hence are believed to be "undifferentiated" or "badly differentiated."

4. Malignant tumors develop very quickly compared to benign tumors. Malignant tumors usually display signs of significant development with the association of neighboring tissue once they reach a clinically detectable stage, over weeks or months, while benign tumors have a slower rate of growth in years.

5. Normal cells need mitogenic growth signals before they can transit from a peaceful tranquil state to a dynamic proliferative state. Cancer cells encourage their own growth. Cancer cells may also change the integrins (extracellular matrix receptors) they express, favoring those that transmit pro-growth signals.

6. Cancer cells fight inhibitory signals that would otherwise halt their growth; however, anti-proliferative signals in normal tissues promote cell quiescence and tissue homeostasis. Cells could be forced out of the active proliferative cycle and into a peaceful (G0) state, from which they could reemerge when extracellular

signals allow. If cancer cells are to thrive inside the body, they must be able to evade these anti-proliferative signals.

7. When a cell is activated by a variety of physiologic signals, apoptosis is triggered in a series of steps in which cell membranes are disrupted, the cytoplasmic and nuclear skeletons are broken down, the cytosol is removed, the chromosomes are debased, and the nucleus is fragmented, all within 30–120 minutes. Cancer cells can develop resistance to apoptosis through a variety of methods. Cancer cells that have lost proapoptotic segments are more likely to hold others that are identical.

8. To keep dividing indefinitely, cancer cells need a mechanism to maintain their telomeric DNA (immortalization). Telomeres, like the rest of a chromosome that contains its genes, are DNA sequences — chemical code chains. Cells can divide 50 to 70 times on average, with telomeres becoming shorter and shorter before the cells become senescent or die. Before a cell may differentiate, it duplicates its chromosomes so that the genetic material of both new cells is indistinguishable. A chromosome's two DNA strands must unwind and split in order to be repeated. Telomerase is a naturally occurring enzyme that promotes the repair of telomeres. It is active in stem cells, germ cells, hair follicles, and 90% of tumor cells, but its expression in somatic cells is poor or non-existent. Telomerase adds bases to the ends of telomeres to make them longer. Telomere maintenance is evident in a wide range of cancer cells.

9. Blood vessels provide oxygen and nutrients, which are critical for cell capacity and survival. Angiogenesis, or the development of blood vessels, may be aided or hindered by the balance of positive and negative signals.

10. Metastases are responsible for 90% of cancer deaths in humans. Cancer cells with the ability to invade and metastasize can escape the primary tumor mass and colonize new territories in the body, where nutrients and space are not restricted at first.

Cancer cells have been shown to exploit angiogenesis to improve blood supply to the tumors. This represents a key step in tumor expansion.

Epidemiology of Cancer

The epidemiology of cancer is defined as the study of cancer's classification based on various aspects such as sex, age, economic status, *etc.,* and these features determine its dominance. In the past decade, the mortality from cancer has altered from a trivial to a major. In addition, it could be clearly seen that it differs from country to country and changes the cancer risk; variants of disease among geographic landscape shift significantly [13]. Causes of cancer vary based on personal hygiene to life style, for example, cigarette smokers proclaim to have a higher risk of cancer than non-smokers. One of the basic characteristic necessities for effective epidemiology classification is population-based cancer archives which provide the required graphic information on the population [14].

Cancer is already a major problem in different geographic locations, and lifestyle changes fundamentally mark the increasing rates. The available data projections show a rise in aging together with accelerating growth of population; this forecasts that the problem will emerge bigger in the future [15].

Cancer Epidemiology in the World

Classical epidemiologic studies have enlightened with various facts that gave influential aids to classifying the etiology of commonly known cancers. These contributions show there has been a substantive impact on public health. The best-known associations are smoking and lung cancer, and this has motivated cancer prevention initiatives and policy changes widely and spread successfully. In northern parts of America and Western parts of Europe in the midst of the last century, various studies based on lung cancer were published, leading to the assumption that smoking was a significant reason for lung cancer in 1950. Similarly, the chemical industry based in Brittan studied the influence of chemical exposure at the start of the 1950s [8]. At the same time, Cornfield [16] and Mantel *et al.* [17] influenced the methodologic and investigative objectives of the case-control study design. Subsequently, Substantial data on the etiologic roles of explicit lifestyle, viral, work-related, and dietary risk influences in a range of cancers have been provided through many group and case-control studies. The International Agency for Research on Cancer (IARC) weighed the potential of 900 likely candidates for the cancer-causing and classified them into the following clusters (IARC- Report 9) [18]:

- Cluster A: Carcinogenic to humans
- Cluster B1: Possibly carcinogenic to humans
- Cluster B2: Possibly a category of carcinogenic to humans
- Cluster C: Cannot be classifiable as carcinogenicity in humans
- Cluster D: Possibly not carcinogenic to humans

Even though there are a lot of recognized developments in this field of study, we still have a long way to go, as we are on the verge of developing molecular tools to discover these relations. Furthermore, environmental challenges have a direct effect on the genes due to interactions and might modulate genetic properties. DNA damaging could be caused due to environmental exposures and in addition to may also modify gene expression through epigenetic reversible mechanisms is increasingly being recognized as a fact.

Cancer Epidemiology in the Kingdom of Saudi Arabia

Cancer is the 2nd largest cause of death worldwide and is accountable for more than 9.6 million deaths in about 185 countries [19]. Studies reported in the past 25 years on cancer incidence in Saudi Arabia were limited because of the small number of cases 1-12 available in most investigations [20, 21].

The first epidemiological study of cancer which includes over 11,000 consecutive cases seen in one institution in Saudi Arabia (Table **1.1**). In 2018, there were 10,518 cancer-related deaths, and to add on, new cases found were 24,485 in Saudi Arabia amongst the whole population of 33,554,333 [22]. The commonly known cancers comprise breast cancer, colon-rectum (CRC), and prostate. The various cancers accounted for in the region of Saudi Arabia; some cancers magnitude epidemiology has risen drastically in recent years. This escalation might be endorsed to new policies and lifestyle adaptations in the Saudi population. Lack of knowledge and awareness of cancer, deficiency in screening & timely detection programs, and social barriers on the road to cancer investigations could be looked into with great importance. Apparently, risk factors for cancer in Saudi Arabia are due to obesity, iodine & Vit-D deficiency, genetics, use of tobacco, inactive lifestyle and viral infection [23, 24].

Table 1.1. First epidemiological study of cancer.

Duration of Study	Year	Author Reference	Region	No. of Cases Analyzed	Significant Findings
1950-1961	1963	Taylor	Eastern	264	Gastric cancer
1958-1962	1965	Froede & Mason	Western	106	Skin, thyroid
1953-1967	1970	Gelpi	Eastern	43	Lymphomas
1962-1973	1975	Perrine & Juma'a	Eastern	215	Thyroid, lung
10 years	1977	Sayigh *et al.*	Central	3251	Lymphomas, skin, gastrointestinal
3 years	1979	Sayigh *et al.*	Western	1000	Skin, breast, Lymphomas
1978-1981	1982	Amer	Central	1000	Lymphomas, gastrointestinal
1975-1978	1983	El-Akkad	Central	1696	Lymphomas, breast, esophagus
1974-1979	1983	Seraj & Sabbah	Central	136	Esophagus
1981-1982	1984	Koreich & Al-Kuhaymi	Central	297	Hodgkin's disease, thyroid
1981-1984	1985	Amer *et al.*	Central	68	Oral cancer and shamma usage

(Table 1.1) cont.....

Duration of Study	Year	Author Reference	Region	No. of Cases Analyzed	Significant Findings
1979-1984	1986	El-Akkad *et al.*	Nation	7251	Lymphomas, lung, esophagus, breast, thyroid

In recent years, Saudi Arabia has evolved tremendously due to rapid technological and economic development. The health resources have increased dramatically, and with enhancements in the national vaccination program and eventual control and reduction of communicable diseases, life expectancy is increasing and with it, the number of older people in the population. Hence, the incidence of chronic disease and cancer in Saudi Arabia will increase concurrently [25 - 27].

Cancer Registries

Cancer registries extract cancer-related clinical data from patient medical records. These registries provide data to state and national public health organizations in order to monitor cancer diagnosis and care patterns [28]. In the Kingdom of Saudi Arabia, Cancer Incidence Report is published annually by The Saudi Health Council (SHC), which is a collaborative effort by the team of the Saudi Cancer Registry (SCR). SCR is a population-based registry that seeks to identify cancer incidence, prevalence, and patterns in Saudi Arabia in order to aid clinical and epidemiological research and facilitate the assessment of appropriate national programs and activities such as cancer screening and early detection [29].

CONCLUSION

Cancer is a complex disease that usually involves alterations or mutations in the cell genome (carcinogenesis), leading eventually to uncontrolled growth, then invasion and metastasis. During recent decades, there has been a steep increase in cancer rates in most countries, making cancer one of the major health issues for health service providers. By exploiting the recent advances in cell and molecular biology technologies, many cancer development mechanisms can be revealed and understood, leading to the establishment of novel cancer therapeutic approaches.

CONSENT FOR PUBLICATION

Not applicable.

CONFLICT OF INTEREST

The author declares no conflict of interest, financial or otherwise.

ACKNOWLEDGEMENTS

The authors are thankful to Syed Nasrullah for his valuable help in writing this chapter.

REFERENCES

[1] Watson JD, Crick FHC. Molecular structure of nucleic acids; a structure for deoxyribose nucleic acid. Nature 1953; 171(4356): 737-8.
[http://dx.doi.org/10.1038/171737a0] [PMID: 13054692]

[2] Watson JD. The Double Helix: A Personal Account of the Discovery of the Structure of DNA. New York: Athenaeum Press 1968.

[3] Watson JD, Crick FHC. Genetical implications of the structure of deoxyribonucleic acid. Nature 1953; 171(4361): 964-7. https://www.nature.com/articles/171964b0
[http://dx.doi.org/10.1038/171964b0] [PMID: 13063483]

[4] Re'camier JC. Recherchessur le traitement du cancer sur la compression methodique simple oucombineeetsurl'histoiregenerale de la meme maladie. 2nd ed., 1829.

[5] Hart IR, Fidler IJ. Role of organ selectivity in the determination of metastatic patterns of B16 melanoma. Cancer Res 1980; 40(7): 2281-7.
[PMID: 7388794]

[6] Talmadge JE, Fidler IJ. AACR centennial series: the biology of cancer metastasis: historical perspective. Cancer Res 2010; 70(14): 5649-69.
[http://dx.doi.org/10.1158/0008-5472.CAN-10-1040] [PMID: 20610625]

[7] Hanahan Douglas, Weinberg Robert A. Hallmarks of cancer: the next generation 2011.
[http://dx.doi.org/10.1016/j.cell.2011.02.013]

[8] Case RAM, Hosker ME, McDonald DB, Pearson JT. Tumours of the urinary bladder in workmen engaged in the manufacture and use of certain dyestuff intermediates in the British chemical industry. I. The role of aniline, benzidine, alpha-naphthylamine, and beta-naphthylamine. Occup Environ Med 1954; 11(2): 75-104.
[http://dx.doi.org/10.1136/oem.11.2.75] [PMID: 13149741]

[9] Quintana E, Shackleton M, Sabel MS, Fullen DR, Johnson TM, Morrison SJ. Efficient tumour formation by single human melanoma cells. Nature 2008; 456(7222): 593-8.
[http://dx.doi.org/10.1038/nature07567] [PMID: 19052619]

[10] Loeb LA. Human cancers express mutator phenotypes: origin, consequences and targeting. Nat Rev Cancer 2011; 11(6): 450-7.
[http://dx.doi.org/10.1038/nrc3063] [PMID: 21593786]

[11] DeGregori J. Evolved tumor suppression: why are we so good at not getting cancer? Cancer Res 2011; 71(11): 3739-44.
[http://dx.doi.org/10.1158/0008-5472.CAN-11-0342] [PMID: 21610109]

[12] Yachida S, Jones S, Bozic I, *et al.* Distant metastasis occurs late during the genetic evolution of pancreatic cancer. Nature 2010; 467(7319): 1114-7.
[http://dx.doi.org/10.1038/nature09515] [PMID: 20981102]

[13] Watson A, Kent P, Alam M, *et al.* GLI1 genotypes do not predict basal cell carcinoma risk: a case control study. Mol Cancer 2009; 8(1): 113.
[http://dx.doi.org/10.1186/1476-4598-8-113] [PMID: 19948058]

[14] Helikar T, Konvalina J, Heidel J, Rogers JA. Emergent decision-making in biological signal transduction networks. Proc Natl Acad Sci USA 2008; 105(6): 1913-8.
[http://dx.doi.org/10.1073/pnas.0705088105] [PMID: 18250321]

[15] Natarajan M, Lin KM, Hsueh RC, Sternweis PC, Ranganathan R. A global analysis of cross-talk in a mammalian cellular signalling network. Nat Cell Biol 2006; 8(6): 571-80. [http://dx.doi.org/10.1038/ncb1418] [PMID: 16699502]

[16] Cornfield J. A method of estimating comparative rates from clinical data; applications to cancer of the lung, breast, and cervix. Am J Public Health Nations Health 1951; 41: 654-61. [http://dx.doi.org/10.2105/AJPH.41.6.654] [PMID: 18017295]

[17] Mantel N, Haenszel W. Statistical aspects of the analysis of data from retrospective studies of disease. J Natl Cancer Inst 1959; 22(4): 719-48. [PMID: 13655060]

[18] International Agency for Research on Cancer (IARC). Report of an IARC Working Group to Review the Approaches and Processes Used to Evaluate the Carcinogenicity of Mixtures and Groups of Chemicals. IARC Internal Technical Report No. 89/004, IARC, Lyon.

[19] Taylor JW. Cancer in saudi arabia. Cancer 1963; 16(12): 1530-6. [http://dx.doi.org/10.1002/1097-0142(196312)16:12<1530::AID-CNCR2820161204>3.0.CO;2-Q] [PMID: 14085266]

[20] Froede RC, Mason JK. Malignant disease of Aden Arabs. Cancer 1965; 18(9): 1175-9. [http://dx.doi.org/10.1002/1097-0142(196509)18:9<1175::AID-CNCR2820180917>3.0.CO;2-R] [PMID: 14332546]

[21] Gelpi AP. Malignant lymphoma in the Saudi Arab. Cancer 1970; 25(4): 892-5. [http://dx.doi.org/10.1002/1097-0142(197004)25:4<892::AID-CNCR2820250422>3.0.CO;2-1] [PMID: 4910127]

[22] Perrine RP, Juma'a A. Changing trends in cancer in Saudi Arabs. ARAMCO Medical Services Organization Epidemiology Bulletin 1975; (January): 1-4.

[23] Sayigh AA, Sebai ZA, Haleem A. Preliminary study of the solar radiation effect on skin cancer. Proceedings of the First Conference on the Biological Aspects of Saudi Arabia. Riyadh. 1977; pp. 185-95.

[24] Stirling G, Khalil AM, Nada GN, Saad AA, Raheem MA. Malignant neoplasms in Saudi Arabia. Cancer 1979; 44(4): 1543-8. [http://dx.doi.org/10.1002/1097-0142(197910)44:4<1543::AID-CNCR2820440456>3.0.CO;2-N] [PMID: 498028]

[25] Amer MH. Pattern of cancer in Saudi Arabia: a personal experience based on the management of 1,000 patients (part I). King Faisal Spec Hosp Med J 1982; 2(4): 203-15.

[26] El-Akkad S. Cancer in Saudi Arabia: a comparative study. Saudi Med J 1983; 4(2): 156-64.

[27] Amer MH. Epidemiologic aspects of esophageal cancer in Saudi Arabian patients. Ann Saudi Med 1985; 5(2): 69-77. [http://dx.doi.org/10.5144/0256-4947.1985.69]

[28] National Cancer Institute, "What is a Cancer Registry?" https://seer.cancer.gov/registries/cancer_registry/cancer_registry.html Last Viewed on May 10, 2021

[29] Saudi Health Council - National Health Information Center: Saudi Cancer Registry Cancer Incidence Report, Saudi Arabia 2015. https://nhic.gov.sa/eServices/Documents/E%20SCR%20final %206%20NOV.pdfLast Viewed on May 10, 2021

CHAPTER 2

Cancer Traits; Present and Future

Khalid A. Asseri[1,*] and **Afaf Ahmed Aldahish**[2]

[1] *College of Pharmacy, King Khalid University, Abha 62529, Asir, Saudi Arabia*

[2] *Pharmacology & Toxicology Department, College of Pharmacy, King Khalid University, Abha 62529, Asir, Saudi Arabia*

Abstract: This chapter on "Cancer Traits; Present and Future" begins with a description of the process of carcinogenesis and, finally, the abnormal process leading to carcinogenesis.

Cancer is a multi-step mechanism in which cells undergo biochemical and behavioral changes, causing them to proliferate in an unnecessary and untimely manner. These changes occur from modifications in mechanisms that regulate cell proliferation and longevity, relationships with neighboring cells, and the ability to escape the immune system. Modifications that contribute to cancer require genetic modifications that alter the DNA sequence. Another way to alter the program of cells is to adjust the conformation of chromatin, the matrix that bundles up DNA and controls its access through DNA reading, copying and repair machinery. These modifications are called "epigenetic. The abnormal process that leads to carcinogenesis includes early mutational events in carcinogenesis, microRNAs in human cancer and cancer stem cell hypothesis, Contact inhibition of proliferation, autophagy, necroptosis, signaling pathways, telomere deregulation, microenvironment, growth suppressors evasion, resisting cell death and sustained cell survival, enabling replicative immortality through activation of telomeres, inducing angiogenesis, ability to oppose apoptosis, and activating invasion and metastasis. Intensive research efforts during the last several decades have increased our understanding of carcinogenesis and have identified a genetic basis for the multi-step process of cancer development. Recognition and understating of the prevalent applicability of cancer cell characterization will increasingly affect the development of new means to treat human cancer.

Keywords: Angiogenesis, Apoptosis, Metastasis, Proliferation, Telomerase.

* **Corresponding author Khalid A. Asseri:** Pharmacology & Toxicology Department, College of Pharmacy, King Khalid University, Abha 62529, Asir, Saudi Arabia; E-mail: kaasseri@kku.edu.sa

Faris Q.B. Alenzi (Ed.)

INTRODUCTION

Mechanisms of Contact Inhibition and its Evasion

The term 'contact inhibition' denotes two separate but carefully related processes in cell biology, proliferation contact inhibition and locomotive contact inhibition, established by fibroblasts while in connection with each other. Fibroblasts, until they come into contact with a neighboring cell, they move about the culture dish surface. It leads to the inhibition of further cell migration, and regular cells attach each other, making a collection of cells on the culture dish. Around the surface of the culture dish, standard fibroblasts travel until they meet a neighboring cell. Regular cells bind to each other, and further cell migration is inhibited [1].

The elementary property (Contact inhibition of Proliferation (CIP)), by which cells stop to multiply and differentiate as allotted space is filled at the confluence point. CIP is upturned under conditions including augmented cell growth and proliferation, such as healing wounds or tissue regeneration and development of the embryo. However, CIP is absent in cancer cells, and the absence of this factor leads to tumorigenesis [2].

CIP is a regulatory process that helps prevent cells from expanding into a single cell layer of thickness. If the usable substrate space in the cell is more, it duplicates easily and travels liberally. This process will last until the cells surmount the entire substratum. Regular cells would avoid replicating at this stage. When motile cells come across the confluent cultures, they display diminished mitotic activity and mobility over time. Further, though mitotic inhibition occurs later, the ascending growth occurs between colonies in contact for several days. This delay between cell interaction and the initiation of inhibition of proliferation decreases as the culture becomes more mingled. Therefore, cell-cell contact is a necessary prerequisite for preventing the spread of contact but for mitotic inhibition, it is inadequate. In addition to interaction with further cells, under the restrictions and mechanical tension exerted by neighboring cells, the cell area of the contact-inhibited cell, reduces. Mechanical stress has also been proposed to serve as an inhibitory indication for mitosis. Also, mitotic inhibition is a spatial phenomenon that happens among a small number of cells in a potentially diverse population [3].

Unchanged human cells display natural cell activity and mediate their development and spread through interactions between signaling of growth factor, cell density and environmental nutrients. As cell density rises and uniform culture is formed, cell cycle arrest is activated, and mitogen signaling pathways are regulated independently of cell metabolism or external factors. This effect is known as CIP and is important for the suitable development of the embryo as well as for differentiation, morphogenesis and tissue recovery; CIP is one of the main deregulation mechanisms in transformed cells during tumorigenesis. Many cancer cells are unaffected by confluence-tempted proliferation. Several theories were suggested to clarify the beginning of contact-reliant development arrest, like the discharge of inhibitory composites, the part of cell form on nutritional fatigue or growth aspects or growth or in the culture medium. This results in the migration of adjacent tissues, their metastases to adjacent organs, and ultimately tumorigenesis [1].

Cell-cell interactions influence intracellular signaling trails, such as ERK and Akt, and cell cycle growth is inhibited. To receptors that ease cell bonds, such as E/VE-Cadherin, growth factor receptors, interact themselves. Also, by automatically bonding adjacent cells and disturbing the spreading of traction powers, cadherins avoid interaction in multicellular clusters. Family proteins of ERM, Atypical Cadherin, Fat and Merlin, are also a part of the Hippo pathway that has developed as unique key regulators for the determination of organ size in both mammalian systems and drosophila, and contact inhibition. The lack of immunity related to malignant cell contact suppression will be affected by a reduction in the bond between the disk surface and malignant cells. Also, it could be from a rise in adhesion amid the regular and malignant cells, representing the *vitro* substitute as contact inhibition to the method to keep normal tissue homeostasis *in vivo*. When faced with normal cells, the movement of malignant cells in a given direction is not inhibited. The passage of regular cells, on the other hand, is obstructed when it is met by cells of malignancy. The cells are more rounded and extended than the malignant ones, which are spindle-made. Rounding of the cell is perhaps the index of the cell absence of adhesion to the substrate. Gene activation is caused by Cell-cell contact [1].

Recently, the NF2 gene product has been recognized by Merlin that it is involved in the suppression of the binding of adhesion molecules to the tyrosine kinase transmembrane receptor. The adhesivity of Merlin improves Cadherin-linked cell-to-cell bonding, and by recapturing receptors of growth factors, its ability to produce mitogenic signals is condensed. The other way of inhibition includes the epithelial polarity protein (LKB1), which escapes the mitogenic properties of enhanced Myc oncogene in ordered epithelial structures; on the other side, when expression LKB1 is inhibited, epithelial reliability is weakened, leading to Myc-induced renovation.

Cell adhesion affects a variety of cell behaviors by providing a wide range of mechanical and biochemical signals for cells. The Hippo-YAP pathway, which is primarily responsible for hindering cell formation in mammals, is one such pathway. Mainly, this pathway consists of a phosphorylation cascade, which is serine kinases-based and controlled by regulatory proteins that regulate cell growth by attributing to growth-control genes. However, that contact inhibited cells experience cell cycle arrest, but do not become senescent. It has now been shown that contact-inhibited (CI) cells, when substituted in a less confluent culture, restore natural proliferation and mitogen signaling. CIP can therefore be seen as a reversible mode of cell cycle arrest [4].

In addition, the cells of CI must arouse growth-activating paths such as mTOR to move to senescence from cell cycle arrest. The adhesion formations activate mechanisms that control mitogen signaling and cell proliferation until cells in cultures of high-density converge adequate such that the cell area decreases below a critical value. Therefore, the mTOR pathway of growth-promotion is blocked, and the CI cells do not change from cell cycle arrest to senescence. In cancer therapy, this has important implications; while cancer cells are not CI, their senescence machinery is still suppressed by convergent cancer cell cultures [5].

MALIGNANCY SUPPORTED BY THE DEFECTS OF THE TGF-β PATHWAY

The transforming growth factor (TGF) pathway is a key participant in metazoan biology, and its disruption can lead to tumor formation. TGF-β evolved to control neural tissue, epithelial processes, the immune system, and the healing of wounds. Tumorigenesis is related to these critical regulatory roles of TGF-β. Virtually all forms of human cells are TGF-β sensitive. By controlling not only cellular differentiation proliferation, adhesion and survival, but also the cellular microenvironment. The incipient tumors are prevented by TGF-β from moving to malignancy by preserving tissue homeostasis. However, cancer cells can possibly resist the TGF-β pathway's oppressive effect as genetically dysfunctional entities. Abnormal types of TGF-β signaling ease immune surveillance evasion, tumor growth invasion, and metastasis and dissemination of cancer cells [6 - 8]. The risk factor for colorectal neoplasia can also be serum TNF-β since it is linked with many recognized risk factors such as smoking, adiposity, age, and an augmented occurrence of colorectal adenomas (Table **2.1).**

Table 2.1. TNF supporter polymorphisms and expression sites linked to malignant cancers.

TNF Expression	Type of Cancer
Tumor progression	cervical carcinoma, prostate cancer, and breast cancer
Reduced therapy response	breast and prostate cancer
Higher cancer risk	Barrett's adenocarcinoma
Decreased cancer risk	Lymphoma of B-cell

The inhibitory effects of TGF-β can be circumvented by malignant cells either by inactivating the main mechanism of the pathway, either by TGF-β receptors, or by changes that restrict specific ways of tumor-suppression. If the above form of bypassing is used, tumor cells can freely take advantage of the lasting TGF-β regulatory functions, acquire invasion ability, generate autocrine mitogens, or discharge premetastatic cytokines. Through receptor inactivation, decapitation of the TGF-β pathway will remove tumor inhibition, whereas amputation of the path that involves the growth-suppressive arm, not only eliminates growth suppression, but also makes additional tumor progression probability. The importance of TGF-β on the tumor stroma is also important, for the growth of cancer; TGF-β is a vital executor of tolerance of immune power and protects from immune surveillance by tumors that contain this cytokine in high levels. Faulty TGF-β responsiveness in immune cells, on the other hand, may result in chronic inflammation and the development of a pro-tumorigenic environment. Tumor-based TGF-β may utilize osteoclasts and myofibroblasts [6, 9].

For the entire TGF-β family, the receptor system is provided by five receptors of type II and seven receptors of type I paired in various mixtures. In the cytoplasmic area of these receptors, there is a serine/threonine kinase field. A switch for kinase activation is given by a small segment N-terminal only to the type I receptors kinase domain. The lively kinase core in the fundamental state is pushed against by the GS domain, repressing catalytic competence. The GS domain will be switched from the repressor portion to the substrate Smad protein-docking site by ligand-based phosphorylation by the receptors of the type II category. Only TBRII can bind to TGF-β. In addition, TBRI can be unified into this TBRII-TGF-B (Fig. **2.1**) [6, 10].

The inactivation of Bi-allelic TGF-βRII happens in gastric, colon, biliary, respiratory, esophageal, ovarian, and head and neck carcinomas through the mutational changes that shorten the receptor protein or deactivate its kinase area. In tumors with microsatellite variability, TGF-βRII mutations are highly represented through a genetic disease initiated by mutations in replication healing genes. A polyadenine repeat with 10-base in the TGF-βRII coding region, susceptible to replication errors, is found. In microsatellite instability tumors, these poly (A) mistakes remain unrepaired, causing in mutant TGF-βRII alleles that encrypt receptors that are inactive. This TGF-βRII mutation style is commonly seen when the second TGFβRII allele is inactivated. In most biliary and gastrointestinal carcinomas with dysfunction in microsatellite and lung adenocarcinomas and gliomas, TGF-βRII mutations in the poly (A) tract accumulate. These mutations are available in patients of colon cancer with hereditary faults in improper repair genes. Remarkably, endometrial tumors and breast tumors do not add TGF-βRII mutations with microsatellite instability.

Unstable Colon tumors in microsatellite mutations in TGF-βRII, and biallelic mutations in type II receptor of poly (A) area occur, representing that ACVR2 also has importance in tumor suppression [6].

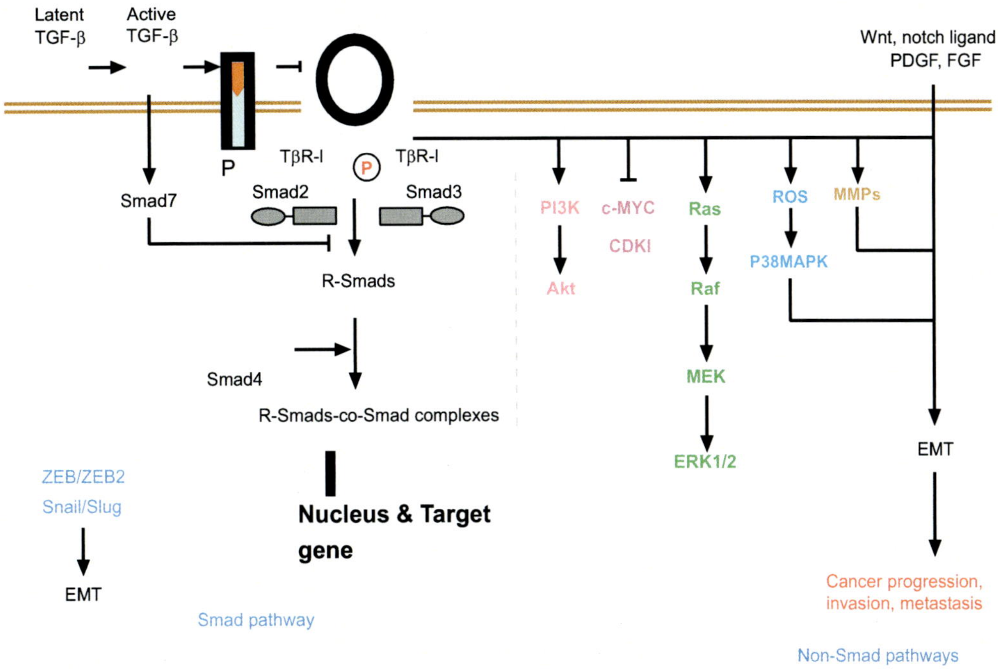

Fig. (2.1). TGF- transmits signals over both non-Smad and Smad pathways. TGF attaches to TRII, which, after phosphorylation of TRI and stimulate Smad2 and Smad3 in the Smad pathway (left) (Smads).

Other mutations, such as missense and frameshift, are found in the TGF-βRI coding area in subdivisions of neck and head, ovarian and esophageal cancers. A specific TGFBRI*6A which is a hypomorphic allele in some types of cancer, is linked with amplified risk [11]. At the epigenetic stage, receptor alterations may also occur. Reduced appearance of TGF-βRI or TGFβRII happens in bladder, prostate, gastric and lung cancers. The defect in gastric cancers is associated with the methylation of the promoter of TGF-βRI. Finally, in Juvenile Polyposis Syndrome (JPS), which is predisposed to gastrointestinal polyps and cancer, mutations of type I BMP receptor occur [6].

Sustained discharge of TGF-β may be necessary for the maintenance of homeostasis in normal, unstressed tissue. However, TGF-β can be abundantly produced by various stromal components and blood platelets under tissue damage to inhibit inflammation and runaway regenerative cell proliferation. Truly, TGF-β also exists in the microenvironment of tumors, originally as a sign to hinder the development of pre-malignancy, but finally used by malignant cells for their selfbenefit. Many tumor types have reported the existence of TGF-β demonstrating that this cancer is mostly associated with cytokine [12]. The three different tumor bases of TGF-β involve the the cancer cells as well as different tumor stroma cells, with each basis contributing to purposeful effects that depend on the context. Myeloid precursor cells, macrophages, bone marrow-derived mesenchymal, leukocytes, and endothelial cells intrude the tumors. The incidence of tumor-infiltrating cells relates to the discharge of TGF-β and, therefore a mistrusted source of TGF-β build-up at the tumor-invasion front [13]. The presence of TGF-β at this site is linked with the progression of tumors in metastasis; TGF-β of specialized local sources is also significant. TGF-β is stored by the bone matrix, which, during osteolytic metastasis, is organized [14].

Latent TGF-β activation involving many enzymatic and non-enzymatic actions is expected to differ in different tumors. With rising clinical evidence that TGF-B works as a tumor-centered immunosuppressor and stimulates tumor mitogens, which controls carcinoma invasion and a cause for the production of prometastatic cytokine, there is growing interest in TGF-B as a treatment area. Despite the sobering concerns, the pleiotropic cytokine path, compounds of anti-TGF-β, have been recognized, proving effectiveness in animal studies and clinical studies of these compounds that are in development [15].

The inhibitors of the TGF-β pathway established to date include many groups. These include TGF-β growth inhibitors hosted into immune cells or tumors. They also contain receptor-ligand interaction inhibitors like anti-receptor antibodies, antibodies of anti-TGF-β, TGF-β receptor kinases aimed by small-molecule inhibitors, and ectodomain proteins of the TGF-β duping receptor. Members of both collections of inhibitors have reached at clinical trial phase for effectiveness against cancers (breast, glioma cancer, melanoma) and alongside fibrosis, scarring, and other disorders arising from the unwarranted activity of TGF-β.

In melanoma, renal cell carcinoma and glioma tumors, therapeutic targeting of the pathway of TGF-β is focused on the basis that TGF-β employs significant properties of immunosuppression in these tumors. By blocking the TGF-β action, could also empower the immunity against the tumor. Additional tumor-specific advantages may also be available to block TGF-β action. Inhibition of TGF-β in gliomas, for instance, may decrease the development of autocrine survival issues, such as PDGF-β. Contrarily, hindering TGF-B in ER cancer of the breast can prevent the seeding and reseed metastases by primary or metastatic tumors.

Finally, blocking TGF-β in osteolytic bone metastasis could disrupt the cycle of osteoclastogenic factors induced by TGF-β and halt tumor development. While these cases illustrate the main importance of the pathway as a mark for therapeutics, negative effects are also likely. Suppression of TGF-βmay result in autoimmune and inflammatory responses, though this has not yet occurred in systemic TGF-β blockers in preclinical or clinical trials. Inhibition of TGF-β receptor activity by other Smad pathway activators can also direct to runaway compensatory tools, comparable to what happens in individuals with deactivating TGF-βRI or TGF-βIII mutations [16]. Lastly, TGF-β signaling inhibition may boost the development of lesions of premalignancy. This will be a minor pain in cancer patients whose malignancies thrive on vTGF-β.

To determine the possibility of TGF-β based therapy, improvement in mechanisms and protumorigenic effects of TGF-β in many tumor types and in various stages of cancer progression is important. The recent development of prognostic tools for TGF-β gene expression and biomarkers for TGF-B response can offer a way to choose patients for the intervention of anti-TGF-β in assessing the successful pharmacological targeting of this path. In experimental models and human models, a study of the TGF-β signaling pathway has provided much-needed clarification about the significance of TGF-β in human cancer and clinical compliance.

TUMOR CELL SURVIVAL AND DEATH MEDIATES AUTOPHAGY

For programmed cell death (PCD), multicellular organisms rely on multiple types to kill damaged or unwanted cells. PCD is an evolutionary process, and apoptosis is the best-studied type of PCD. However, several cancers are unaffected to apoptosis that are alternate, non-apoptotic types of PCD, and some may be active therapeutic avenues, particularly for apoptosis-refractory cancer treatment. The apoptosis-independent cell death process is the result of autophagy over-activation, a response that normally acts as a mechanism based on quality-control [17]. The word "autophagy" was named by Christian de Duve, the Nobel Laureate, during the Symposium of Ciba Foundation on Lysosomes, held in London from February 12 to 14, 1963.

Autophagy is an intracellular degradation mechanism that takes place under many stressful conditions, including organ damage, metabolic stress, abnormal protein presence, and lack of nutrients [18]. These trigger cellular adaptation mechanisms that are necessary for cells to either withstand adverse conditions or to cause cell suicide mechanisms to kill damaged and potentially dangerous cells. Stress promotes autophagy, in which proteins, cytoplasm, protein aggregates and organelles are formed and swallowed by double-membrane vesicles that are then transported to lysosomes where they are degraded, thereby providing energy [19]. Depending on the various mechanisms, autophagy is divided into three major types: chaperone, microautophagy and macroautophagy-mediated autophagy.

Macroautophagy with autophagosome and autolysosome formation is the most commonly investigated autophagic process. Double-membrane cytoplasmic vesicles are autophagosomes, which overcome various cellular constituents, containing cytoplasmic organelles. Autolysosomes in lysosomes were made by combining autophagosomes, where sequestered cell materials are digested [19].

Tumorigenesis and Tumor Progression Autophagy

Autophagy is multifaceted in tumorigenesis and tumor development. It is believed that autophagy employs a tumor-suppressive role in the beginning stages of tumorigenesis. The autophagy path relates to oxidative stress and better genomic stability to ensure that stable, untransformed cells live. Instead, autophagy has recently been suggested to promote cancer development by promoting the survival and fitness of tumor cells under replication stress, a feature of many malignancies. ACD (autophagic cell death) can act as the last obstacle for oncogenic alteration through a replicative crisis by introducing another layer of complexity. Autophagy inhibition has led to constant progress and increased genomic variability in this climate. Furthermore, core constituents of autophagic machinery are known to be tumor suppressors, such as BECN1 (Beclin1) and AMBRA1 (beclin1 regulator 1 and autophagy). In particular, in many cancers like prostate, breast, and ovarian cancer, BECN1 is monoallelically deleted. Monoallelic mutations often happen in UVRAG (UV irradiation resistance-associated gene) in human colon cancers.

As spontaneous tumor growth is caused by Bif-1 knockout in mice, extra Bif-1 (Endophilin B1) and BECN1-binding protein, may have tumor-oppressive functions. AMBRA1 deficiency also contributes to unrestrained cell increase, and AMBRA1 could also communicate with BECN1, over-promoting autophagy-suppressive tumor action. There is a change to autophagy of tumor-promotion from tumor suppression through the course of tumor growth. Autophagy is believed to be able to relieve stressful environmental factors, such as hypoxia or nutritional deficiency. Since chronic inflammation is another main characteristic of cancer, it will be significant to appreciate the interplay between inflammation and autophagy. There is an indication that autophagy can either prevent or facilitate cancer inflammation. Likewise, in a context-dependent way, inflammatory pathways may suppress or induce autophagy. A dynamic scenario that will allow studies to translate the exact function of autophagy in moulding the inflammatory microenvironment and immunity of tumors has recently emerged. Likewise, in a context-dependent way, inflammatory paths may either suppress or make autophagy. Recently, a complex scenario that will enable future studies to decode the precise part of autophagy in the modelling of the immunity of tumors and inflammatory microenvironment has emerged [17].

Autophagy Inhibits Tumor Progression

A significant mechanism that cells use to preserve genomic steadiness and cellular integrity is autophagy. Naturally, homeostasis will interrupt by the loss of autophagy genes, leading to tumor formation in the cell. In this respect, in addition to the remark that BECN1 hemizygosity is connected with human cancers, a variety of other autophagy regulatory regulators have found tumor-associated deletions or mutations. Gastric and colorectal cancers have been confirmed to have frameshift-type of mutations in ATG12, ATG9B, ATG2B, and ATG5. Bif-1 is an autophagy effector that is active in autophagosome development, as illustrated above. In gastric and prostate cancers, their expression is downregulated and mice missing Bif-1 are vulnerable to tumorigenesis. In major colon cancers, monoallelic UVRAG mutations have also been identified, but autophagy does not seem to be hindered by the manifestation of wild-type UVRAG depletion or mutant UVRAG in cell lines, suggesting that this influence on tumor growth could happen by an autophagy-independent mechanism. Various pathways lead to autophagy's tumor-suppressing effect. Autophagy is triggered under stress conditions to eliminate ruined proteins and organelles, including mitochondria [20, 21].

Inhibition or nonexistence of autophagy contributes to a higher amount of reactive oxygen species, leading to DNA damage accumulation, which is expressed as gene amplification, higher polyploid nuclei and double-strand breaks. This augmented DNA damage could lead to a better vulnerability to the initiation and growth of cancer. A signaling scaffold and protein chaperone inside the cytoplasm is p62. In human cancers, p62 levels are upregulated, and this is believed to facilitate tumorigenesis. P62 aggregation leads to DNA harm and increased endoplasmic reticulum (ER) pressure and also leads to modification in cancer pathways and antioxidant nuclear factor erythroid-2 related factor and nuclear factor kappa β (NF- kβ). P62 works on misfolded proteins as a connector protein that connects LC3 with ubiquitin moieties in the sense of autophagy, Therefore, autophagy facilitates p62 clearance along with ubiquitylated proteins. Autophagy conquest thereby results in the aggregation of p62, leading to oncogenesis.

In this regard, it's worth noting that the benign tumors formed by mice with either a liver-targeted deletion of Atg7 or mosaic deletion of Atg5 show an accumulation of p62. In addition, p62 deletion in these mice suppresses tumor development, suggesting a relevant link between the buildup of p62 and the forming of adenoma. Moreover, oncogenic signal activation leads to autophagy, and this has a part to play in the formation of senescence produced by the oncogene. As senescence in several cancers is considered a significant barrier to tumor growth, this may be another mechanism in which tumor suppression involves autophagy [20, 21].

NECROSIS HAS PRO-INFLAMMATORY AND TUMOR-PROMOTING POTENTIAL

Cell death may occur either through an aggressive, regulated phase called apoptosis (programmed cell death), or through necrosis (a passive, uncontrolled path). Apoptosis is marked by caspase activation, and necrosis is believed to be independent of caspase function. Necrosis is also characterized by cellular swelling, dysfunction of the organelle, severe mitochondrial disturbance and breakup of the plasma membrane. As necrotic cells, including proteins and nucleic acids, release their cell material, necrosis is a great inflammatory relative to apoptosis [22]. Tumor necrosis is commonly linked to aggressive tumor development and spread in patients with lung, breast, and kidney cancer, and it is seen as an indication of poor prognosis. Molecular mechanism-based studies have shown that MLKL (mixed lineage kinase domain) phosphorylation occurs in tumor necrotic areas of dying cells and have shown that during tumor necrosis, necroptosis is also involved [23]. Specifically, tumor necrosis is successfully decreased by deletion of the MLKL gene after necroptosis blocking, and the residual death of the tumor in MLKL-null tumors is apoptotic, which is unexpected [23]. Therefore, tumor cell necroptosis seems to be the key reason for tumor necrosis and delivers a viable method for determining the part of tumor necrosis in tumor necrosis.

However, the influence of necroptosis in tumor development is not well understood since both promoting effects and tumor-suppressing have been reported. In many cancer forms and several tumor cell lines, RIPK3 expression is inhibited. More precisely, necroptosis' immune-boosting impact would increase the immunity in the microenvironment of tumor, because necroptotic cell death activates inflammatory responses. In specific, the anti-tumor immunity is improved by chemotherapy or irradiation for massive acute necroptosis. For example, radiation-induced tumor cell necroptosis, and HMGB1 (high mobility group box 1), which are pro-inflammatory mediators, can improve prognosis and enhance anti-tumor immunity. Interestingly, cell death by necroptosis induces robust cross-priming of cytotoxic CD8+ T lymphocytes in an NF-k and RIPK1-dependent manner, despite the fact that DAMPs released from dead cells alone are not required [24]. Therefore, during tumor development, inflammatory pathway-induced necroptosis can present a tumor suppressor role. Necroptosis can have a positive impact on tumor development, as the important players inRIPK1, necroptosis, and RIPK3 are vital for the development of tumors.

The necroptotic pathway was discovered in the pancreatic ductal adenocarcinoma (PDA), which promotes suppression of immunity in the tumor microenvironment by releasing chemokine (C-X-C motif) ligand 1 (CXCL1) and 130 kDa Sin3-associated polypeptide (SAP-130). CXCL1 is free in a RIPK3-dependent way from PDA cells, and CXCL1 obstruction activates tumor degeneration by diminishing the attack of myeloid-derived suppressor cells (MDSCs) and M2-like macrophages. Meanwhile, the SAP-130 nuclear factor interacts with the Ca^{2+}-dependent lectin receptor inducible Macrophage, which is seen on the cell surface of macrophages, inhibiting cytotoxic T-cell activation and infiltration [25].

Necroptosis occurs in the necrotic regions of the tumor and changes to tumor apoptosis by hindering necroptosis. Importantly, necroptosis occurs only in the final stage of tumor formation, necroptosis inhibition decreases tumor growth in the late stage and does not affect tumor origination and early growth. RIPK3 expression falls in the early stages of mouse MMVT-PyMT breast cancers, and significant alterations in the expression of RIPK3 have been identified in tumors of late-stage. MLKL expression was also greatly improved. Therefore, as tumors undergo metabolic stress, the expression of these main necroptosis mediators has possibly been reprogrammed to reestablish the necroptotic machinery in tumor cells. Taken together, the supportive role of necroptosis is apparent in the growth of tumors [23].

NECROPTOSIS: A PRO- OR ANTI-INFLAMMATORY MODE OF CELL DEATH

Due to the discharge of intracellular damage-associated molecular pattern molecules (DAMPs), classical necrosis is usually pro-inflammatory, and it is also hypothesized that the switching to necroptosis by TNF-induced signaling, *via* inhibition or caspase-8 exclusion, aggravates inflammation through the discharge of DAMP. First, TNF stimulation is fundamentally extremely pro-inflammatory to start the creation of many pro-inflammatory chemokines and cytokines, to facilitate necroptosis in the absence of any action. Indeed, in a varied of cell types, one of the greatest important causes of inflammatory cytokine synthesis is TNF which has been involved as a significant stimulator of basic diseases of inflammation, involving inflammatory bowel disease, psoriasis, rheumatoid arthritis, Crohn's disease and other conditions. Second, TNF stimulation rarely causes cell death in many cell types, with maximum cells demanding TNF-induced NF-k initiation of the blockage before TNF-induced apoptosis may occur [26].

In most types of cells, however, the primary outcome of TNF stimulation is the development of a large range of cytokines and chemokines. Therefore, shifting an inflammatory TNF-dependent reaction to a necroptotic TNF-dependent reaction is not necessarily fluctuating to a necrotic one from an apoptotic response. Instead, because of the multitude of cytokines and chemokines production, the transition from a vigorous TNF-driven pro-inflammatory response to a necroptotic one is also pro-inflammatory but contributes to the early closure of the transcriptional response caused by TNF. Here, the problem is whether the latter reaction is almost pro-inflammatory compared to the previous one [26].

In comparison, since other factors encouraging necroptosis, like TLR3 or TLR4 involvement, are often intensely pro-inflammatory lacking the use of necroptosis, moving the effects of these paths to necroptosis has related repercussions. Therefore, since necroptosis leads to fast lysis of the responding cell, due to early cessation of inflammatory cytokine development induced by TNF/LPS, this type of cell death could be very less pro-inflammatory related to another outcome of TNF or LPS stimulation. In certain cases, it is probable that the discharge of DAMP by virtue of necroptosis can replace or even surpass the damage of inflammatory cytokines caused by TNF/LPS due to the primary loss of TNF-stimulated cells. However, it is unlikely that necroptosis is constantly inflammatory when compared to the alternative effects of stimulation by TLR or TNFR; this is expected to rest on the net equilibrium of or lack of production involving pro-inflammatory cytokine due to the necroptosis against the discharge of DAMPs has an outcome of cell lysis induced by necroptosis.

Because of the early shutdown of inflammatory cytokine development induced by TNF/TLR, the switching of TLR-facilitated signaling or TNF to necroptosis in some locations could finally overturn inflammation. Therefore, whether necroptosis is more or less inflammatory than other effects of TNF virtue of R/TLR stimulus is more likely to be context reliant.

NEW FUNCTION OF TELOMERASE

Human telomeres perform as a protective structure covering the chromosome's two ends. They contain long, repeated TTAGGG sequences, associated with many proteins that attach to telomeres. Telomeres, activate all that can end in cell death, shield the chromosomes, recombination, and decay. Telomeres cannot be fully repeated during cell replication. They are eventually reduced, and cell reproduction in what is termed "replicative senescence." is halted until the telomeres exceed a critical level. Hence, telomeres function as an internal "counting" system in the ageing phase of the cell. Telomerase is a complex of enzymatic ribonucleoproteins, which perform in telomere elongation as a reverse transcriptase. The activity of Telomerase is not present in somatic cells but is seen in many of tumor cells and embryonic stem cells. In reality, tumor cells contain small and steady telomeres, which confer immortality on cancer cells and are thus skillful at replicating forever. Telomere deregulation thus shows a vital role in the interaction between the syndrome of premature aging and cancer (Table **2.2**) [27, 28].

Table 2.2. Telomerase modulation has both advantages and disadvantage (adapted from Ref. [29]).

Telomerase OFF	
PROS	**CONS**
Over 90% of all cancers have a universal target. Specificity is predicated on the fact that cancer cells have considerably greater telomerase expression and activity. Development and survival of tumors are dependent on this component.	Unwanted effects in normal/stem cell. Immune system dysfunction. Destabilization ofgenome in non-target tissues. Telomerase independent cancer cells selection (*e.g.* induction of the ALT pathway).
Telomerase ON	
PROS	**CONS**
Regeneration/Proliferative effect. DNA repair pathways inductionin normal cells. Oxidative species reduction. Improvement of mitochondrial function. Anti-premature age-related diseases.	Mitogenic pathways induction. Cancer development induction in patients with lack in tumor suppressor mechanisms. Non-specific side effects.

This enzyme consists of two major ingredients, a share of reverse transcriptase telomere (TERT) and telomere RNA (TERC). A variety of experiments has shown that in usual somatic cells, the production of telomerase is almost not there. However, in mitotically lively cells, including blood, lymphocytes, and endometrium, a low grade of telomerase action was seen. In these proliferating cells, growth regulates telomerase activity. To sustain telomere length during their life cycle, stem cells release telomerase. Short telomeres and raised levels of telomerase activity are seen in about 90% of cancer cells. For example, 98% of bladder cancers, 95% of colorectal cancers, 80% of lung cancers, 75% of oral carcinomas, 84% of prostate cancers, 93% of breast cancers, 85% of liver cancers and 94% of neuroblastomas have observable telomerase activity [30, 31].

Whether telomerase can be an approachable biomarker for primary recognition of cancer, prognosis and diagnosis remains to be known. Normal human cells with Telomerase-negative transfected with human (h) TERT encoding vectors, such as foreskin fibroblasts and retinal pigment epithelial cells, display telomere elongation, while telomere-negative directive cells display telomere senescence and shortening. Likewise, telomerase-lacking mice showed chromosome ends worn-out by telomere, end-to-end fusion, and viability failure. All of these events were prevented by the implementation of telomerase, suggesting that telomerase can boost longevity, encourage proliferation and prolong the life span [30, 31].

Telomere length performs as an intrinsic biological clock that control the life period of the cell until it undergoes replicative senescence. Thus, by causing senescence as a kind of tumor suppressing process, telomeres impair a cell's ability to replicate. As discussed, telomeres are increasingly reduced with successive cell divisions [32, 33].

Senescence induction is related to the stimulation of a variety of pathways, including the Rb/p16INK4A cell-cycle control point path, p53 and p21, as they exceed a crucial length. Cell growth is then detained, and apoptosis happens as a result. There are long telomeres in the human fibroblasts of young adults, whereas older individuals have shorter telomeres. Likewise, relative to stable adults of the same age, patients with premature aging syndrome have shorter telomeres. The injection into normal cells of humans of the catalytic subunit of hTERT contributes to indefinite and uncontrolled proliferation. Thus, telomere shortening tends to culminate in cellular MI or senescence [32, 33].

Tumorigenesis Due to Malfunction of Telomere

The cells face two conflicting fates as telomeres get too small and break the binding of the defensive shelter in the complex. In cells with preserved control points, degradation of the telomere contributes to senescence. In addition, telomere dysfunction causes genomic instability in p53 absence and fuels tumor development. The development of human cancers is also driven by telomere dysfunction. Several solid tumors, like those of the prostate and colon of the breast, have shorter telomeres relative to those of normal tissue.

In the hyperplasia-to-carcinoma conversion, which overlaps with telomerase reactivation, anaphase bridges are found. This type of tumor provides a rare ability for patients at various stages of the disease to conduct high-resolution measurements of telomere length in B cells. The findings suggest that telomere shortening is closely associated with telomere fusions, and disease progression has been identified in the earlier stages of the disease, possibly setting the stage for gross genomic rearrangements that drive CLL (chronic lymphocytic leukemia) progression [34].

Telomeres as Suppressors of Tumors

Divisions in human cells deficient in telomerase action contribute to telomeres being reduced and broken in their spatial arrangement. Telomere shortening due to the 'end replication dilemma' is a normal consequence of cell division and leads to condensed telomeres that lead to DDR (DNA damage response). DNA damage-finding pathways are caused by chromosomal variability and activation of the p53 or p16-RB path, and the cell arrives at a state called replicative senescence. By obstructing multiplying and genetic mutations originating from DNA repetition, this is thought to be an efficient protection against cancer [35].

If the cells develop a mutation that is accountable for sensing small telomeres or other control point proteins in the p53 encoding gene, they may resolve senescence. Until telomeres are dangerously small, the cells will begin to proliferate and then will be guided to apoptosis. Any cells (~1/107) that activate ALT or telomerase and change the ability for infinite replication as virtue of different disorders, render them immortal. Very commonly, this state is accomplished by telomerase upregulation or reactivation.

In order to preserve telomeres, the occasional telomerase-negative immortalization process requires DNA recombination [35].

Telomeresas a Potential Target for Therapy

In certain cancer stem cells and cancer types, telomerase is stated and is the objective of cancer therapies. Generally, human cells have less action of the telomerase and typically have telomeres extended than cancer cells. Selective killing of cancer cells, thus diminishing the outcome on human cells, is the main feature of anti-telomerase therapy.

To accomplish this aim, many therapeutic techniques have been introduced, including oligonucleotides, anti-telomerase immunotherapy, TERT-targeted peptide vaccines, TERT-targeted dendritic cell (DC) immunotherapy, DNA vaccines, gene-modified T-cell therapy, nucleosides, small molecule inhibitors, G quadruplex stabilization, gene therapy, telomere targeting and telomerase-associated proteins, inhibitors of telomerase originating from natural and microbial products and causes of telomerase and oxidative stress [36].

THE NEXT GENERATION OF INDUCING ANGIOGENESIS

Tumors, like regular tissues, require nutrition and oxygen, and the ability to eliminate carbon dioxide and metabolic wastes. These criteria are located by neovasculature associated with tumors, which is created using the angiogenesis technique. According to a growing amount of data, the switch of angiogenesis is mediated by neutralizing factors that promote or inhibit the angiogenic switch.

Any of these angiogenic controllers indicate proteins that fix to the stimulatory or inhibitory cell superficial receptors on vascular endothelial cells. Thrombospondin-1 (TSP-1) and vascular endothelial growth factor-A (VEGF-An) are two well-known angiogenesis inhibitors and inducers, respectively [17 - 19].

Angiogenesis, or the creation of novel capillaries from current vessels, is a critical biological process involved in reproduction, wound healing, and embryonic development [37]. It is triggered by protease release from active endothelial cells, which causes the basement membrane to degrade, allowing endothelial cells to migrate into the space of the interstitial part, where they multiply to differentiate into matured blood vessels. Proteolytic enzymes are formed after endothelial cells are triggered by angiogenic stimuli, which tear down the ECM (perivascular extracellular matrix) and basement membrane, leading to the development of capillary loops (Fig. **2.2**) [38].

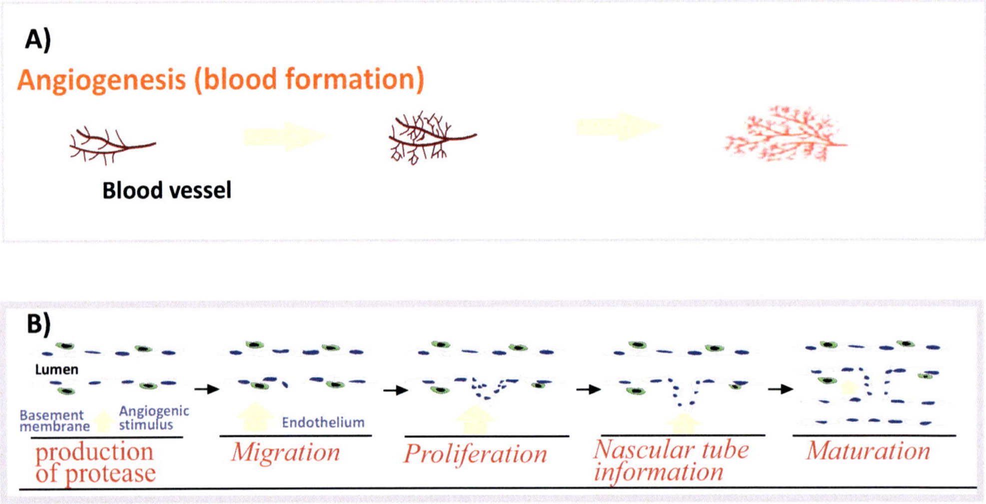

Fig. (2.2). (A) From pre-existing vessels, the procedure of development of new blood vessels is angiogenesis, and it allows tumor to grow. **(B)** Angiogenesis process.

Angiogenesis is normally restricted to particular tissues in humans, but it is widely understood that it plays a serious role in the development of cancer and is the rate-defining stage in tumor growth. Tumors produce a diffusible material that promotes cancer angiogenesis, according to research published in 1968 [39].

Several chemical signals promote blood production; however, an additional type of chemical signal recognized as an angiogenesis inhibitor inhibits blood formation. The messages may impair blood vessel development or encourage the discard of existing vessels on a systemic level. Angiogenic activators such as angiogenin, VEGF, transforming growth factor (TGF- and TGF-ß), basic fibroblast factor, growth placental factor growth (bFGF, factor, FGF2), tumor necrosis factor (TNF), platelet-derived endothelial growth factor, and the epidermal growth factor have been identified as inhibitors. The balance between activators and inhibitors, which is regulated by vascular hemostasis, is critical [40]. The strongest and most potent angiogenic agent is VEGF, and its receptors have been extensively investigated in neoplastic vascularization [41].

Vascular Endothelial Growth Factor (VEGF) Role in Angiogenesis

Vascular endothelial growth factors are a 34-42 kD homodimeric protein that improves skin vascular permeability [42]. The most prominent factor promoting angiogenesis is VEGF and its corresponding receptor (VEGFR), which stimulates cellular pathways that promote fast tumor growth and enable metastatic potential [43]. VEGF is a group of ligands that bind to the VEGFR tyrosine kinase (VEGF-A to D and placental growth factor (PIGF) [44]. VEGF-A & B and PIGF are important factors in angiogenesis because they have the highest affinity for VEGFR-1 and -2, which are responsible for the bulk of angiogenic effects. Because VEGFR-1 adversely controls the VEGF-A/VEGFR2 interaction, it is considered to operate as a receptor by limiting the amount of unrestricted VEGF-A existing to activate VEGFR-2 [45].

Hypoxia, which increases VEGF mRNA and is facilitated by the hypoxia-inducible factor-1, stimulates VEGF production (HIF-1). Tumor cells require vascular supply to deliver nutrition and oxygen in order to develop beyond 2-3 mm^3, which they do by secreting angiogenic growth factors like VEGF. The HIF-1 is a heterodimeric basic helix-loop-helix transcription factor that is made up of two units: HIF-1a and HIF-1h (ARNT), with HIF-1a being the more important regulatory component. Prolyl hydroxylases hydroxylate HIF-a on conserved prolyl remainders in the oxygen-reliant degradation domain, which attaches to von Hippel-Lindau protein and aims it for destruction by the ubiquitin pathway of the proteasome. Inactivation of prolyl hydroxylase, on the other hand, results in HIF1a stability in hypoxic circumstances. HIF-1 transcriptional activity is increased in hypoxia by "factor-inhibiting HIF-1," an oxygen-sensitive enzyme that hydroxylates asparagine residues at the C-terminal transactivation domain of HIF-1a to displace p300/CBP coactivator proteins [46].

VEGF levels and vascularization indicators were dramatically decreased in xenograft models using stem cells of an embryo from HIF-1a -/- mice [47]. The role of HIF-1 in human cancers could be better understood, if researchers used cells that were genetically targeted for HIF-1 in an *in vivo* xenograft model. Surprisingly, short interfering RNA (siRNA) knockdown of HIF-1a in a DLD-1 cell xenograft of colon cancer inhibited the growth of the tumor but not tumor angiogenesis. HIF-1 deficient xenograft microvessels density was similar to that of HIF-1-expressing xenografts. Interestingly, the stimulation of VEGF in HIF-1–lacking xenograft tissue and HIF-1–deficient cells *in vitro* was not eliminated. VEGF intensities were decreased by around 50 percent, indicating that significant quantities of VEGF were generated [48].

Cancer Therapy and HIF-1 Inhibitors

Several studies reported that chemical agents can inhibit tumor xenograft development and inhibit HIF activity through diverse molecular pathways. The medicines listed below, whether authorized for cancer therapy or other diseases, or still in clinical trials, are meant to serve as examples rather than exhaustive lists. Reduced HIF-1a mRNA levels; the active ingredient in AFP-464 that is now being tested in Phase-1 cancer trials, largely abolishes mRNA expression of HIF-1a while nearly entirely inhibiting the expression HIF-1a protein [49]. This suggests that aminoflavone reduces HIF-1a mRNA stability and translation. mTORC1 inhibitors, such as temsirolimus (CCI-779) and rapamycin, block the translation of HIF-1a mRNA into protein and decrease tumor burden [50].

Enhanced HIF-1a degradation; 17 allylamino-17-demethoxygeldanamycin is an HSP90 inhibitor that reduces HIF binding to DNA, HIF subunit heterodimerization, and HIF transcriptional activity by causing RACK1-dependent ubiquitination, VHL independent, and degradation of proteasomal HIF-1a. HIF heterodimerization; Acriflavine, an antibacterial medication, binds straightly to the PAS-B subdomain of HIF-1a & 2a and reduces their contact with HIF1b, preventing HIF-dependent gene transcription and causing tumor development and vascularization problems [51].

Anthracyclines, such as daunorubicin and doxorubicin (Adriamycin), fix to DNA and limit HIF-1 & 2 binding, as well as prevent HIF-1-dependent production of angiogenic growth factors, resulting in decreased development of tumor and vascularization [51]. Bortezomib, a proteasome inhibitor authorized for the treatment of multiple myeloma and mantle cell lymphoma by the FDA, and by targeting HIF-1a's C-terminal transactivation region reduces HIF-1 transcriptional activity, which relates with the coactivator p300. Bortezomib decreases HIF-1a protein expression in cancer cells of the prostate by obstructing ERK signaling and phosphatidylinositol-3-kinase/AKT/mTOR [52]. However, there is a lot of proof that HIFs have a role in radiation and chemotherapy resistance [53]. However, there is growing proof that HIF-1 activation might lead to resistance to new targeted treatments like imatinib, which is used for the treatment of chronic myeloid leukemia. Several studies using mouse models identified that treatment with the small molecule tyrosine kinase inhibitor sunitinib, or the anti-VEGFR2 antibody DC-101 condensed primary tumor development and vascularization but amplified metastasis, most likely because inhibited angiogenesis caused increased intertumoral hypoxia and increased HIF activity [54]. On the other hand, HIF inhibitors significantly reduced the natural metastasis of breast cancer cells to the lungs of orthotopic transplant types of mice by inducing multiple stages in the metastatic process [55]. Therefore, research from mouse models suggests that combining antiangiogenic medicines with HIF inhibitors may increase their effectiveness (Fig. **2.3**).

New information and developments of specific connection between tumour physiology and HIF inhibitors are highlighted here [56 - 59].

- Angiogenic Switch Progression: Despite the fact that the result is a normal inductive sign, the angiogenic switching process will change in shape.
- Natural Barriers to Tumor Angiogenesis: Endogenous Angiogenesis Inhibitors have been discovered to function as endogenous regulators of angiogenesis.
- Pericytes Play an Important Function in Tumor Neovasculature: The tumor neovasculature is made up of pericytes, which are essential components.
- Tumor Angiogenesis Involves Bone Marrow-Derived Cells: It is well understood that a variety of cell types that emerge from the bone marrow perform important roles in pathological angiogenesis.

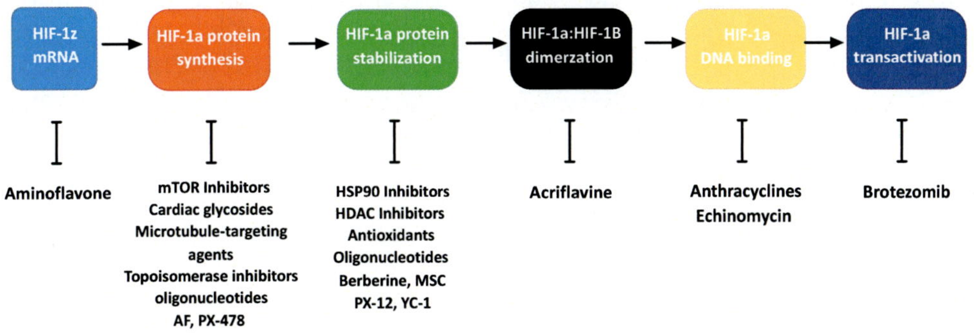

Fig. (2.3). Molecular mechanism of action of drugs that inhibit HIF-1.

THE NEXT GENERATION OF ACTIVATING INVASION AND METASTASIS

Invasion and Migration

The hallmarks cascades (Cancer invasion and metastasis) transform the growing localized tumor into a systemic metastatic, and life-threatening disease. Invasion occurs through single-cell or collective groups of cell migration. Detachment of individual cells and moving from the primary site and invading adjacent, which delivers high numbers of circulating cells, leads to metastatic cascade. The basic steps for local invasion contain activation of signaling pathways, which regulate cytoskeletal mechanisms in cell-matrix, cell-cell junctions and the tumor, monitored by exaggerated tumor cell migration into the nearby tissue.

Tumor cells are first detached from the extracellular matrix, followed by ECM deprivation by several proteolytic enzymes, intravasation into the bloodstream, attack of neighboring tissues and the basal lamina, transport and survival through the bloodstream, extravasation from the distal site, migration, and development of a metastatic lesion [60]. For an epithelial cancer cell to separate from the main tumor and achieve motility, it must lose its E-cadherin activities (Fig. **2.4**). The adherent's junction (AJ most's) prevalent transmembrane protein, E-cadherin, initiates intercellular connections *via* trans-pairing among cadherins on opposite cells [61].

E-cadherin function of downregulation is frequently related to tumor development, followed by a shift to a more invasive and motile phenotype. E-cytoplasmic cadherin's domain interacts with affiliates of the catenin protein family, P120-catenin and ß-catenin, which form a protein complex with the cytoskeleton of actin *via* a-catenin; the catenin-cadherin complexes on adjacent cells cause localized actin remodeling, which is essential for the formation of AJs.

ß-catenin binds to E-cadherin immediately after its production and transports it to the membrane of plasma, where it forms a p120-catenin complex, which stabilizes and at the plasma membrane, it controls E-cadherin [62]. Upregulation of transcriptional repressors SLUG, SNAIL, and SIP1 or methylation of E-cadherin promoters (also known as GEMIN2) are an utmost common reason for the damage of E-cadherin look in human tumors [63].

The E-cadherin function loss aids the invasiveness of epithelial-derived malignancies, allowing the basement membrane to disseminate and spread. The reintroduction or overexpression of E-cadherin in cell lines results in the reversal of poorly differentiated carcinoma phenotypes, whereas silencing expression results in the reversal of poorly differentiated cancer phenotypes. The loss of E-cadherin stimulates carcinogenic pathways of signaling, such as rat sarcoma viral oncogene (Ras) and mitogen-activated kinase (MAPK) [64].

To diffuse *via* blood arteries and populate micrometastases, primary tumor cells must have invasive properties. Cadherins and catenins work together to provide a junction between the cytoskeleton and the extracellular space. Another cadherin molecule, N-cadherin, is expressed by mesenchymal cells. In tumor cells, E-cadherin is usually reduced, but N-cadherin is up-regulated [65].

Epithelial-to-Mesenchymal Transition (EMT) and Metastasis

The initial phase for tumor metastasis is epithelial-to-mesenchymal transition (EMT), which involves a cadherin switch and the production of markers of mesenchyme, such as N-cadherin and vimentin [66]. EMT is a potentially significant step in the metastatic tumor cells spreading because it involves the instability of cell–cell connections and the attainment of a more invasive and migratory mesenchymal character, as well as alterations in gene expression patterns. In adherence and tight junctions, the downregulation of epithelial markers [67], the cytokeratin filament network and the mesenchymal markers upregulation of (vimentin, N-cadherin, fibronectin, integrins, fibroblast specific protein 1 and tenascin C) were all observed [68]. Because N-cadherin has a high affinity for stroma cells, upregulation of the protein enhances the likelihood of migration to the stroma. Cancer-associated fibroblasts (CAFs), Tumor-associated endothelial cells (TECs), and tumor-associated macrophages were all found in the tumor stroma (TAMs).

These cells have important roles in boosting motility and invasion by producing inflammatory, growth, angiogenic, and proteolytic factors. They can also create a tumor-friendly milieu by redundantly producing EMC proteins, including collagen, fibronectin, and periostin [69]. Intrinsic oncogenic activity, such as Her2 overexpression or K-Ras mutation, can govern EMT. External stimuli such as cancer-associated fibroblasts, extracellular matrix ECM (hyaluronic acid, collagen type I), immune cells and myofibroblasts can also be motivated by signaling pathways such as Notch, Wnt, Hedgehog, NFkB, TGF, FGF, EGF, HGF, or MMP3 [60]. Slug, ZEB1 and 2, Snail1 and 2, and Twist are among the intracellular transcription factors controlled by these signaling pathways. Several of the mechanisms that cause EMT also play a role in stem cell self-renewal.

The Epithelial-Mesenchymal Transition Generates Cells with Properties of Stem Cells

The epithelial-mesenchymal transition (EMT) is an example of cellular plasticity, which refers to a cell's ability to acquire new phenotypes and change its shape and characteristics, in which an epithelial cell develops a phenotype similar to mesenchyma that improves its invasive and migratory properties, whereas the mesenchymal-epithelial transition (MET), which happens during embryonic development, allows the cells to differentiate into various organs and tissues. Stemness refers to stem cells' ability to proliferate uncontrollably along an asymmetric pattern, allowing them to act as a cell reservoir, preserve stem cell identity, and generate new, more differentiated cells. Evidence suggests a direct molecular connection between EMT and stemness, with the same genes that drive EMT potentially influencing stemness pathways [70]. The T-cell Factor 4 (TCF4)/catenin complex fixes to the Zeb1 promoter directly and stimulates its transcription. Wnt stemness-linked signaling paths have been in various elements of the EMT program [71].

The emergence of a less differentiated phenotype is linked to the EMT process prompted by TGF- in epithelial cells. Activation of the EMT in non-transformed epithelial cells, imparts SC (stem cell) characteristics. Excessive TGF- treatment of human embryonic hepatocytes makes a mesenchymal phenotype linked with poor expression of certain hepatic genes and the SC markers development, resembling progenitor-like cells. Because the mesenchymal stem-like cells re-differentiate to bile duct cells or hepatocytes under strict control of experimental circumstances that promote MET and re-expression of liver-specific genes, this process is reversible [72].

EMT also confers stem-like qualities to tumor cells; numerous reports have shown that EMT is responsible for the cells' stem and tumorigenic properties. With the help of a sensitive technique to track epithelial cells of the pancreas is in a rat model of pancreatic cancer, it was discovered that detached tumor cells exhibited stem cell characteristics and had a mesenchymal phenotype [73]. This would demonstrate the concept of a circulating (migratory) cancer stem cell (CSC) and back up the hypothesis that the EMT program and the stemness phenotype are linked. In the setting of a cirrhotic liver, TGF- stimulates the growth of tumor-initiating cells. TGF-induced EMT in tumor cells of liver is also associated with alterations in the stem markers expression such as CD44 and CD133 [74]. Overexpression of CD44 has been linked to E-cadherin downregulation, vimentin overexpression, and a poor prognosis in prostate cancer [75]. Another theory is that stemness and EMT are separate routes. For example, in normal glands, Sox9 and Slug incorporate the stem cell state; however, although Slug is primarily engaged in EMT stimulation, Sox9 is required for entrance into the phenotype of stem cells [76]. Several studies recommend that the EMT process is critical for entering the stem, but it is inadequate to tempt this change in differentiated luminal cells on its own; therefore, additional genetic program activation is mandatory to induce stemness in differentiated luminal cells by working in tandem with the EMT program.

The transitory stages of EMT in cancer, allow cancer cells in mesenchyma to re-proliferate and colonize in new tissues or organs by partially reverting to an epithelial phenotype. During metastasis, there are two distinct frameworks for EMT. (i) Stemness and EMT are intertwined procedures that result in the development of migratory cancer stem cells, which are activated by Twist1 (Fig.

2.4). (ii) Prxx1 confers EMT and migratory phenotypes but suppresses stemness, and Prxx1 downregulation is required for the gaining of stem properties, suggesting that only the initial EMT process would link with stemness phenotype *via* the acquisition of epithelial properties, but late EMT process may lead to decrease in the flexibility of mesenchymal phenotype (Fig. **2.4**) [77].

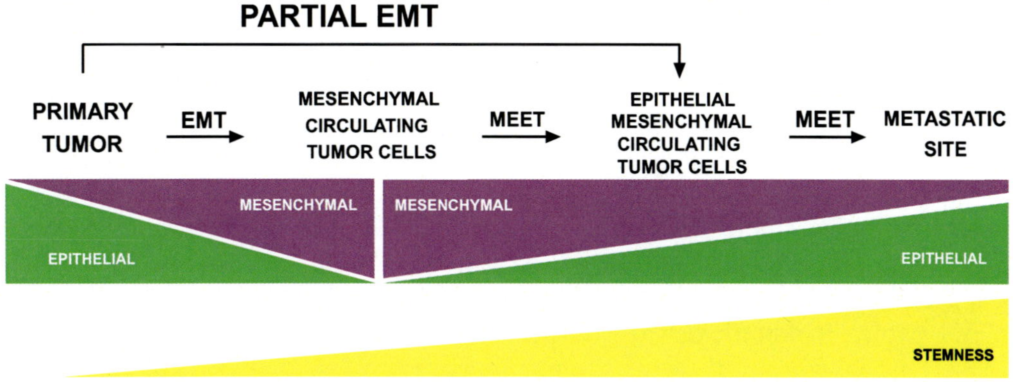

Fig. (2.4). The activation of the EMT program may present various threshold levels that may or may not integrate EMT from stemness ability.

Cancer Cells Promote their Own Growth

Most human cancers include mutations that disrupt the cell cycle's early stages. Cells have created many checkpoints to guarantee proper passage through the cell cycle. These checkpoints stop cells from entering a new phase of the cycle until the previous one has been properly completed. Cell size, Extracellular growth signals, and DNA integrity are all assessed by the numerous checkpoints (Fig. **2.5**). The somatic cells are split into four oscillation periods. The cells divide into two phases, each of which includes the creation of a sole copy of its genetic material and the separation of all cellular parts among the two similar daughter cells (M phase or mitosis). Gap periods (G1 and G2) occur in the other two stages of the cell cycle, where the cells make themselves for the effective completion of the M and S phases, respectively. The most important stages are S phase, when DNA replication occurs, and M phase, when the cell splits into two daughter cells. The cyclin-dependent kinase (CDK) family of serine/threonine kinases and their regulatory partners of the cyclins, serve as the core of the regulatory apparatus during cell cycle progression. Cyclin D-CDK4, cyclin D-CDK6, and cyclin E-

CDK2 are proteins that promote G1 advancement by preventing the cell from completing the cycle.

The right order of events is maintained by sensor systems known as checkpoints, which govern cell cycle development. If sensor tools detect incomplete or abnormal cell cycle events (for example, DNA damage), checkpoint pathways send a signal to effectors, which can lead to a cell cycle halt until the problem is solved. CDK inhibitors (CDKIs) are harmed by effector proteins, which can stop cell cycle progression reversibly [38]. The Cip/Kip family andINK4 family are two distinct CDK inhibitor families that have been identified. P15 (INK4b), p16 (INK4a), p18 (INK4c), and p19 (INK4d) are members of the INK4 family, which deregulate and deactivate G1 CDK (CDK4 and CDK6). Before cyclin binding, these CKI form stable complexes with the CDK enzyme, blocking cyclin D interaction. The Cip/Kip family of inhibitors includes p21 (Waf1, Cip1), p27 (Cip2), and p57 (Kip2), which block G 1CDKcyclin complexes, as well as CDK1-cyclin B complexes to a lesser extent. The production of p21 is under transcriptional control of the p53 tumor suppressor gene, and CKIs are controlled by a variety of internal and external cues [78, 79].

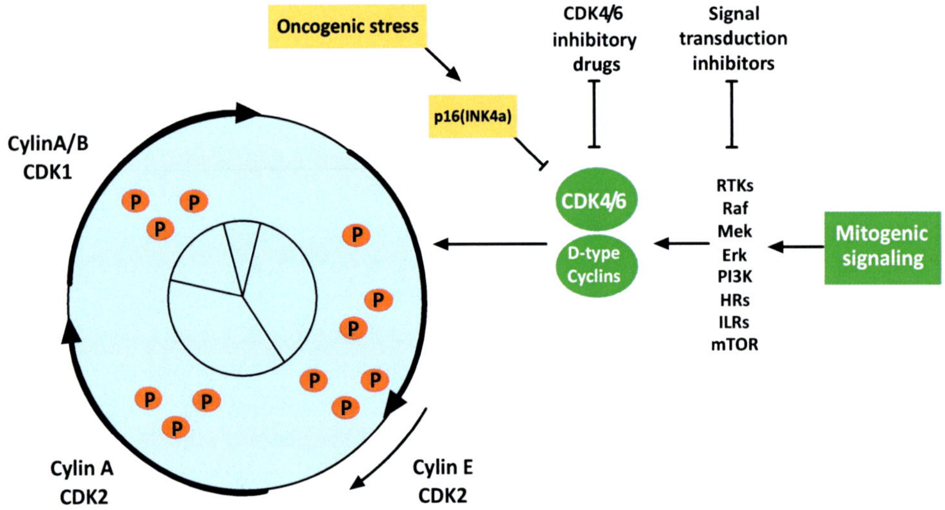

Fig. (2.5). Cell cycle dynamic.

Abnormalities in the Cell Cycle Control Proteins in Cancer

Essential modulation in the genetic regulation of cell division occurs in cancer, resulting in unrestrained cell proliferation. Tumor suppressor genes and proto-oncogenes are the most often mutated genes. Tumor development can be triggered by a mutated model of proto-oncogenes or oncogenes. When tumor suppressor genes like pRb and p53 are inactivated, proteins that usually impede cell cycle progression become dysfunctional and deregulated. Cell cycle dysregulation is linked to cancer and is affected by mutations in proteins that are vital at different stages of the cell cycle. CDK-activating enzymes, CDK, cyclins, CDK substrates, CKI, and checkpoint protein genes have all been shown to have mutations in cancer [80].

CDK and CDK Activating Enzyme

CDK molecule abnormalities in cancer have been investigated, but infrequently. In cell lines, sarcoma, melanoma, and glioma, CDK4 overexpression have been seen [81]. Following that, evidence of cyclin involvement in additional human cancer cells was discovered, including breast, gastric, B cell lymphoma, esophageal and colon carcinomas, as well as a variety of other malignancies [82]. Increased cyclin D1 expression is one of the most common anomalies in human cancer, occurring in 40% of colorectal cancers, 60% of breast malignancies, 20% of prostate cancer, and 40% of head and neck squamous carcinoma [83]. But the role of CDKs in cancer in general has yet to be known.

Members of the Cdc25 phosphatase family control CDK activation by dephosphorylating it. Cdc25A is required for theCdc25B to be activated during S-phase, G1/S phase transition, and Cdc25C activates CDK1-cyclin B during the mitotic entrance. Uncontrolled or upregulated Cdc25 allows for unscheduled CDK-cyclin activation, which has been linked to tumor development. Cdc25B is overexpressed in around 32% of primary breast tumors, and c-myc, an oncogene shown to be frequently mutated in human malignancies, activates transcription of the Cdc25A and Cdc25B genes [79].

CKI

CKI has an inhibitory action, meaning it inhibits growth by activating pRb, which reflects CKI's tumor suppressor role. The p16 gene is altered in a large percentage of human cancers, and its function can be inhibited by a variety of methods, including point mutations, deletion, and hypermethylation. Cells with the p16 mutation will be uncontrollable in their progress through the G1 phase. The p16 protein is a CDK-cyclin D inhibitor that inhibits phosphorylation of the pRb protein, causing cells to enter G1 phase. Because p16 and CDK/cyclin D are functionally linked in the same way as pRb is, any disruption in one of these cell cycle regulators is expected to have a comparable impact, and changes in at least one of these regulators are seen in virtually all human malignancies [79]. In addition to the p16 gene, the p19 transcript regulates p53 stability independently of p16. The p19 gene may be manipulated by big deletions of the ARF-INK4 region, leading to a mutant p19 and p53 dysregulation. Loss of p27 expression has been related to poor prognosis, tumor aggressiveness, and recurrence in a variety of human tumor types (lung, breast, bladder). Promoting proteolysis that is proteasome-dependent, rather than gene loss, has been linked to the downregulation of p27 in colorectal carcinomas [84]. The tumor suppressor protein p53 regulates p21, which has been implicated in carcinogenesis. The p53 gene is the maximum altered gene in human cancer, and when p53 is inactivated, the control of p21 in reaction to DNA damage is reduced [85].

Cell Cycle Control and Cancer Treatment

Instead of discovering medicines that inhibit tumor cell growth, researchers are now concentrating on more mechanistic techniques that target molecular targets that underpin cell creation. CDK activity can be controlled in a number of ways, including an indirect method that targets the major regulators of CDK activity or a direct technique that inhibits the catalytic activity of CDK kinases. The indirect method comprises upregulating CKI, synthesizing peptides that mimic CKI's actions, lowering cyclin levels, and controlling the phosphorylated state of CDK and associated enzymes. The most effective method for developing robust cell cycle inhibitors has been to block CDK kinase activity directly [79].

CANCER OPPOSE APOPTOSIS

A disruption of the natural stability between cell death and proliferation, which is required to preserve tissue homeostasis, is a hallmark of human malignancies. Apoptosis is a form of programmed cell death that regulates cell proliferation in answer to DNA damage and tissue development. Apoptosis is related to a cell death mechanism that occurs when DNA is broken and cannot be repaired. The extrinsic-death receptor pathway and the intrinsic-mitochondrial pathway are the two key pathways that leading to apoptosis [86].

The Extrinsic Pathway

The themembrane-bound Fas ligand, death receptors, Fas-associated death domain (FADD), caspases 8 and 10 and Fas complexes are all components of the extrinsic pathway, which influence the rate of downstream caspases leading to apoptosis (Fig. **2.6**). TNF receptors include DR3 (Apo 2), TNF R1, DR5 (TRAIL R2), DR4 (tumor necrosis factor-related apoptosis-inducing ligand receptor 1 [TRAIL R1]), and DR6 (tumor necrosis factor-related apoptosis-inducing ligand receptor 1 [TRAIL R1]), DR5 (TRAIL R2), and DR6 [87]. Because Fas signals are important for immune monitoring of altered cells, any deficiency or mutation in this system has been linked to a variety of cancers and autoimmune diseases.

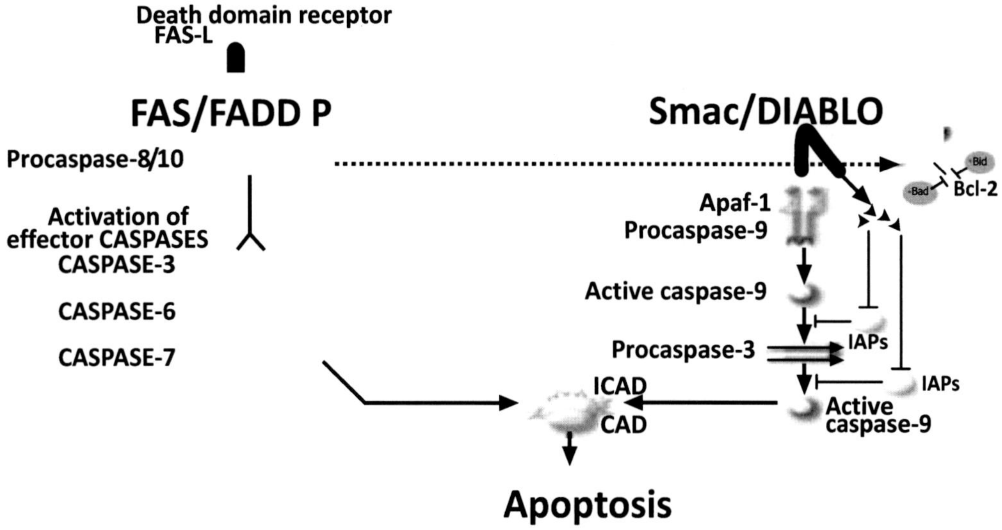

Fig. (2.6). Pathways of apoptosis the death receptor triggers the extrinsic pathway, which releases cytochrome-c from the mitochondria, and the intrinsic pathways, which release cytochrome-c from the mitochondria.

The death-related activities of the Fas ligand (FasL)-Fas system are revealed. The membrane-bound FasL binds the dormant Fas complexes and creates the death-inducing signaling pathways when death initiates the route. Caspases 8 and 10 trigger death signaling pathways, which cause Caspases 8 to activate, which then activates the remainder of the downstream Caspases. With some intrinsic apoptotic pathways, Caspase 8 interacts by cleaving Bid (a proapoptotic member of the Bcl-2 family) and then releasing cytochrome-c in specific types of cells. Whether deletions or mutations of the Fas gene were seen in some hematologic malignancies, dysregulation of the extrinsic pathway led to malignant transformation [88]. Because the FasL gene is a transcriptionally dormant gene, pathways regulators include transcription factors like NFk and activating protein 1. Other inhibitory pathways include Fas-associated death-domain protein-like, FAP-1, and other soluble decoy receptors such as TRAIL R-3/DcR1 and DcR2, which compete with ligands to block FasL activation.

The Intrinsic Pathway

One of the greatest significant regulators in this system, the Bcl-2 family, is increased in a variety of cancer cells [55]. Overexpression of Bcl-2 contributes to chemotherapeutic medicines resistance and radiation treatment, whereas reduced Bcl-2 expression may start apoptotic reactions to anticancer medications. The Bcl-2 family is made up of two sets of proteins that control the pathway. Anti-apoptotic members such as Bcl-W, Bfl-1, Bcl-2, Bcl-XL, and Mcl-1, as well as pro-apoptotic members such as Bad, Bcl-XS, Bax, Bak, and Bid [50]. Anti-apoptotic proteins (which function as repressors) block the discharge of cytochrome-c from mitochondria, whereas pro-apoptotic proteins (which act as promotors) escalate it. A balance of anti and pro-apoptotic proteins is needed for apoptosis to begin. In the cytoplasm, when the cytochrome protein is released, it produces an apoptosome and activates caspase-3.Omi/high-temperature requirement protein A (HtrA2), Apoptosis-inducing factor (AIF), direct IAP Binding protein with Low pI (DIABLO), and second mitochondria-derived activator of caspase (Smac) are all apoptotic factors that are released into the cytoplasm from the mitochondrial intermembrane gap.

Smac/DIABLO or Omi/HtrA2 connect to an inhibitor of apoptosis proteins (IAPs) and activate caspases, causing IAP interaction to be disrupted and caspase-9 proenzymes to be activated. Caspases 9 and 3 are activated by active caspase-9, which then activates the rest of the caspase cascade, resulting in apoptosis [89 - 91].

The Final Pathway: Caspases

The triggering of a group of proteases known as caspases is the last step that leads to the execution of the signal death. For the intrinsic pathway, the upstream caspase is Caspase-9, whereas for the extrinsic pathway, the upstream caspase is caspase-8, and caspase-3 converges both pathways. Caspase-3 cleaves the Deoxy Ribo Nuclease inhibitor, which is required for nuclear apoptosis. Protein kinases, DNA repair proteins, cytoskeletal proteins, and inhibitory components of the endonucleases family are all cleaved by downstream caspases. All of these factors combine to create morphological alterations in apoptosis, such as changes in cell cycle control, cytoskeletal structure and signaling pathways, eventually leading to morphologic changes in apoptosis, including fragmentation of DNA and condensation [91].

INHIBITORY SIGNALS THAT MAY GENERALLY STOP CANCER DEVELOPMENT

Immune Checkpoint Inhibitors

Immune checkpoint proteins can be found in both immune cells and tumor. Immune surveillance is based on the immune system's capacity to recognize and eliminate cells that have the potential to develop cancerous features. This notion is based on the idea of immune editing, which is a process in which the tumor immunogenicity is altered as a result of the immune response's pressure on tumor cells. The cancer cell may manipulate the immune system through a variety of methods, including boosting cell death resistance pathways, avoiding immune-cell identification, and generating an immunosuppressive environment.

The capacity of cancer cells to escape immune-mediated elimination is the disease's characteristics. In response to the diversity of immune mechanisms, many immunotherapy methods have been developed, including cancer vaccines to improve immune system antigen identification and adoptive cell therapy to replenish cytotoxic immune cells and boost the immune response of anti-tumors [92]. As a negative consequence of the immune response to reduce additional peripheral tissue damage, immunological checkpoints are over-expressed due to continuous immune-cell activation Programmed cell death-1 (PD-1). Cytotoxic T-lymphocyte antigen-4 (CTLA-4) and Programmed cell death ligand-1 (PD-L1), inhibitor treatments are the most therapeutically developed of these immunological checkpoint proteins [93].

PD-1 Inhibitors

T cells, B cells, and natural killer (NK) cells all express PD-1, which is a member of the CD28 family. The PD-1 cytoplasmic domain consists of immune receptors, immune receptor tyrosine-based switch motif and inhibitory motif based on tyrosine. PD-1 is a protein of transmembrane type with just one variable domain of extracellular Ig [94]. PD-1 expression inhibited cytokine production and had a detrimental effect on the cytotoxic capability of NK cells. Furthermore, monocytes and macrophages have been found to be inhibited by PD-1 expression [95].

The clinically licensed inhibitors for the programmed cell death ligand-1 (PD-1) are pembrolizumab (Keytruda®) and nivolumab (Opdivo®). Pembrolizumab and nivolumab have drastically changed how many advanced unresectable and metastatic solid tumors are treated. These therapies appear to have potent benefits in many cancers. The L1/PD-1 pathway has been therapeutically explored with significant success in several clinical studies (over 1500), including PD-1 inhibition, and is presently sponsored by the National Cancer Institute, with a rate of response ranging from 20% to 50% in diverse kinds of cancer [96].

Pembrolizumab reduces immune-cell suppression and deactivation by obstructive communication between PD-1 and its ligands. The first FDA-approved PD-1-targeted medication is Pembrolizumab, and also the first immune-type checkpoint inhibitor to be used as a first-line melanoma treatment [97]. Also, it is the first anti-cancer treatment based on a biomarker that has been approved for all cancer types: pembrolizumab has been approved for anti-tumor effects in many cancers, including but not limited to breast, bladder, gastric, colorectal, and ovarian cancers [98].

By binding to the PD-1 epitope, nivolumab inhibits PD-1's capacity to adversely regulate T-cell proliferation and activation. The FDA has authorized Nivolumab for the treatment of renal cell carcinoma (RCC), melanoma, non-small cell lung cancer (NSCLC), urothelial carcinoma (UC), and squamous cell carcinoma of the neck and head [99, 100].

As different studies employed low thresholds for PD-L1 positive, uneven interpretations of PD-L1 staining/positivity thresholds, and different statistical methods, using PD-L1 as a biomarker of response is difficult [92].

CTLA-4 Inhibitors

CTLA-4 is a kind of immunological checkpoint protein, also known as CD152. CTLA-4 is a protein that controls T-cell activity and protects against immune cell-mediated harm. In 2011, after studies in metastatic melanoma, ipilimumab (Yervoy®) was approved by the Food and Drug Administration (FDA) as the first immune checkpoint inhibitor [94]. In antigen-presenting cells (APCs) and also T cells, Ipilimumab blocks CTLA-4's inhibitory power by inhibiting the interaction of CTLA-4's with CD80 and CD86. By this, CD80/CD86 is connected to CD28, and T cell is triggered. Ipilimumab, in grouping with the PD-1 inhibitor nivolumab, has been accepted for the advanced treatment of naive renal cell unresectable melanoma, carcinoma (RCC), and mismatch repair deficient (dMMR) colorectal cancer or metastatic microsatellite instability-high (MSI-h) that has spread after previous treatment [101].

The human IgG2 monoclonal antibody, Tremelimumab (AstraZeneca), inhibits the interaction among CTLA-4 and CD28, reducing the inactivation of CTLA-4-mediated immune cell [102]. It works in the same way as ipilimumab, inhibiting CTLA-4-mediated immune-cell inactivation. Tremelimumab is now being tested in conjunction with other immunoediting medicines to see whether it has any therapeutic advantage in other cancer types [92].

CONCLUSION

Cancer is a multi-step process in which cells undergo biochemical and behavioral alterations that cause them to multiply excessively and prematurely. Recognizing and comprehending the widespread applicability of cancer cell characterisation will have a growing impact on the development of innovative treatments for human cancer. Because growth-promoting pathways like mTOR are inhibited, CI cells do not progress from cell cycle arrest to senescence. While cancer cells are not CI, convergent cancer cell cultures decrease their senescence machinery, which has crucial implications in cancer therapy. Furthermore, improving the mechanisms and protumorigenic effects of TGF- β in a variety of tumor types and stages of cancer growth is critical in determining the possibility of TGF- β based therapy. The recent development of predictive tools for TGF- β gene expression and biomarkers for TGF-B response may provide a mechanism to select patients for anti-TGF-B intervention and measure the success of this path's pharmaceutical targeting. The investigation of the TGF-signaling pathway in both experimental and human models has offered much-needed clarification concerning the role of TGF in human cancer and therapeutic compliance. Furthermore, autophagy has a variety of roles in carcinogenesis and tumor progression. Autophagy is thought to play a tumor-suppressive role in the early stages of carcinogenesis. A complex scenario has recently developed that will allow future studies to unravel the specific role of autophagy in the modeling of tumor immunology and the inflammatory milieu. Furthermore, oncogenic signal activation causes autophagy, which plays a role in the creation of oncogene-induced senescence. Senescence is thought to be a significant barrier to tumor growth in several malignancies, therefore, this could be another method in which autophagy is involved in tumor suppression.

Cell death can take place in two ways: as an aggressive, regulated process called apoptosis or as a necrotic process. The expression of these primary necroptosis mediators may have been altered to reconstruct the necroptotic machinery in tumor cells as tumors endure metabolic stress. Human telomeres also serve as a protective structure at the ends of the chromosomes. Telomere shortening has been linked to cellular MI or senescence, according to studies. Furthermore, telomerase is expressed in some cancer stem cells and cancer types and is the primary target of cancer therapy. Many therapeutic techniques have been developed to achieve this goal, including oligonucleotides, anti-telomerase immunotherapy, TERT-targeted peptide vaccines, TERT-targeted dendritic cell (DC) immunotherapy, DNA vaccines, gene-modified T-cell therapy, nucleosides, small molecule inhibitors, G quadruplex stabilization, gene therapy, telomere targeting and telomerase-associated proteins, a telomerase inhibitor

Tumors, like other tissues, require nutrition and oxygen, as well as the ability to expel carbon dioxide and metabolic waste. The neovasculature linked with malignancies is used to locate these criteria. VEGF is the most powerful and potent angiogenic agent, and its receptors have been studied extensively in the field of neoplastic vascularization. Furthermore, pharmacologic treatments have been shown to decrease tumor xenograft development and HIF activity *via* a variety of molecular pathways in various investigations. The hallmark pathways (Cancer invasion and metastasis) that turn a localized tumor into a systemic metastatic, life-threatening disease. Invasion happens when a single cell or a group of cells migrates. Furthermore, an epithelial cancer cell must lose its E-cadherin activities in order to split from the primary tumor and acquire mobility. The role of E-cadherin downregulation is usually linked to tumor growth. The epithelial-to-mesenchymal transition (EMT), which involves a cadherin switch and the generation of mesenchymal markers, including N-cadherin and vimentin, is the first step in tumor metastasis. The epithelial-mesenchymal transition (EMT) is an example of cellular plasticity, which refers to a cell's ability to acquire new phenotypes and change its shape and characteristics, in which an epithelial cell develops a phenotype similar to mesenchyma, which improves its invasive and migratory properties, whereas the mesenchymal-epithelial transition (MET), which occurs during embryonic development, allows cells to differentiate into various organs and tissues. In cancer, essential modification in the genetic regulation of cell division occurs, resulting in unregulated cell proliferation. The most frequently mutated genes include tumor suppressor genes and proto-oncogenes. A mutant model of proto-oncogenes or oncogenes can cause tumor formation. CDK molecule anomalies in cancer have been studied, albeit only on a small scale. CKI has an inhibitory effect, which means it suppresses growth by activating pRb, indicating that it is a tumor suppressor.

Researchers are increasingly focusing on more mechanistic strategies that target molecular targets that underpin cell development, rather than finding drugs that impede tumor cell proliferation. Apoptosis is a type of programmed cell death that controls cell proliferation and tissue growth in response to DNA damage. The two main routes that lead to apoptosis are the extrinsic-death receptor pathway and the intrinsic-mitochondrial pathway. The extrinsic route includes membrane-bound Fas ligand, death receptors, Fas-associated death domain (FADD), caspases 8 and 10, and Fas complexes, which impact the rate of downstream caspases leading to apoptosis. The intrinsic pathway is one of the most important regulators in this system, and the Bcl-2 family is upregulated in many cancer cells. In both immune cells and tumors, immune checkpoint proteins can be detected. The most therapeutically developed immunological checkpoint proteins are Cytotoxic T-lymphocyte antigen-4 (CTLA-4) and Programmed cell death ligand-1 (PD-L1), which have inhibitor therapies. PD-1, a member of the CD28 family, is expressed by T cells, B cells, and natural killer (NK) cells. Immune receptors, a tyrosine-based switch motif, and an inhibitory motif based on tyrosine make up the cytoplasmic domain of PD-1. Pembrolizumab (Keytruda®) and nivolumab (Opdivo®) are two clinically approved inhibitors of programmed cell death ligand-1 (PD-1). Pembrolizumab and nivolumab have revolutionized the treatment of advanced unresectable and metastatic solid cancers. CTLA-4, also known as CD152, is an immune checkpoint protein. CTLA-4 is a protein that regulates T-cell activity and protects immune cells from injury. CTLA-4-mediated immune-cell inactivation is inhibited by apilimumab. Tremelimumab is now being studied in combination with other immunoediting drugs to see if it has any therapeutic benefits in cancers other than lung cancer. Immunological checkpoint proteins are found in both immune cells and malignancies. Cytotoxic T-lymphocyte antigen-4 (CTLA-4) and Programmed cell death ligand-1 (PD-L1) inhibitors are the most therapeutically developed immunological checkpoint proteins. T cells, B cells, and natural killer (NK) cells all express PD-1, a CD28 family member. The cytoplasmic domain of PD-1 is made up of immune receptors, an immune receptor tyrosine-based switch motif, and a tyrosine-based inhibitory motif.

CONSENT FOR PUBLICATION

Not applicable.

CONFLICT OF INTEREST

The author declares no conflict of interest, financial or otherwise.

ACKNOWLEDGEMENT

Declared none.

REFERENCES

[1] Ribatti D. A revisited concept: Contact inhibition of growth. From cell biology to malignancy. Exp Cell Res 2017; 359(1): 17-9. [http://dx.doi.org/10.1016/j.yexcr.2017.06.012] [PMID: 28642051]

[2] Pavel M, Renna M, Park SJ, *et al.* Contact inhibition controls cell survival and proliferation *via* YAP/TAZ-autophagy axis. Nat Commun 2018; 9(1): 2961. [http://dx.doi.org/10.1038/s41467-018-05388-x] [PMID: 30054475]

[3] Shraiman BI. Mechanical feedback as a possible regulator of tissue growth. Proc Natl Acad Sci USA 2005; 102(9): 3318-23. [http://dx.doi.org/10.1073/pnas.0404782102] [PMID: 15728365]

[4] Pavel M, Renna M, Park SJ, *et al.* Contact inhibition controls cell survival and proliferation via YAP/TAZ-autophagy axis. Nat Commun 9, 2018; Article No. 2961. [http://dx.doi.org/10.1038/s41467-018-05388-x]

[5] Leontieva OV, Blagosklonny MV. DNA damaging agents and p53 do not cause senescence in quiescent cells, while consecutive re-activation of mTOR is associated with conversion to senescence. Aging (Albany NY) 2010; 2(12): 924-35. [http://dx.doi.org/10.18632/aging.100265] [PMID: 21212465]

[6] Levy L, Hill C. Alterations in components of the TGF-β superfamily signaling pathways in human

cancer. Cytokine Growth Factor Rev 2006; 17(1-2): 41-58.
[http://dx.doi.org/10.1016/j.cytogfr.2005.09.009] [PMID: 16310402]

[7] Colak S, ten Dijke P. Targeting TGF-β Signaling in Cancer. Trends Cancer 2017; 3(1): 56-71. [http://dx.doi.org/10.1016/j.trecan.2016.11.008] [PMID: 28718426]

[8] Wang X, Lin Y. Tumor necrosis factor and cancer, buddies or foes? Acta Pharmacol Sin 2008; 29(11): 1275-88.
[http://dx.doi.org/10.1111/j.1745-7254.2008.00889.x] [PMID: 18954521]

[9] Syed V. TGF-β Signaling in Cancer. J Cell Biochem 2016; 117(6): 1279-87.
[http://dx.doi.org/10.1002/jcb.25496] [PMID: 26774024]

[10] Liu S, Chen S, Zeng J. TGF-β signaling: A complex role in tumorigenesis (Review). Mol Med Rep 2018; 17(1): 699-704.
[PMID: 29115550]

[11] Kaklamani V, Baddi L, Rosman D, *et al.* No major association between TGFBR1*6A and prostate cancer. BMC Genet 2004; 5(1): 28.
[http://dx.doi.org/10.1186/1471-2156-5-28] [PMID: 15385056]

[12] Xie W, Mertens JC, Reiss DJ, *et al.* Alterations of Smad signaling in human breast carcinoma are associated with poor outcome: a tissue microarray study. Cancer Res 2002; 62(2): 497-505.
[PMID: 11809701]

[13] Yang L, Huang J, Ren X, *et al.* Abrogation of TGF beta signaling in mammary carcinomas recruits Gr-1+CD11b+ myeloid cells that promote metastasis. Cancer Cell 2008; 13(1): 23-35.
[http://dx.doi.org/10.1016/j.ccr.2007.12.004] [PMID: 18167337]

[14] Kingsley LA, Fournier PGJ, Chirgwin JM, Guise TA. Molecular biology of bone metastasis. Mol Cancer Ther 2007; 6(10): 2609-17.
[http://dx.doi.org/10.1158/1535-7163.MCT-07-0234] [PMID: 17938257]

[15] Wrzesinski SH, Wan YY, Flavell RA. Transforming growth factor-beta and the immune response: implications for anticancer therapy. Clin Cancer Res 2007; 13(18): 5262-70.
[http://dx.doi.org/10.1158/1078-0432.CCR-07-1157] [PMID: 17875754]

[16] Loeys BL, Schwarze U, Holm T, *et al.* Aneurysm syndromes caused by mutations in the TGF-beta receptor. N Engl J Med 2006; 355(8): 788-98.
[http://dx.doi.org/10.1056/NEJMoa055695] [PMID: 16928994]

[17] Linder B, Kögel D. Autophagy in Cancer Cell Death. Biology (Basel) 2019; 8(4): 82.
[http://dx.doi.org/10.3390/biology8040082] [PMID: 31671879]

[18] Yun C, Lee S. The Roles of Autophagy in Cancer. Int J Mol Sci 2018; 19(11): 3466.
[http://dx.doi.org/10.3390/ijms19113466] [PMID: 30400561]

[19] Bhutia SK, Mukhopadhyay S, Sinha N, *et al.* Autophagy. Adv Cancer Res 2013; 118: 61-95.
[http://dx.doi.org/10.1016/B978-0-12-407173-5.00003-0] [PMID: 23768510]

[20] Alenzi FQ. Links between apoptosis, cell cycle and proliferation (REVIEW). Br J Biomed Sci 2004; 61(2): 99-102.
[http://dx.doi.org/10.1080/09674845.2004.11732652] [PMID: 15250676]

[21] Alenzi FQB, Warrens AN. Cellular and molecular themes in apoptosis. Wien Klin Wochenschr 2003; 115(15-16): 563-74.
[http://dx.doi.org/10.1007/BF03040450] [PMID: 14531169]

[22] Alenzi F. Cell type specific expression of the apoptosis stimulating protein (ASPP-2) in human tissues. Acta Microbiol Immunol Hung 2010; 57(4): 419-29.
[http://dx.doi.org/10.1556/AMicr.57.2010.4.8] [PMID: 21183427]

[23] Alenzi FQ, Lotfy M, Wyse R. Swords of cell death: caspase activation and regulation. Asian Pac J Cancer Prev 2010; 11(2): 271-80.

[PMID: 20843101]

[24] Liu EY, Ryan KM. Autophagy and cancer – issues we need to digest. J Cell Sci 2012; 125: 2349. [http://dx.doi.org/10.1242/jcs.093708] [PMID: 22641689]

[25] White E. The role for autophagy in cancer. J Clin Invest 2015; 125(1): 42-6. [http://dx.doi.org/10.1172/JCI73941] [PMID: 25654549]

[26] Liu Z, Jiao D. Necroptosis, tumor necrosis and tumorigenesis. Cell Stress 2020; 4(1): 1-8. [http://dx.doi.org/10.15698/cst2020.01.208] [PMID: 31922095]

[27] Jiao D, Cai Z, Choksi S, *et al.* Necroptosis of tumor cells leads to tumor necrosis and promotes tumor metastasis. Cell Res 2018; 28(8): 868-70. [http://dx.doi.org/10.1038/s41422-018-0058-y] [PMID: 29941926]

[28] Yatim N, Jusforgues-Saklani H, Orozco S, *et al.* RIPK1 and NF-κB signaling in dying cells determines cross-priming of CD8$^+$ T cells. Science 2015; 350(6258): 328-34. [http://dx.doi.org/10.1126/science.aad0395] [PMID: 26405229]

[29] Seifert L, Werba G, Tiwari S, *et al.* The necrosome promotes pancreatic oncogenesis *via* CXCL1 and Mincle-induced immune suppression. Nature 2016; 532(7598): 245-9. [http://dx.doi.org/10.1038/nature17403] [PMID: 27049944]

[30] Kearney CJ, Martin SJ. An Inflammatory Perspective on Necroptosis. Mol Cell 2017; 65(6): 965-73. [http://dx.doi.org/10.1016/j.molcel.2017.02.024] [PMID: 28306512]

[31] Wai LK. Telomeres, telomerase, and tumorigenesis-a review. MedGenMed 2004; 6(3): 19. [PMID: 15520642]

[32] Wang Y, Sušac L, Feigon J. Structural Biology of Telomerase. Cold Spring Harb Perspect Biol 2019; 11(12): a032383. [http://dx.doi.org/10.1101/cshperspect.a032383] [PMID: 31451513]

[33] Romaniuk A, Paszel-Jaworska A, Totoń E, *et al.* The non-canonical functions of telomerase: to turn off or not to turn off. Mol Biol Rep 2019; 46(1): 1401-11. [http://dx.doi.org/10.1007/s11033-018-4496-x] [PMID: 30448892]

[34] Blasco MA. Mammalian telomeres and telomerase: why they matter for cancer and aging. Eur J Cell Biol 2003; 82(9): 441-6. [http://dx.doi.org/10.1078/0171-9335-00335] [PMID: 14582532]

[35] Bodnar AG, Ouellette M, Frolkis M, *et al.* Extension of life-span by introduction of telomerase into normal human cells. Science 1998; 279(5349): 349-52. [http://dx.doi.org/10.1126/science.279.5349.349] [PMID: 9454332]

[36] Reddel RR. The role of senescence and immortalization in carcinogenesis. Carcinogenesis 2000; 21(3): 477-84. [http://dx.doi.org/10.1093/carcin/21.3.477] [PMID: 10688868]

[37] Shay JW, Zou Y, Hiyama E, Wright WE. Telomerase and cancer. Hum Mol Genet 2001; 10(7): 677-85. [http://dx.doi.org/10.1093/hmg/10.7.677] [PMID: 11257099]

[38] Sfeir A. Telomeres at a glance. J Cell Sci 2012; 125(18): 4173-8. [http://dx.doi.org/10.1242/jcs.106831] [PMID: 23135002]

[39] Kowalska A, Kowalik A. Telomeres and telomerase in oncogenesis. Contemp Oncol (Pozn) 2006; 10: 485-96.

[40] Trybek T, Kowalik A, Góźdź S, Kowalska A. Telomeres and telomerase in oncogenesis (Review). Oncol Lett 2020; 20(2): 1015-27. [http://dx.doi.org/10.3892/ol.2020.11659] [PMID: 32724340]

[41] Hyder SM, Stancel GM. Regulation of angiogenic growth factors in the female reproductive tract by

estrogens and progestins. Mol Endocrinol 1999; 13(6): 806-11.
[http://dx.doi.org/10.1210/mend.13.6.0308] [PMID: 10379879]

[42] Koch AE, Distler O. Vasculopathy and disordered angiogenesis in selected rheumatic diseases: rheumatoid arthritis and systemic sclerosis. Arthritis Res Ther 2007; 9 (Suppl. 2): S3.
[http://dx.doi.org/10.1186/ar2187] [PMID: 17767741]

[43] Ehrmann RL, Knoth M. Choriocarcinoma. Transfilter stimulation of vasoproliferation in the hamster cheek pouch. Studied by light and electron microscopy. J Natl Cancer Inst 1968; 41(6): 1329-41.
[PMID: 5750121]

[44] Bharali DJ, Rajabi M, Mousa SA. Anti-Angiogenesis Strategies in Cancer Therapeutics. Cancer Cell 2017; 165-78.

[45] Winkler F. Hostile takeover: how tumours hijack pre-existing vascular environments to thrive. J Pathol 2017; 242(3): 267-72.
[http://dx.doi.org/10.1002/path.4904] [PMID: 28390068]

[46] Senger H D DR, Galli SJ, Dvorak AM. Tumor cells secrete a vascular permeability factor that promotes accumulation of ascites fluid. Science 1983; 219: 983–5.
[http://dx.doi.org/10.1126/science.6823562]

[47] Schito L. Bridging angiogenesis and immune evasion in the hypoxic tumor microenvironment. Am J Physiol Regul Integr Comp Physiol 2018; 315(6): R1072-84.
[http://dx.doi.org/10.1152/ajpregu.00209.2018] [PMID: 30183339]

[48] Zhao Y, Adjei AA. Targeting Angiogenesis in Cancer Therapy: Moving Beyond Vascular Endothelial Growth Factor. Oncologist 2015; 20(6): 660-73.
[http://dx.doi.org/10.1634/theoncologist.2014-0465] [PMID: 26001391]

[49] Phung TL, Ziv K, Dabydeen D, *et al.* Pathological angiogenesis is induced by sustained Akt signaling and inhibited by rapamycin. Cancer Cell 2006; 10(2): 159-70.
[http://dx.doi.org/10.1016/j.ccr.2006.07.003] [PMID: 16904613]

[50] Mizukami Y, Kohgo Y, Chung DC. Hypoxia inducible factor-1 independent pathways in tumor angiogenesis. Clin Cancer Res 2007; 13(19): 5670-4.
[http://dx.doi.org/10.1158/1078-0432.CCR-07-0111] [PMID: 17908955]

[51] Semenza GL. Hypoxia-inducible factors: mediators of cancer progression and targets for cancer therapy. Trends Pharmacol Sci 2012; 33(4): 207-14.
[http://dx.doi.org/10.1016/j.tips.2012.01.005] [PMID: 22398146]

[52] McMahon G. VEGF receptor signaling in tumor angiogenesis. Oncologist 2000. 5 (Suppl. 1): 3-10.
[http://dx.doi.org/10.1634/theoncologist.5-suppl_1-3] [PMID: 10804084]

[53] Terzuoli E, Puppo M, Rapisarda A, *et al.* Aminoflavone, a ligand of the aryl hydrocarbon receptor, inhibits HIF-1α expression in an AhR-independent fashion. Cancer Res 2010; 70(17): 6837-48.
[http://dx.doi.org/10.1158/0008-5472.CAN-10-1075] [PMID: 20736373]

[54] Li J, Wang L, Chen X, *et al.* CD39/CD73 upregulation on myeloid-derived suppressor cells *via* TGF-β-mTOR-HIF-1 signaling in patients with non-small cell lung cancer. OncoImmunology 2017; 6(6): e1320011.
[http://dx.doi.org/10.1080/2162402X.2017.1320011] [PMID: 28680754]

[55] Pang Y, Yang C, Schovanek J, *et al.* Anthracyclines suppress pheochromocytoma cell characteristics, including metastasis, through inhibition of the hypoxia signaling pathway Oncotarget 2017; 8(14): 22313–24.
[http://dx.doi.org/10.18632/oncotarget.16224]

[56] Ferris RL, Blumenschein G Jr, Fayette J, *et al.* Nivolumab for Recurrent Squamous-Cell Carcinoma of the Head and Neck. N Engl J Med 2016; 375(19): 1856-67.
[http://dx.doi.org/10.1056/NEJMoa1602252] [PMID: 27718784]

[57] Motzer RJ, Tannir NM, McDermott DF, *et al.* Nivolumab plus Ipilimumab *versus* Sunitinib in Advanced Renal-Cell Carcinoma. N Engl J Med 2018; 378(14): 1277-90. [http://dx.doi.org/10.1056/NEJMoa1712126] [PMID: 29562145]

[58] Overman MJ, Kopetz S, Lonardi S, *et al.* Nivolumab ± ipilimumab treatment (Tx) efficacy, safety, and biomarkers in patients (Pts) with metastatic colorectal cancer (mCRC) with and without high microsatellite instability (MSI-H): results from the CheckMate-142 study. Ann Oncol 2016; 27: vi158. [http://dx.doi.org/10.1093/annonc/mdw370.27]

[59] Calabrò L, Morra A, Fonsatti E, *et al.* Tremelimumab for patients with chemotherapy-resistant advanced malignant mesothelioma: an open-label, single-arm, phase 2 trial. Lancet Oncol 2013; 14(11): 1104-11. [http://dx.doi.org/10.1016/S1470-2045(13)70381-4] [PMID: 24035405]

[60] Vriend J, Reiter RJ. Melatonin and the von Hippel-Lindau/HIF-1 oxygen sensing mechanism: A review. Biochim Biophys Acta 2016; 1865(2): 176-83. [PMID: 26899267]

[61] Zhang H, Wong CCL, Wei H, *et al.* HIF-1-dependent expression of angiopoietin-like 4 and L1CAM mediates vascular metastasis of hypoxic breast cancer cells to the lungs. Oncogene 2012; 31(14): 1757-70. [http://dx.doi.org/10.1038/onc.2011.365] [PMID: 21860410]

[62] Ebos JML, Lee CR, Cruz-Munoz W, Bjarnason GA, Christensen JG, Kerbel RS. Accelerated metastasis after short-term treatment with a potent inhibitor of tumor angiogenesis. Cancer Cell 2009; 15(3): 232-9. [http://dx.doi.org/10.1016/j.ccr.2009.01.021] [PMID: 19249681]

[63] Wong CCL, Gilkes DM, Zhang H, *et al.* Hypoxia-inducible factor 1 is a master regulator of breast cancer metastatic niche formation. Proc Natl Acad Sci USA 2011; 108(39): 16369-74. [http://dx.doi.org/10.1073/pnas.1113483108] [PMID: 21911388]

[64] Perlikos F, Harrington KJ, Syrigos KN. Key molecular mechanisms in lung cancer invasion and metastasis: A comprehensive review. Crit Rev Oncol Hematol 2013; 87(1): 1-11. [http://dx.doi.org/10.1016/j.critrevonc.2012.12.007] [PMID: 23332547]

[65] Hartsock A, Nelson WJ. Adherens and tight junctions: Structure, function and connections to the actin cytoskeleton. Biochim Biophys Acta Biomembr 2008; 1778(3): 660-9. [http://dx.doi.org/10.1016/j.bbamem.2007.07.012] [PMID: 17854762]

[66] Ireton RC, Davis MA, van Hengel J, *et al.* A novel role for p120 catenin in E-cadherin function. J Cell Biol 2002; 159(3): 465-76. [http://dx.doi.org/10.1083/jcb.200205115] [PMID: 12427869]

[67] Canel M, Serrels A, Frame MC, Brunton VG. E-cadherin–integrin crosstalk in cancer invasion and metastasis. J Cell Sci 2013; 126(2): 393-401. [http://dx.doi.org/10.1242/jcs.100115] [PMID: 23525005]

[68] Rodriguez FJ, Lewis-Tuffin LJ, Anastasiadis PZ. E-cadherin's dark side: possible role in tumor progression. Biochim Biophys Acta 2012; 1826(1): 23-31. [PMID: 22440943]

[69] Kondo T, Oka T, Sato H, *et al.* Accumulation of aberrant CpG hypermethylation by *Helicobacter pylori* infection promotes development and progression of gastric MALT lymphoma. Int J Oncol 2009; 35(3): 547-57. [PMID: 19639175]

[70] Shah GV, Muralidharan A, Gokulgandhi M, Soan K, Thomas S. Cadherin switching and activation of β-catenin signaling underlie proinvasive actions of calcitonin-calcitonin receptor axis in prostate cancer. J Biol Chem 2009; 284(2): 1018-30. [http://dx.doi.org/10.1074/jbc.M807823200] [PMID: 19001380]

[71] Thomas S, Chigurupati S, Anbalagan M, Shah G. Calcitonin increases tumorigenicity of prostate cancer cells: evidence for the role of protein kinase A and urokinase-type plasminogen receptor. Mol Endocrinol 2006; 20(8): 1894-911. [http://dx.doi.org/10.1210/me.2005-0284] [PMID: 16574742]

[72] Xiao D, He J. Epithelial mesenchymal transition and lung cancer. J Thorac Dis 2010; 2(3): 154-9. [PMID: 22263037]

[73] Morra L, Moch H. Periostin expression and epithelial-mesenchymal transition in cancer: a review and an update. Virchows Arch 2011; 459(5): 465-75. [http://dx.doi.org/10.1007/s00428-011-1151-5] [PMID: 21997759]

[74] Pradella D, Naro C, Sette C, Ghigna C. EMT and stemness: Flexible processes tuned by alternative splicing in development and cancer progression. Mol Can. 2017; 16(8): 1-19. [http://dx.doi.org/10.1186/s12943-016-0579-2]

[75] Sánchez-Tilló E, de Barrios O, Siles L, Cuatrecasas M, Castells A, Postigo A. β-catenin/TCF4 complex induces the epithelial-to-mesenchymal transition (EMT)-activator ZEB1 to regulate tumor invasiveness. Proc Natl Acad Sci USA 2011; 108(48): 19204-9. [http://dx.doi.org/10.1073/pnas.1108977108] [PMID: 22080605]

[76] Valdés F, Alvarez AM, Locascio A, *et al.* The epithelial mesenchymal transition confers resistance to the apoptotic effects of transforming growth factor β in fetal rat hepatocytes. Mol Cancer Res 2002; 1(1): 68-78. [PMID: 12496370]

[77] Herman DS, Lam L, Matthew RG, *et al.* NIH Public Access. Bone 2010; 23(1): 1–7.

[78] Fernando J, Malfettone A, Cepeda EB, *et al.* A mesenchymal-like phenotype and expression of CD44 predict lack of apoptotic response to sorafenib in liver tumor cells. Int J Cancer 2015; 136(4): E161-72. [http://dx.doi.org/10.1002/ijc.29097] [PMID: 25053293]

[79] Omara-Opyene A L, Qiu J, Shah G V, Iczkowski K A. Prostate cancer invasion is influenced more by expression of a CD44 isoform including variant 9 than by Muc18. Lab Investig 2004, 894-907.

[80] Guo W, Keckesova Z, Donaher JL, *et al.* Slug and Sox9 cooperatively determine the mammary stem cell state. Cell 2012; 148(5): 1015-28. [http://dx.doi.org/10.1016/j.cell.2012.02.008]

[81] Ocaña OH, Córcoles R, Fabra Á, *et al.* Metastatic colonization requires the repression of the epithelial-mesenchymal transition inducer Prrx1. Cancer Cell 2012; 22(6): 709-24. [http://dx.doi.org/10.1016/j.ccr.2012.10.012] [PMID: 23201163]

[82] Bahassi M. The cell cycle and cancer. Med Cell Biol 2007; 273–289.

[83] Vermeulen K, Van Bockstaele DR, Berneman ZN. The cell cycle: a review of regulation, deregulation and therapeutic targets in cancer. Cell Prolif 2003; 36(3): 131-49. [http://dx.doi.org/10.1046/j.1365-2184.2003.00266.x] [PMID: 12814430]

[84] Sherr CJ. G1 phase progression: Cycling on cue. Cell 1994; 79(4): 551-5. [http://dx.doi.org/10.1016/0092-8674(94)90540-1] [PMID: 7954821]

[85] Wölfel T, Hauer M, Schneider J, *et al.* A p16INK4a-insensitive CDK4 mutant targeted by cytolytic T lymphocytes in a human melanoma. Science 1995; 269(5228): 1281-4. [http://dx.doi.org/10.1126/science.7652577] [PMID: 7652577]

[86] Hunter J. Pines T. Cyclins and cancer. II: Cyclin D and CDK inhibitors come of age. Cell 1994; 79: 573–82.

[87] Park MT, Lee SJ. Cell cycle and cancer. J Biochem Mol Biol 2003; 36(1): 60-5. [PMID: 12542976]

[88] Pagano M. Control of the Cell Cycle by the Ubiquitin System 2006; 15: 162-5.

[89] Deng C, Zhang P, Wade Harper J, Elledge SJ, Leder P. Mice Lacking p21CIP1/WAF1 undergo normal development, but are defective in G1 checkpoint control. Cell 1995; 82(4): 675-84. [http://dx.doi.org/10.1016/0092-8674(95)90039-X] [PMID: 7664346]

[90] Ouyang L, Shi Z, Zhao S, *et al.* Programmed cell death pathways in cancer: a review of apoptosis, autophagy and programmed necrosis. Cell Prolif 2012; 45(6): 487-98. [http://dx.doi.org/10.1111/j.1365-2184.2012.00845.x] [PMID: 23030059]

[91] Ghobrial IM, Witzig TE, Adjei AA. Targeting apoptosis pathways in cancer therapy. CA Cancer J Clin 2005; 55(3): 178-94. [http://dx.doi.org/10.3322/canjclin.55.3.178] [PMID: 15890640]

[92] Landowski TH, Moscinski L, Burke R, *et al.* CD95 antigen mutations in hematopoietic malignancies. Leuk Lymphoma 2001; 42(5): 835-46. [http://dx.doi.org/10.3109/10428190109097702] [PMID: 11697638]

[93] Llambi F, Green DR. Apoptosis and oncogenesis: give and take in the BCL-2 family. Curr Opin Genet Dev 2011; 21(1): 12-20. [http://dx.doi.org/10.1016/j.gde.2010.12.001] [PMID: 21236661]

[94] Wong RSY. Apoptosis in cancer: from pathogenesis to treatment. J Exp Clin Cancer Res 2011; 30(1): 87. [http://dx.doi.org/10.1186/1756-9966-30-87] [PMID: 21943236]

[95] Sankari SL, Masthan KMK, Babu NA, Bhattacharjee T, Elumalai M. Apoptosis in cancer-an update. Asian Pac J Cancer Prev 2012; 13(10): 4873-8. [http://dx.doi.org/10.7314/APJCP.2012.13.10.4873] [PMID: 23244073]

[96] Gaynor N, Crown J, Collins D M. Immune checkpoint inhibitors: Key trials and an emerging role in breast cancer Semin Cancer Biol 2022; 79: 44-57. [http://dx.doi.org/10.1016/j.semcancer.2020.06.016]

[97] Pardoll DM. The blockade of immune checkpoints in cancer immunotherapy. Nat Rev Cancer 2012; 12(4): 252-64. [http://dx.doi.org/10.1038/nrc3239] [PMID: 22437870]

[98] Quezada SA, Peggs KS. Exploiting CTLA-4, PD-1 and PD-L1 to reactivate the host immune response against cancer. Br J Cancer 2013; 108(8): 1560-5. [http://dx.doi.org/10.1038/bjc.2013.117] [PMID: 23511566]

[99] Asai A, Yasuoka H, Tsuchimoto Y, *et al.* PD-L1 expression of monocytes may be used a new marker of the classification for the cancer progression in hepatocellular carcinomale. J Immunol 2018; 200 (1_Supplement): 56.8.

[100] Topalian SL, Hodi FS, Brahmer JR, *et al.* Safety, activity, and immune correlates of anti–pd-1 antibody in cancer. New Eng J Med 2012: 2443–54.

[101] Robert C, Schachter J, Long GV, *et al.* Pembrolizumab *versus* Ipilimumab in Advanced Melanoma. N Engl J Med 2015; 372(26): 2521-32. [http://dx.doi.org/10.1056/NEJMoa1503093] [PMID: 25891173]

[102] Webb ES, Liu P, Baleeiro R, Lemoine NR, Yuan M, Wang YH. Immune checkpoint inhibitors in cancer therapy. J Biomed Res 2018; 32(5): 317-26. [PMID: 28866656]

CHAPTER 3

Exogenous Factors and Cancer

Baraa T. Alhajhussein[1,*], **Majed H. Wakid**[2], **Najwa Mohamad Alsawi**[3], **Hesham Hamdy Amin**[3,4] and **Fahad Nasser Alonazi**[5]

[1] *King Saud Bin Abdulaziz University for Health Sciences (KSAUHS), Jeddah, Saudi Arabia*

[2] *Department of Medical Laboratories Technology, Faculty of Applied Medical Sciences, King Abdulaziz University, Jeddah, Saudi Arabia*

[3] *Hotat Bani Tamim General Hospital, Riyadh, Saudi Arabia*

[4] *Al Azhar Faculty of Medicine, Egypt*

[5] *Saudi Public Health Authority, Riyadh, Saudi Arabia*

Abstract: The causation of cancer, whether exogenous or endogenous, is a cornerstone of cancer prevention and treatment. Many intrinsic factors are discussed in other chapters of this book; this chapter will shed light on exogenous factors influencing cancer with detailed specific examples of microbial, physical and chemical factors.

Microbial role in cancer has been debated over many centuries, whether as an antagonist or a cause, since Imhotep's time through the mid-17th century when cancer was considered contagious, and later cancer hospitals were forcefully moved out of the cities as isolation camps. There are now vivid evidences that specific microbial pathogens are causing up to 25% of cancer cases (lymphoma, solid or others), and in some cases, a single pathogen was found in association with many types of cancer, such as HPV and EBV, to a lesser extent.

Also, several non-biological factors are classified as carcinogens as humans are exposed to millions of chemicals whether in environment or smoke processed food.

Keywords: Bacterial carcinogen, Free Radicals, Microbial carcinogenesis, Parasitic carcinogen, Radioactive cancer, Smoke and cancer, Viral carcinogen.

* **Corresponding author Baraa T. Alhajhussein:** King Saud Bin Abdulaziz University for Health Sciences (KSAUHS), Jeddah, Saudi Arabia; E-mail: alhajhusseinbt@gmail.com

INTRODUCTION

Since cancer was first described as a human disease in 2600 BC., microbes were thought to play a role in cancer but rather as an antagonist than a cause. This was reflected by the practice of the Egyptian physician Imhotep who would incise the area of tumor to infect such location so that infection, would cause tumor regression [1].

Centuries later, Zacutus Lusitani and Nicholas Tulp promoted the contagion theory in 1649 and 1652, respectively, concluding that cancer was contagious based on their experiences with breast cancer in members of the same household in the Netherlands. They further proposed patient isolation, that has been officially adopted later in France in 1779 when cancer hospitals were moved by force out of the cities as the public belief was that cancer is contagious [2, 3].

In addition to many theories attributing cancer to intrinsic factors discussed in the other chapters of this book, the role of exogenous causes of cancer was still active. In 1921, after discovering the active cancer-causing agents (carcinogens) in cigarette smoke, the Institute of Cancer Research assigned Sir Ernest Kennaway to investigate the carcinogenic properties of tars and oils [4].

Only a few years after describing Burkitt lymphoma in 1958, it was the first time ever to associate a specific microbe with human cancer when Burkitt lymphoma was linked to Epstein-Barr virus (EBV) in 1964 [5]. In 1980s, human papillomavirus DNA of HPV types 16 and 18 were linked to cervical carcinogenesis after being identified in a high proportion of cervical cancer biopsies [6], and soon after, other types of cancer were identified in association with HPV [7].

On the other hand, a century after the first successful surgical treatment of gastric cancer in 1881, *C. pyloridis* (later named *H. pylori*) has been proved to be causing gastric ulcer in 1983 [8] and soon after a cause of gastric cancer [9].

As humans and other living beings have potential exposure to millions of environmental chemicals worldwide, controlling inflammation and its resolution will be a critical component of successful cancer prevention and treatment of cancer [10]. Epidemiological studies guided the resolution of the World Health Organization's International Agency for Research on Cancer to classify processed meat as a group I carcinogen of which the risk category is similar to that of alcohol and cigarettes [11]. Currently, around 25% of human cancers are associated with infectious diseases, of which some have been confirmed as the cause [12].

BACTERIA AND CANCER

Although microbial infections have been associated with cancer for centuries but not specifically among the leading causes of cancer. However, nominating *H. pylori* as the first bacteria to be identified as a cause of human cancer in humans, followed by the discovery of its inflammatory mechanism of carcinogenesis in the early 1990s, by which bacteria cause cancer made the proof of causation [13]. *Chlamydophila pneumoniae* is an intracellular Gram-negative bacillus that has been detected in a number of chronic lung diseases, most commonly in adults. However, there is more evidence that links *C. pneumoniae* infection and lung carcinomas, especially in heavy smokers [14]. In addition, studies on survivors of colorectal cancer (CRC) have concluded the causative role of *Streptococcus bovis* in colon malignancy where *S. bovis* bacteremia was the strongest signal [15].

Direct Bacterial Carcinogenesis

Microbial Carcinogenesis is a multistep process orchestrated by both host genetic and epigenetic changes in either the oncogenes, tumor suppressor genes or different molecules involved in cell adhesion in addition to microbial toxins or metabolites that also modulate host cell transformation [16].

This is reflected classically in *H. pylori* infection, where the bacteria release reactive nitrogen species (RNS) and reactive oxygen species (ROS), where both strongly trigger "stem cell" hyperplasia followed by increased telomerase activity and, therefore, telomere reduction in parallel with overexpression of hTRT. Consequently, DNA replication errors, DNA hypermethylation, and p53 mutations, along with CD44 abnormal transcripts composing the early steps of well-differentiated gastric cancer [17].

In addition, the risk is considerably driven by *H. pylori* strain virulence variation exacerbated by the host immunogenetics governing the resulting inflammatory response. Such interactions can directly cause specific tissue damage, leading to gastric cancer development [18]. Because of underreporting tumor-associated clinical symptoms prior to diagnosing the disease, nearly half of cases end up being advanced complicated type gastric cancer upon the first visit and therefore, the prognosis is poor [19].

Indirect Bacterial Carcinogenesis

The second bacterial oncogenesis mechanism is driven by the oncogenic metabolites of bacteria. The best example is the microbiota-associated colon cancer in the presence of bile salt metabolites that intensifies colonic cell proliferation [20, 21].

Due to the natural function of the gallbladder in concentrating molecules, it is likely to augment carcinogenesis mediators. *Salmonella typhi* is significantly associated with the gallbladder Carcinoma CaGB along with Chronic persistence typhoid, where the production of chronic inflammation mediators and a distinct cytotoxic distending toxin, CdtB; a genotoxic toxin. Along with *S. typhi*, some *Helicobacter* species (*H. bilis* and *H. hepaticus*) and *Escherichia coli* have carcinogenic roles [22].

In parallel, exogenous compounds such as rutin may be metabolized into mutagens by resident colonic flora. This could be represented by producing high concentrations of the potent mutagens; fecapentaenes by Bacteroides species [23].

Furthermore, not only *Helicobacter pylori* has been closely associated with the most common haematologic malignancy ; Non-Hodgkin's lymphoma (NHL), but also *Chlamydia psittaci*, *Coxiella burnetii*, *Borrelia burgdorferi* and *Campylobacter jejuni* were found in NHL tissue samples. Such a phenomenon is under investigation to establish grounds for detecting certain bacteria as early biomarkers for lymphoma progression [24].

Other Roles for Bacteria in Cancer

The complexity of the microbial role in cancer isn't limited to causation or synergistic interactions but also to antagonising certain steps in the ontogenesis process. Some of these roles are referred to in Tables **3.1** and **3.2**, with the specific role of each organism [25].

Several thorough reviews of bacterial toxins implicated in carcinogenesis, and the involved carcinogenic pathways have been represented in informative figures and tables. In summary, bacterial toxins either directly attack the host DNA or interfere with the key eukaryotic processes, such as cellular signalling components. Enzymatic attack, DNA damage or impairing DNA damage repair mechanisms could cause direct host cell damage. While the indirect action is caused by free radicals' production or chronic inflammatory reaction induction [26, 27].

Table 3.1. Bacteria causing cancer [25].

Helicobacter pylori	Gastric cancer
Salmonella typhi	Gallbladder cancer
Mycobacterium tuberculosis	Lung cancer
Streptococcus bovis	Lung cancer
Chlamydia pneumonia	Lung cancer
Fusobacterium nucleatum	Colorectal cancer
Campylobacter jejuni	Small intestinal lymphomas
Bacteroides fragilis	Colon cancer
Porphyromonas gingivalis	Oral cancer
Streptococcus bovis	Colorectal neoplasia
Citrobacter rodentium	Human colorectal cancer
Chlamydia psittaci	Ocular lymphomas
Chlamydia trachomotis	Cervical cancer
Escherichia coli	Colon cancer
Helicobacter pylori	Gastric cancer
Salmonella typhi	Gallbladder cancer

Table 3.2. Bacteria antagonising cancer [25].

Clositridum novi	Removes the letal toxin gene
Streptococcus pyogenes	Coley vaccine regression of tumor
Serratia marcescens	Coley vaccine
Bacillus calmette-guerin	Reduces cancer
Clostridium spp	Regression of tumor
Salmonella typhimurium	Antitumor agent
Listeria monocytogenes	Regression of tumor
Clostridium acetobutylicum	Increases the production of IL-2
Bifidobacterium longum	Increases the gene vectors in tumor
Salmonella enterica	Vaccines against tumor
Corynebacterium diphtheriae	Enhanced apoptosis
Clostridium perfringens	Rapid cytolysis
Clostridium botulinum	Botulinum neurotoxin effect on tumor

Bacterial Cancer Therapy

Since the beginning of cancer gene therapy, the key obstacle has been selective delivery into tumor cells [28]. Building on the old hypotheses [1], some clostridia were found to flourish in oxygen-poor cancerous tissue and consequently deplete and kill neoplastic cells [29]. Further work identified other bacterial anti-cancer roles [30], as detailed in Fig. (**3.1**).

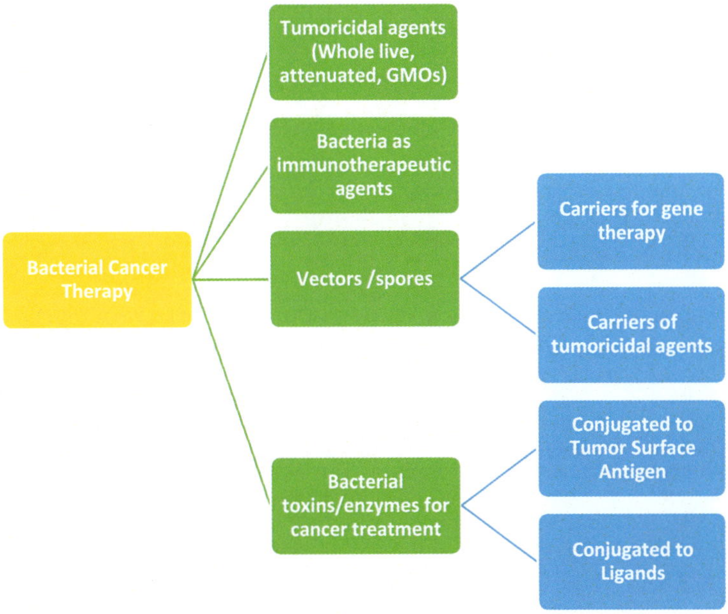

Fig. (3.1). Roles of bacteria anti-cancer.

Since several solid tumors, lymphomas and immunoproliferative diseases have been convincingly linked to underlying bacterial infections that could be cured with antibiotics, identification of bacterial oncogenesis is essential for the prevention of some cancer [31]. This is more obvious in the gastrointestinal tract from the mouth and larynx to the colon and rectum [32, 33]. Therefore, examining the microbiomes in cancer patients should become a cornerstone for understanding the aetiology, pathogenesis and prognosis of these diseases in order to plan better preventative measures as well as therapeutic interventions [34].

PARASITES AND CANCER

A parasite is an organism that depends on other organisms (the hosts) for its survival. Some blood and liver fluke helminths can directly cause cancer in humans, and thus, IARC classified them among Group 1 carcinogens [35]. On the other hand, some other parasitic infections may have an indirect role and increase the risk for carcinogenesis.

Blood Flukes

Human schistosomiasis (Bilharziasis) is among the neglected disease caused mainly by *Schistosoma* species (*S. haematobium, S. mansoni* and *S. japonicum*), representing blood fluke trematodes.

S. haematobium is common in many African and Middle East countries. The adult worms inhabit the venous plexuses around the urinary bladder, causing urogenital schistosomiasis.

Interaction of the infected host with parasite-derived products and eggs can lead to the induction of carcinogenesis [36 - 42].

S. mansoni infection was associated with several types of cancer [43 - 49]. On the other hand, several East and Southeast Asian studies suggested that *S. japonicum* may lead to hepatocellular and other carcinomas [50 - 53].

Mechanism

Host schistosomiasis initiates the pathway to cancer signalling through somatic mutations in the cancer genome and control of immune responses.

The strong immunogenic activity of the soluble antigens from schistosome eggs activates T helper cell subpopulations and stimulates chronic inflammation, which then contributes to carcinogenesis by targeting oncogenes (Fig. **3.2**) [54]. Arginine missense mutations in the gene of tumor protein p53 were detected in colorectal cancer during schistosomiasis [47, 55]. In addition, B-cell lymphoma 2 (Bcl-2) and cellular Myelocytomatosis (C-Myc) oncogenes are linked with the formation of schistosomal colorectal cancer [48].

Intestinal bilharziasis depresses cell-mediated responses in relation to developing hepatosplenomegaly. Immune responses during chronic schistosomiasis are modulated by the production of anti-idiotype (Anti-ID) antibodies (Fig. **3.2**) [56, 57].

Urogenital bilharziasis is strongly linked to bladder cancer because of various factors, such as the damage of the epithelium, chronic inflammatory mechanism, and oxidative stress (Fig. **3.2**) [38, 40, 58, 59]. Eggs can induce carcinogenesis through fibrosis, which increases host cell proliferation, hyperplasia, and metaplasia. Adult worms' production of nitrosamines, β-glucuronidase (GUSB) and cyclooxygenase-2 (COX-2) are confirmed as bladder carcinogens [58, 59].

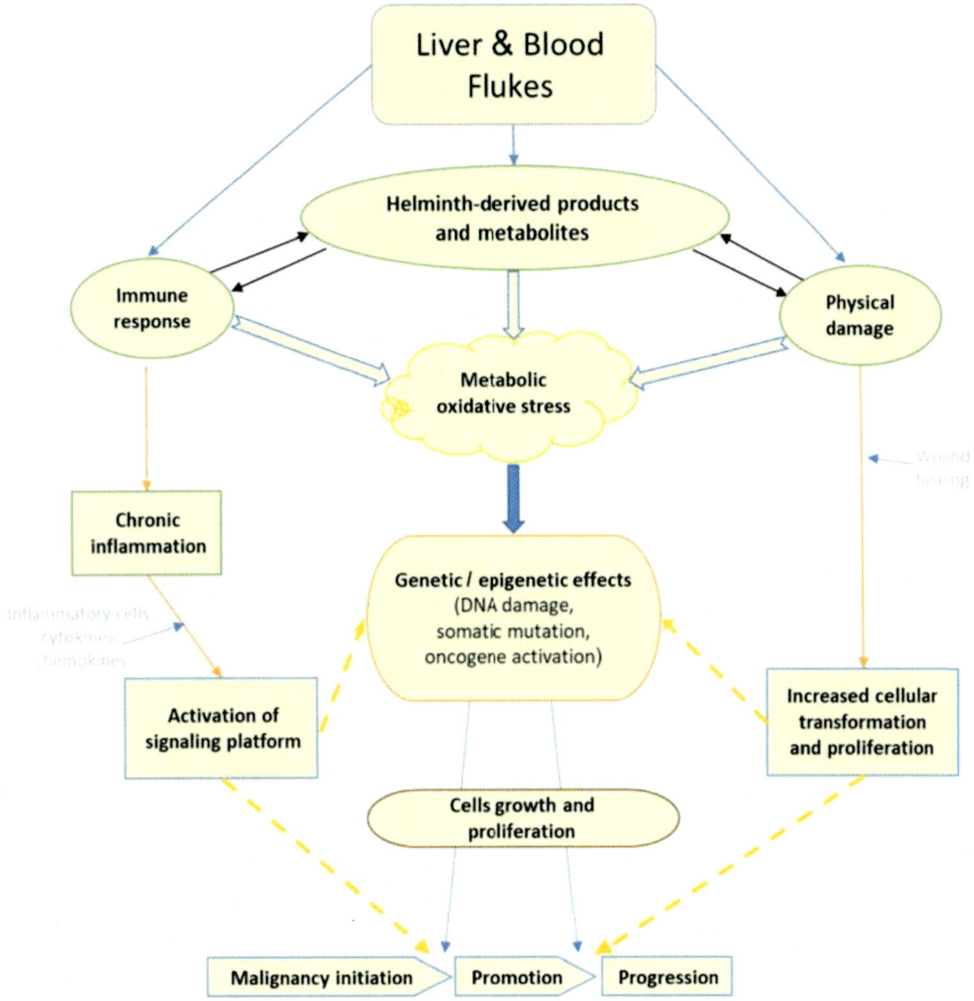

Fig. (3.2). Summary of the carcinogenicity mechanisms induced by liver and blood flukes.

The carcinogens from *S. haematobium* metabolites can trigger chronic inflammation by DNA damage and somatic mutations because of the immune responses, and the oxidative stress. Such stress was related to several oncogenes, mainly p53, RB tumor suppressor protein, EGFR, and ERBB2 [36, 37, 39, 41, 42, 60].

Liver Flukes

The common liver flukes include *Opisthorchis viverrini* and *Clonorchis sinensis*. They are fish-borne found in Eastern and Southeastern Asia. Opisthorchiasis and Clonorchiasis are mainly responsible for cholangiocarcinoma aggressive malignancy (cancer of the bile ducts) [38, 61 - 65].

Mechanism

Sever opisthorchiasis and clonorchiasis can damage the biliary epithelium. In addition, the enduring immune-mediated pathogenesis, impacts of Dimethylnitrosamine, granulin, and oxysterol production on the bile duct proliferation, IL-6 production, strong stimulation of Th2, and fibrosis can collectively promote cholangiocarcinoma [38, 62, 63, 66 - 68].

Apoptosis is prevented by thioredoxin (TRX) and thioredoxin peroxidase (TPX), which are both produced by parasites [69 - 71].

Opisthorchiasis has several effects on the regulation and expression of several proteins (such as p16INK4, RB1, CDK4 and cyclin D1). These proteins are involved in the RB tumor suppressor protein pathway [72]. Chronic inflammatory adjusts the signalling pathways of PI3K/AKT and Wnt/β-catenin correlated with tumorigenesis [73]. During the early stages of cholangiocarcinoma related to opisthorchiasis, the 14-3-3η protein is upregulated [74], and somatic mutations appear in the p53 and SMAD4 genes (Fig. **3.2**) [75, 76].

Clonorchiasis-derived products can enhance the gathering and invasion process of bile duct cancer cells into the surrounding extracellular matrix [77] and activate NF-κB with an inverse expression of Prdx6 (peroxiredoxin 6) [78]. In addition, the parasite activates the expressions of several lipid peroxidation carcinogenic products and plasma proinflammatory cytokines, proving that the parasite has a strong immunogenic effect and metabolic oxidative stress induction.

Indirect Carcinogenic Parasites

Several human parasitic infections are risk factors that can cause different types of cancers. These parasites could be protozoa or helminths.

The main protozoan parasites are *Plasmodium falciparum* [79, 80], *Toxoplasma gondii* [81 - 85], *Entamoeba histolytica* [86, 87], *Cryptosporidium parvum* [88 - 91] and *Trichomonas vaginalis* [92 - 95].

Strongyloides stercoralis [96 - 98], and *Taenia solium* [99, 100] are the two main helminths considered indirect carcinogenic parasites.

VIRAL ONCOGENESIS

Viruses are intracellular pathogens that reproduce only in living cells by manipulating the cellular machinery to produce more viruses. Viruses are made up of a small number of genes in the form of DNA or RNA surrounded by a protein coating [101]. Since viral replications influence host cellular genes in different cancerous ways, around 20% of all human cancers are caused by oncoviruses through chronic inflammation leading to cell death, uncontrollable proliferation, and modulated expression of some of the regulatory proteins [102].

Viral Oncogenesis is a multistep phenomenon in which normal host cells are transformed into cancerous cells on the basis of host genetic variability. Oncogenic viruses encode genes that cause viral replication and transformation of the host cells to produce viral proteins and protein complexes. The phenomenon from basic viral infection to tumorigenesis is lengthy due to the involvement of factors like immunity complications, cellular mutations, and exposure to other cancerous agents. The viruses that are involved in human cancer development are Hepatitis B virus (HBV), Hepatitis C virus (HCV), Epstein-Barr virus (EBV), Human papillomavirus (HPV), Kaposi's sarcoma herpes virus (KSHV), and Human T lymphotrophic virus 1 (HTLV-1) [103].

Epstein-Barr Virus (EBV)

EBV is a herpes virus that is best known for causing infectious mononucleosis and transmitted *via* droplet, and most people in the United States are infected with EBV by the end of their teen years but mostly asymptomatic [104].

Similar to other herpes viruses, EBV infection is persistent although asymptomatic for the first few weeks after infecting *B lymphocytes*. Generally, EBV isn’t associated with serious complications in most people [105].

Sustained EBV infection increases a person’s risk of developing nasopharyngeal and stomach cancer along with Burkitt’s and Hodgkin’s lymphoma or other fast-growing lymphomas but still not very common worldwide. Nevertheless, Africa and parts of Southeast Asia exhibit the majority of EBV-related cancers [106].

EBV proteins BHRF1 and BALF1 are orthologs of the cellular anti-apoptotic protein Bcl-2, which has been extensively described to negatively regulate both apoptosis and autophagy. In addition, viral EBNA-1 is involved in carcinogenesis by acting on cellular environment and inducing genomic instability EBNA-2 deregulates c-Myc expression increasing cell proliferation, and EBNA3A and EBNA3C repress both BIM and p16 and prevent differentiation into plasma cells [107].

Human Papillomaviruses (HPVs)

Human papillomaviruses (HPVs) are a group of more than 150 related viruses called *papillomaviruses* because some cause papillomas, more commonly known as warts. Some types of HPV only grow in the skin, while others grow in mucous membranes such as the mouth, throat, or vagina [108].

All types of HPV are spread by contact (touch). More than 40 types of HPV can be passed on through sexual contact. Most sexually active people are infected with one or more of these HPV types at some point in their lives. At least a dozen of these types are known to cause cancer [109].

While HPV infections are very common, cancer caused by HPV is not. Most people infected with HPV will not develop a cancer related to the infection. However, some people with long-lasting infections of high-risk types of HPV, are at risk of developing cancer [7, 110].

HPV infections of the mucous membranes can cause genital warts, but they usually have no symptoms. There are no effective medicines or other treatments for HPV, other than removing or destroying cells that are known to be infected. But in most people, the body's immune system controls the HPV infection or gets rid of it over time [111, 112].

Cervical cancer is the second most common cancer among women worldwide and is caused mainly by a few types of HPV of which E6 and E7 oncogenes deregulate the host cell cycle by binding and inactivating tumor suppressor genes p53 and pRb. Binding of E6 gene to p53 causes degrades p53 while the E7 gene binds to pRb and disrupts the pRb and E2F complex leading to uncontrolled proliferation. Early cervical screening using Pap smear test does reveal pre-cancerous lesions that can be destroyed or removed as means of early prevention of cancer [113]. With the lack of effective treatment, the HPV vaccine remains the key to prevention. In addition to causing cervical cancer, HPV also has been reported as a cause of cancers across the human body, such as the penis, anus, vagina, vulva, mouth and throat [114].

Hepatitis B Virus (HBV) and Hepatitis C Virus (HCV)

Both HBV and HCV cause viral hepatitis, a liver infection. Although other viruses can also cause hepatitis (A & E, for example), only HBV and HCV cause chronic infections that increase the chance of developing liver cancer [115]. Some research also suggests that long-term HCV infection might be linked with some other cancers, such as non-Hodgkin lymphoma [116]. HBV and HCV are transmitted through blood products, sharing needles, unprotected sex, blood transfusions, tissue transplants or childbirth (Fig. **3.3**) [117].

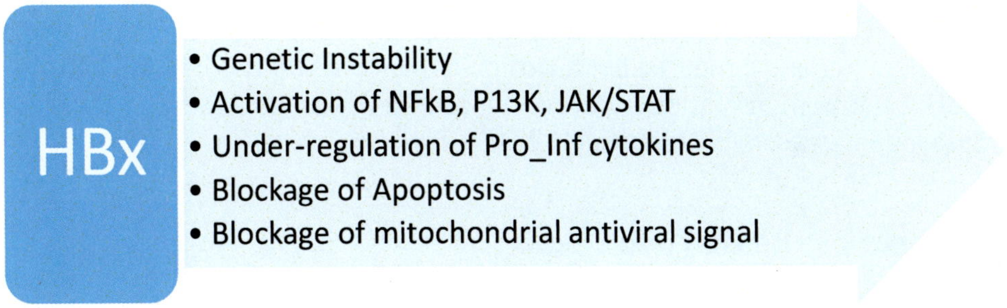

Fig. (3.3). Summary of HBx oncogenes.

Role of HBx in HCC development: Hepatitis B X antigen induces host cell genome instability and altered expression of various cytokines leading to an antiviral state. HCC, hepatocellular carcinoma [118]. HCV is less likely to cause symptoms than HBV, but it is more likely to cause chronic infection, which can lead to liver damage or even cancer resulting from chronic HBV infections [119].

A number of drugs are used to treat chronic hepatitis B. Although they don't cure the disease, they can lower the risk of liver damage and might lower the risk of liver cancer as well. There is a vaccine to prevent HBV infection, but none for HCV [120].

Host cell membranes undergo extensive rearrangements once induced by some of the HCV proteins (such as Core, NS2, NS5B, NS3, and NS5A), leading to the formation of double-membrane vesicles (DMVs) to build a membranous web that contains facilitate viral RNA replication and assembly. Such viral proteins directly mediate HCVcarcinogenesis through stimulating NF-KB activation, genetic instability angiogenesis as well as cell proliferation, or by suppressing tumor suppressors, apoptotic pathway and immune response. In addition to the direct role of oncoviral proteins, alterations of the autophagic pathway have been reported in HCVmediated HCC progression [121, 122].

Human Immunodeficiency Virus

Human Immunodeficiency Virus (HIV) causes Acquired Immune Deficiency Syndrome (AIDS), and directly causes cancers by increasing the host's risk of getting several types of cancer, through either co-infection along with other oncogenic viruses [123, 124] or by damaging helper T-cells and disrupting the host's immune system. Furthermore, HIV infection increases the risk of developing Kaposi sarcoma, cervical cancer and central nervous system lymphoma [125].

Chronic HIV-infected patients have a higher risk of acquiring HPV where anal, mouth, penile, vaginal, throat, or head and neck cancers could develop [126], but that is less common in patients receiving anti-HIV drugs where the risk of developing other cancers is reduced [127].

Human Herpes Virus 8 (HHV-8)

HHV-8 is named the *Kaposi sarcoma–associated herpes virus* (KSHV) since it is commonly detected in patients suffering Kaposi sarcoma (KS). In KS, HHV-8 infects the cells lining blood and lymph vessels, allowing further multiplication and longer survival of the virus leading to the development of cancer cells [128].

HHV-8, as a herpes virus, causes a life-long infection, and although it is transmitted through sexual contact, blood and saliva, it is less likely to cause disease in an immunocompetent host. HHV-8 causation of KS is nearly restricted to immunocompromised patients [129].

HHV-8 infection is also associated with multicentric Castleman disease, primary effusion lymphoma and a few other rare blood cancers and lymphomas [130].

Human T-Lymphotropic Virus-1 (HTLV-1)

Similar to HIV, HTLV-1 is a *retrovirus* of the RNA virus family, Retroviridae. Therefore, some of the newly generated DNA may integrate into the chromosomes of the infected human cell leading to cancer [131]. HTLV-1 is linked with *adult T-cell leukemia/lymphoma* (ATL), which is mostly found in southern Japan, central Africa, the Caribbean and South America, along with some immigrant groups in the southeast of United States [132, 133]. Although very similar to HIV in biology and means of transmission, HTLV-1 cannot cause AIDS [134] and only 5% of people infected with HTLV-1 develop ATL after a long asymptomatic period [135].

Merkel Cell Polyomavirus (MCV)

MCV is a polyomavirus discovered in 2008 in samples of patients suffering *Merkel cell carcinoma* (MCC); an aggressive rare type of skin cancer that develops such symptoms after a very long asymptomatic period [136]. MCV has been confirmed to be transmitted through skin and saliva [137].

How Viruses Cause Cancer?

Most of the viruses associated with human cancer have the capacity to integrate into the host genome and therefore immortalize the target cell in order to secure their own permanent replication [136]. Consequently, the infected cell will end up expressing the viral oncogenes that induce cell growth and proliferation, and inhibit apoptosis. In chronic inflammation, normal cell division is deregulated, where the risk of genetic mutation increases [137].

The key mechanisms are summarized as follows [136 - 140]:

- Evading growth suppressors by distributing anti growth signalling tissue invasion and metastasis by altering extracellular matrix adhesion and remodelling.
- Enabling replicative immortality by uncontrolled cell cycle.
- Sustained angiogenesis by altered metabolism under hypoxia and altered expression of angiogenesis effectors.
- Resisting cell death by acquired resistant to apoptosis.
- Sustained proliferative singling by altering the expression of the growth factor.
- Altering the immune system to protect the malignant cell from attacking by immune cell.
- Directly damage DNA in host cells.

In summary, viral infection can alter almost all the "hallmarks of cancer" mechanisms, whether directly or indirectly, or at the DNA, RNA or epigenome level.

ROLE OF FREE RADICALS, CHEMICALS IN ONCOGENESIS

Free Radicals are defined as unstable molecules with an unpaired electron in their outer orbital [141]. Free radicals are classified into Oxygen containing molecules and Nitrogen containing Molecules. The rapid uptake of oxygen, activation of NADPH oxidase, and Superoxide radical creation is the first step in the production of ROS. Superoxide Dismutase Enzyme (SOD) then quickly converts Superoxide to hydrogen peroxide (H_2O_2). Myeloperoxidase enzyme (MPO) in the cytoplasmic granules of neutrophils. H_2O_2 is transformed into hypochlorous, a powerful oxidant and antibacterial agent, when it comes into contact with the chloride ion [142]. ROS are also produced from superoxide and H_2O_2 *via* Fenton and/or Haber–Weiss reactions during a 'respiratory burst' [143].

Nitric oxide synthase transforms arginine into reactive nitrogen species (RNS) like nitric oxide (NO.). An inducible nitric oxide synthase (iNOS) may continuously create massive amounts of nitric oxide (NO.), which functions as a superoxide quencher. The NO. and the O_2. - Produce peroxynitrite (ONOO-) by reacting together [144]. The aromatic amino acid residues in the enzyme react with peroxynitrite, resulting in the nitration of the aromatic amino acids [145].

Sources of Free Radicals

ROS can be generated both internally and externally. Two key locations where superoxide radicals are formed in the electron transport chain: Complex I (NADH dehydrogenase) and complex III (ubiquinone cytochrome c reductase).

Transportation of electrons from complex I or II to coenzyme Q or ubiquinone (Q) leads to the formation of reduced coenzyme Q (QH_2), which regenerates coenzyme Q through an unstable intermediate semiquinone anion (.Q-).

The produced (.Q-) transfers electrons to molecular oxygen almost instantly, and as a result, superoxide radical is created. Because enzymes do not produce superoxide, the higher the metabolic rate, the larger the creation of ROS [146].

The major metabolic mechanism that produces H_2O_2 in the peroxisomes is the β-oxidation of fatty acids [147].

ROS are produced by the enzymes cytochrome P-450 and b5, as well as diamine oxidase. Electrons Transfer to molecular oxygen from dithiols catalyzed by the Erop1p Oxidase enzyme, resulting in H_2O_2 production [148].

ROS can be generated internally during Prostaglandin synthesis, adrenalin auto-oxidation, phagocytic cells, reduced riboflavin, $FADH_2$, $FMNH_2$, cytochrome P450, immunological cell activation, inflammation, excessive exercise, mental stress, infection, cancer, aging, and ischemia [149] and also externally by Cigarette smoke [150], drunkenness [151], poisons and pharmaceuticals [152], and ionizing radiation [153].

Environmental Carcinogens as a Source of Free Radical

Inorganic arsenic in soil, water, and the air act as a pollutant. In humans, it is easily absorbed and has been proven to cause cancers in the bladder, prostate, liver, and skin [154]. Inorganic arsenic is methylated with S-adenosyl-L-methionine as the active methyl donor, and Arsenic in its methylated form is regarded to be the supreme cancer-causing agent [155].

Inorganic arsenic or its methylated form produces Free Radicals, resulting in an increase in the synthesis of 8-oxo-deoxyguanosine (a biomarker of DNA oxidative damage). The development of oxidized DNA necessitated inorganic arsenic biomethylation, and this DNA oxidation was connected to a faster transition to a cancer phenotype [155].

Haloalkanes, which are generated when chlorine reacts with alkanes, have been used as solvents, cleansers, anesthetics, antiseptics in industry and contaminants in drinking water and chlorinated swimming pools. Carbon tetrachloride's hepatotoxicity is dose- and time-dependent, and most of its metabolism is done by the enzyme cytochrome P-450 (CY2B2, CYPB1, CYP2E1 and CYP3A). Cytochrome P-450-induced carbon tetrachloride biotransformation produces a carbon-centered free radical (trichloromethyl radical), which binds covalently to several biological macromolecules, including DNA and cytochrome P-450, owing to its reactivity (suicidal inactivation). Cancer is thought to be caused by the creation of DNA adducts with carbon tetrachloride metabolites. Carbon tetrachloride radical interacts with lipids to create lipid peroxy radicals when there is oxygen, resulting in lipid peroxidation and degradation (liver steatosis) [156].

Hydrazines are a type of compound found in edible mushrooms that are also employed in medicine. Hydrazines are poisonous in general, causing a wide range of adverse effects such as liver toxicity, mutagenicity and carcinogenicity. Oxidized hydrazine derivatives (mediated by cytochrome P-450, metal ions and peroxidases) produce free radicals, which cause DNA oxidative damage. A nucleophilic attack causes substituted hydrazines to alkylate DNA rather than free radical production. Carcinogenic events have been connected to DNA alkylation [157].

Smog is a type of air pollution caused by sunlight reacting with hydrocarbons, nitrogen compounds, ozone, and other chemicals found predominantly in the exhaust of cars. Nitric oxide interacts quickly with molecular oxygen to form peroxynitrite, a highly reactive compound that damage DNA, proteins, and lipids [158].

Sulfur dioxide combines with water to form sulfite (hydrated sulfur dioxide), is catalyzed by human myeloperoxidases to produce sulfite (• SO_3) and sulfate (• SO_4^-) anion radicals. Food preservatives containing sulfite are also utilized. In susceptible human groups, sulfite exposure causes allergic responses and bronchoconstriction. Free radical production from sulfite is now considered to be involved in damaging (oxidizing) sensitive proteins [158].

Free radicals produced from the breakdown of secondary ozonides, a reaction result of ozone with unsaturated lipids, have been related to lung inflammation and alveolar epithelial injury by ozone. Ozone also causes damage of DNA through free radical-mediated reactions [159].

Development of Cancer and Free Radicals

Oxidative stress develops if the imbalance between free radical production and the detoxifying and repair systems' capability developed. When free radical damage is not corrected, it damages lipids, proteins, RNA, and DNA, This may result in diseases. Cancer, Alzheimer's disease, Parkinson's disease, atherosclerosis, arthritis, diabetes, kidney disease, schizophrenia, bipolar disorder, emphysema, and cataracts have all been linked to oxidative stress.

Chemical Alteration in DNA is produced by Free radicals, making them potentially mutagenic and contributing to cancer aetiology [160]. Cancer cells create more reactive oxygen species (ROS) than healthy cells and are more prone to mitochondrial malfunction due to their higher metabolic rate [161]. Increased oxidative stress cancerous levels of cells are due to the loss of tumor suppressors and activation of oncogenes [162].

ROS induces cancer cells to proliferate indefinitely by changing growth signals and gene expression [163]. Base alterations, deletions, strand breaks, chromosomal rearrangements, and hyper- and hypo-methylation of DNA can all cause damage to the DNA [164].

Exposure of Intestinal mucosa constantly to oxidants from both endogenous and external sources [165], carcinogens from the diet and bacteria, unregulated free radicals generation, redox imbalance, and development of DNA strand break, eventually leading to an altered intestinal metabolic homeostasis with cancer as a result [166]. Nitric oxide [167], 8-Oxo-2'-deoxyguanosine (8-oxo-dG), the major products of DNA oxidation [166], and lipid peroxides [168] are higher in colorectal tumors.

ROS produces damage to breast epithelium and causes fibroblast proliferation, epithelial hyperplasia, The cell's atypia, and breast cancer [169]. Thymidine phosphorylase enzyme overexpression, which catabolizes thymidine to thymine and 2-deoxy-D-ribose-1-phosphate, which is a powerful reducing sugar that rapidly glycates proteins, generating oxygen radicals within the carcinoma cell, can cause Oxidative Stress in the majority of breast carcinomas [170].

Overexpression of the NADPH oxidase 1 (Nox1) protein is a precursor to prostate cancer [171]. The superoxide produced by NOX in cancer cells from the prostate promotes biological longevity by preventing programmed cell death, resulting in cancer promotion [172].

Particulate matter from cigarette smoke has a complex mixture of carcinogens and stable ROS with lengthy half-lives, which causes progressive malignant transformation of cells, which raises the frequency of mutations caused by DNA strand breaks, finally leading to cancer of the lungs [173].

Bladder cancer is the result of oxidative stress caused by cigarette smoking, exposure to industrial carcinogens (aromatic amines), high amounts of arsenic ingestion, and nutrition [174]. High Nitric oxide in bladder cancer induces matrix metalloproteinases (MMPs), particularly prolidase activity, which takes part in the last step of collagen degradation [175].

Initial Stage of Tumor Formation and Free Radicals

ROS acts as a direct DNA mutagen, causing genomic instability, damage to mitochondrial DNA, and activating numerous signalling pathways, all of which can result in malignant transformation [176]. By influencing epigenetic alterations such as methylation or acetylation, ROS may modify the expression of oncogenes or tumor suppressor genes, increasing carcinogenesis, which in turn promotes the production of Reactive Oxygen species and accumulation, leading to further DNA oxidative damage [177].

Proliferation of Tumor Cells and Free Radicals

ROS controls numerous proteins and signalling pathways, allowing tumor cells to proliferate and avoid apoptosis. ROS transiently inactivate the phosphatase and tensin homologue (PTEN) [178], the protein tyrosine phosphatases (PTPs) [179], and the MAPK phosphatases [180] tumor suppressors, promoting the pro-survival MAPK/ERK and PI3K/AKT signalling pathways. Many transcription factors involved in the control of genes in cell proliferation, such as the hypoxia-inducible factor-1 (HIF-1), the nuclear factor-B (NF-B), Nrf2, and the activator protein 1 (AP-1), are likewise regulated by high amounts of ROS [181].

Angiogenesis and Free Radicals

H_2O_2 produced by NOXs promotes the Proliferation and survival of endothelial cells while also preventing apoptosis [182]. Cadherin/catenin phosphorylation by ROS causes the breakdown of endothelial cell junctions and increases cell migration [183]. ROS stimulate VEGF signalling by inducing the main regulator HIF-1, which raises the Expression of VEGFR and VEGF [184], and by inducing the MAPK and the pathways, which activate Cascades of angiogenic signalling for VEGFR expression upregulation. In some cancer cells, a rise in extracellular SOD levels may decrease the hypoxic buildup of HIF-1 and its downstream target gene VEGF [185].

Metastasis and Free Radicals

ROS plays a part in many cellular activities, including cell-to-cell adhesion loss, cell survival after matrix dissociation, migration of cells and penetration of the basement membrane [186]. In the PI3 kinase-dependent way, H_2O_2 increases cell migration by activating FAK [187]. ROS abnormally activates uPA, MMP, and cathepsins, promoting cell motility. ROS modulates a lot of signalling pathways for tumor invasion upstream of MMPs and uPAs, including the PI3K/Akt, MAPK and PKC pathways, as well as regulated by recognized transcription factors (NF-B and AP-1) [188, 189]. The tendency for the spread of cancer and drug resistance resulted from ROS production of the Snail and HIF-1 transcription factors [190].

PHYSICAL ONCOGENIC FACTORS

Physical oncogenic factors are the second most important group of exogenous non-microbial oncogenic factors and can be divided into two main classes: solid physical material and radiations.

Firstly, solid physical oncogenic materials include fibers (*e.g.,* asbestos, erionite and glass wool), particles (*e.g.,* cobalt and nickel and crystals such as silica), metallic alloys used in arthroplasty, and synthetic plastics used in the vascular procedure. The manner by which hard physical oncogenic materials cause cancer is poorly understood. Most likely, implanting solid physical materials can interrupt cellular metabolism leading to cancer. For example, prolonged, continued pressure of a needle on a tailor's hand may trigger and initiate carcinogenesis. In addition, the bridle in the mouth of the horse may cause squamous cell cancer after many years. Furthermore, it is well established that continued inhalation of asbestos fibers leads to serious health issues, including mesothelioma, lung cancer, and asbestosis [191, 192].

The second category of physical risk factor is radiation. Radiation can be defined as energy released from sources such as the sun (light and heat), microwaves oven (microwaves), X-ray generator (x-rays), and radioactive elements (gamma radiations) [192].

There are two general classes of radiations: ionizing and non-ionizing radiations. Ionizing radiations are a group of invisible, high-frequency rays that carry sufficient energy to break chemical bonds and free electrons from atoms or molecules, thus ionizing them (acquiring them a negative or positive charge). Ionizing radiation can alter the electronic composition of the DNA molecules or genes, leading to cancer; cancers triggered by radiation are termed radiogenic [193, 194]. There is a growing body of evidence implying exposure to ionizing radiation, especially at high doses, is a risk factor for cancer. The evidence has been obtained from studies of prolonged medically radiation-exposed people, atomic bomb survivors in Japan, exposed workers in occupation sittings such as nuclear power stations and medical treatment and diagnosis rooms, and people exposed to naturally occurring radiation such as radon. There are two types of ionizing radiations: natural (naturally available cosmic radiation from decay products such as uranium, radon, thorium, and potassium) and artificial (such as x-rays) [194].

Non-ionizing radiations are electromagnetic rays that do not possess sufficient energy to dislodge electrons (ionize) from atoms or molecules. Non-ionizing radiations are located at the low-frequency end of the electromagnetic spectrum (wavelengths > 350 nm). This type of radiation does not modify the electronic conformation of atoms and cannot break chemical bonds. Thus, non-ionizing radiations have minimal harmful effects on human cells. Examples of non-ionizing radiation include radio waves, microwaves, and extremely low-frequency electromagnetic fields [195]. Ionizing and non-ionizing radiations together may be responsible for about 10% of all cancer cases [196]. Radioactive materials, ultraviolet (UV), pulsed electromagnetic fields (*e.g.,* x-rays), ultraviolet light and heat (from sun) radiations are particularly implicated in cancer incidence [197]. A well-known example of cancer risk associated with radiation is the increased number of cancer cases in Sweden following the exposure to radioactive leakage after the Chernobyl nuclear power plant accident in April 1986. Other examples of cancers caused by radiation include skin, thyroid, lung, and breast cancers and some types of leukemia, sarcomas and lymphoma [193].

CONCLUSION

Microbes around- and inside humans are a major part of our ecosystems that govern our health and disease. In addition to causing different types of cancer, use of live, attenuated and bioengineered bacteria, including Salmonella, Mycobacteria, Clostridia, Bifidobacteria, Bacillus and Listeria, have been used as anti-cancer agents by targeting cancer cells as they grow in the hypoxic core region of solid tumors [198].

Higher complexities are also being investigated for cancer therapeutics such as Mangrove sediments-derived microbes (MSM). They are a naturally rich reservoir of diverse products such as alkaloids, lactones, xanthones, quinones, terpenoids, steroids and more than 500 other bioactive compounds. Some of their pharmacological mechanisms revealed significant medicinal potentials, such as anti-cancer, anti-MDR, and antineoplastic activities [199].

CONSENT FOR PUBLICATION

Not applicable.

CONFLICT OF INTEREST

The authors declare that there are no conflicts of interest.

ACKNOWLEDGEMENTS

We would like to thank Dr. Faris Alenzi for his support.

REFERENCES

[1] Jessy T. Immunity over inability: The spontaneous regression of cancer. J Nat Sci Biol Med 2011; 2(1): 43-9.
[http://dx.doi.org/10.4103/0976-9668.82318] [PMID: 22470233]

[2] The American Cancer Society medical and editorial content team 2018. https://www.cancer.org/cancer/cancer-basics/history-of-cancer

[3] The American Cancer Society medical and editorial content team 2014. https://www.cancer.org/cancer/cancer-basics/history-of-cancer/cancer-causes-theories-throughout-history.html

[4] Bailey EJ, Kennaway EL, Urquhart ME. Arsenic content of cigarettes. Br J Cancer 1957; 11(1): 49-53. [http://dx.doi.org/10.1038/bjc.1957.7] [PMID: 13436696]

[5] Epstein MA, Achong BG, Barr YM. Virus particles in cultured lymphoblasts from Burkitt's lymphoma. Lancet 1964; 283(7335): 702-3.
[http://dx.doi.org/10.1016/S0140-6736(64)91524-7] [PMID: 14107961]

[6] Crum CP, Ikenberg H, Richart RM, Gissman L. Human papillomavirus type 16 and early cervical neoplasia. N Engl J Med 1984; 310(14): 880-3.
[http://dx.doi.org/10.1056/NEJM198404053101403] [PMID: 6321986]

[7] Hausen HZ. Charles S. Mott prize papillomaviruses in human cancer. Cancer 1987; 59(10): 1692-6. https://pubmed.ncbi.nlm.nih.gov/3040050/
[http://dx.doi.org/10.1002/1097-0142(19870515)59:10<1692::AID-CNCR2820591003>3.0.CO;2-F] [PMID: 3030526]

[8] Feng YY, Wang Y. *Campylobacter pylori* in patients with gastritis, peptic ulcer, and carcinoma of the stomach in Lanzhou, China. Lancet 1988; 331(8593): 1055-6. [http://dx.doi.org/10.1016/S0140-6736(88)91877-6] [PMID: 2896897]

[9] IARC Monograph Evalaluation Carcinogenic Risks to Humans. Schistosomes, liver flukes and Helicobacter pylori. IARC Working Group on the Evaluation of Carcinogenic Risks to Humans, 1994. https://www.ncbi.nlm.nih.gov/pmc/articles/PMC7681621/

[10] Bleich RM, Arthur JC. Revealing a microbial carcinogen. Science 2019; 363(6428): 689-90. [http://dx.doi.org/10.1126/science.aaw5475] [PMID: 30765550]

[11] Turesky RJ. Mechanistic Evidence for Red Meat and Processed Meat Intake and Cancer Risk: A Follow-up on the International Agency for Research on Cancer Evaluation of 2015. Chimia (Aarau) 2018; 72(10): 718-24. [http://dx.doi.org/10.2533/chimia.2018.718] [PMID: 30376922]

[12] Fishbein A, Hammock BD, Serhan CN, Panigrahy D. Carcinogenesis: Failure of resolution of inflammation? Pharmacol Ther 2021; 218: 107670. [http://dx.doi.org/10.1016/j.pharmthera.2020.107670] [PMID: 32891711]

[13] Nejsum LN, Andersen ÅB. Infection and the role in cancer development. Acta Pathol Microbiol Scand Suppl 2020; 128(2): 71. [http://dx.doi.org/10.1111/apm.13030] [PMID: 31991492]

[14] Littman AJ, Jackson LA, Vaughan TL. *Chlamydia pneumoniae* and lung cancer: epidemiologic evidence. Cancer Epidemiol Biomarkers Prev 2005; 14(4): 773-8. [http://dx.doi.org/10.1158/1055-9965.EPI-04-0599] [PMID: 15824142]

[15] Boleij A, Schaeps RMJ, Tjalsma H. Association between *Streptococcus bovis* and colon cancer. J Clin Microbiol 2009; 47(2): 516. [http://dx.doi.org/10.1128/JCM.01755-08] [PMID: 19189926]

[16] Tahara E. Molecular mechanism of human stomach carcinogenesis implicated in *Helicobacter pylori* infection. Exp Toxicol Pathol 1998; 50(4-6): 375-8. [http://dx.doi.org/10.1016/S0940-2993(98)80019-5] [PMID: 9784010]

[17] Murakami K, Matsubara H. Chronology of gastrointestinal cancer. Surg Today 2018; 48(4): 365-70. [http://dx.doi.org/10.1007/s00595-017-1574-y] [PMID: 28795270]

[18] Romano M, Ricci V, Zarrilli R. Mechanisms of Disease: *Helicobacter pylori*-related gastric carcinogenesis—implications for chemoprevention. Nat Clin Pract Gastroenterol Hepatol 2006; 3(11): 622-32. [http://dx.doi.org/10.1038/ncpgasthep0634] [PMID: 17068500]

[19] Schmidt N, Peitz U, Lippert H, Malfertheiner P. Missing gastric cancer in dyspepsia. Aliment Pharmacol Ther 2005; 21(7): 813-20. [http://dx.doi.org/10.1111/j.1365-2036.2005.02425.x] [PMID: 15801916]

[20] Smyth EC, Nilsson M, Grabsch HI, van Grieken NCT, Lordick F. Gastric cancer. Lancet 2020; 396(10251): 635-48. [http://dx.doi.org/10.1016/S0140-6736(20)31288-5] [PMID: 32861308]

[21] Loke YL, Chew MT, Ngeow YF, Lim WWD, Peh SC. Colon Carcinogenesis: The Interplay Between Diet and Gut Microbiota. Front Cell Infect Microbiol 2020; 10: 603086. [http://dx.doi.org/10.3389/fcimb.2020.603086] [PMID: 33364203]

[22] Tewari M, Mishra RR, Shukla HS. *Salmonella typhi* and gallbladder cancer: report from an endemic region. Hepatobiliary Pancreat Dis Int 2010; 9(5): 524-30. [PMID: 20943463]

[23] Cheng WT, Kantilal HK, Davamani F. The Mechanism of *Bacteroides fragilis* Toxin Contributes to Colon Cancer Formation. Malays J Med Sci 2020; 27(4): 9-21.

[http://dx.doi.org/10.21315/mjms2020.27.4.2] [PMID: 32863742]

[24] Melenotte C, Mezouar S, Mège JL, Gorvel JP, Kroemer G, Raoult D. Bacterial infection and non-Hodgkin's lymphoma. Crit Rev Microbiol 2020; 46(3): 270-87. [http://dx.doi.org/10.1080/1040841X.2020.1760786] [PMID: 32412856]

[25] Al-Hilu SA, Al-Shujairi WH. Dual Role of Bacteria in Carcinoma: Stimulation and Inhibition. Int J Microbiol 2020; 2020: 1-15. [http://dx.doi.org/10.1155/2020/4639761] [PMID: 32908523]

[26] Nath G, Gulati AK, Shukla VK. Role of bacteria in carcinogenesis, with special reference to carcinoma of the gallbladder. World J Gastroenterol 2010; 16(43): 5395-404. [http://dx.doi.org/10.3748/wjg.v16.i43.5395] [PMID: 21086555]

[27] Sheweita SA, Alsamghan AS. Molecular Mechanisms Contributing Bacterial Infections to the Incidence of Various Types of Cancer. Mediators Inflamm 2020; 2020: 1-10. [http://dx.doi.org/10.1155/2020/4070419] [PMID: 32724295]

[28] Liu S-C, Minton NP, Giaccia AJ, Brown JM. Anticancer efficacy of systemically delivered anaerobic bacteria as gene therapy vectors targeting tumor hypoxia/necrosis. Gene Ther 2002; 9(4): 291-6. [http://dx.doi.org/10.1038/sj.gt.3301659] [PMID: 11896468]

[29] Fabricius EM, Schneeweiss U, Schau HP, Schmidt W, Benedix A. Quantitative investigations into the elimination of *in vitro*-obtained spores of the non-pathogenic Clostridium butyricum strain CNRZ 528, and their persistence in organs of different species following intravenous spore administration. Res Microbiol 1993; 144(9): 741-53. [http://dx.doi.org/10.1016/0923-2508(93)90038-4] [PMID: 8191000]

[30] Sedighi M, Zahedi Bialvaei A, Hamblin MR, *et al.* Therapeutic bacteria to combat cancer; current advances, challenges, and opportunities. Cancer Med 2019; 8(6): cam4.2148. [http://dx.doi.org/10.1002/cam4.2148] [PMID: 30950210]

[31] Parsonnet J. Bacterial infection as a cause of cancer. Environ Health Perspect 1995; 103 (Suppl. 8): 263-8. [http://dx.doi.org/10.1289/ehp.95103s8263] [PMID: 8741796]

[32] Eyvazi S, Vostakolaei MA, Dilmaghani A, *et al.* The oncogenic roles of bacterial infections in development of cancer. Microb Pathog 2020; 141: 104019. [http://dx.doi.org/10.1016/j.micpath.2020.104019] [PMID: 32006638]

[33] Chattopadhyay I, Verma M, Panda M. Role of Oral Microbiome Signatures in Diagnosis and Prognosis of Oral Cancer. Technol Cancer Res Treat 2019; 18. [http://dx.doi.org/10.1177/1533033819867354] [PMID: 31370775]

[34] Saus E, Iraola-Guzmán S, Willis JR, Brunet-Vega A, Gabaldón T. Microbiome and colorectal cancer: Roles in carcinogenesis and clinical potential. Mol Aspects Med 2019; 69: 93-106. [http://dx.doi.org/10.1016/j.mam.2019.05.001] [PMID: 31082399]

[35] IARC working group on the evaluation of carcinogenic risks to humans. Biological agents. A review of human carcinogens. IARC Monogr Eval Carcinog Risks Hum 2012; 100(Pt B):1-441.

[36] Bernardo C, Cunha MC, Santos JH, *et al.* Insight into the molecular basis of *Schistosoma haematobium*-induced bladder cancer through urine proteomics. Tumour Biol 2016; 37(8): 11279-87. [http://dx.doi.org/10.1007/s13277-016-4997-y] [PMID: 26951512]

[37] Abd El-Aal AA, Bayoumy IR, Basyoni MMA, *et al.* Genomic instability in complicated and uncomplicated Egyptian schistosomiasis haematobium patients. Mol Cytogenet 2015; 8(1): 1. [http://dx.doi.org/10.1186/s13039-014-0104-5] [PMID: 25628757]

[38] Brindley PJ, Costa JMC, Sripa B. Why does infection with some helminths cause cancer? Trends Cancer 2015; 1(3): 174-82. [http://dx.doi.org/10.1016/j.trecan.2015.08.011]

[39] Honeycutt J, Hammam O, Hsieh MH. *Schistosoma haematobium* egg-induced bladder urothelial abnormalities dependent on p53 are modulated by host sex. Exp Parasitol 2015; 158: 55-60. [http://dx.doi.org/10.1016/j.exppara.2015.07.002] [PMID: 26160678]

[40] Honeycutt J, Hammam O, Fu CL, Hsieh MH. Controversies and challenges in research on urogenital schistosomiasis-associated bladder cancer. Trends Parasitol 2014; 30(7): 324-32. [http://dx.doi.org/10.1016/j.pt.2014.05.004] [PMID: 24913983]

[41] Santos J, Fernandes E, Ferreira JA, *et al.* P53 and cancer-associated sialylated glycans are surrogate markers of cancerization of the bladder associated with *Schistosoma haematobium* infection. PLoS Negl Trop Dis 2014; 8(12): e3329. [http://dx.doi.org/10.1371/journal.pntd.0003329] [PMID: 25502795]

[42] Botelho MC, Veiga I, Oliveira PA, *et al.* Carcinogenic ability of *Schistosoma haematobium* possibly through oncogenic mutation of *KRAS* gene. Adv Cancer Res Treat 2013; 2013: 876585. [PMID: 25221779]

[43] Choto ET, Mduluza T, Mutapi F, Chimbari MJ. Association of schistosomiasis and risk of prostate cancer development in residents of Murehwa rural community, Zimbabwe. Infect Agent Cancer 2020; 15(1): 59. [http://dx.doi.org/10.1186/s13027-020-00327-2] [PMID: 33042215]

[44] Kiremit MC, Cakir A, Arslan F, Ormeci T, Erkurt B, Albayrak S. The bladder carcinoma secondary to *schistosoma mansoni* infection: A case report with review of the literature. Int J Surg Case Rep 2015; 13: 76-8. [http://dx.doi.org/10.1016/j.ijscr.2015.05.038] [PMID: 26125519]

[45] Toda KS, Kikuchi L, Chagas AL, *et al.* Hepatocellular carcinoma related to Schistosoma mansoni infection: case series and literature review. J Clin Transl Hepatol 2015; 3(4): 260-4. [http://dx.doi.org/10.14218/JCTH.2015.00027] [PMID: 26807381]

[46] Salim OEH, Hamid HKS, Mekki SO, Suleiman SH, Ibrahim SZ. Colorectal carcinoma associated with schistosomiasis: a possible causal relationship. World J Surg Oncol 2010; 8(1): 68. [http://dx.doi.org/10.1186/1477-7819-8-68] [PMID: 20704754]

[47] Madbouly KM, Senagore AJ, Mukerjee A, *et al.* Colorectal cancer in a population with endemic *Schistosoma mansoni*: is this an at-risk population? Int J Colorectal Dis 2006; 22(2): 175-81. [http://dx.doi.org/10.1007/s00384-006-0144-3] [PMID: 16786317]

[48] Zalata KR, Nasif WA, Ming SC, *et al.* p53, Bcl-2 and C-Myc expressions in colorectal carcinoma associated with schistosomiasis in Egypt. Cell Oncol 2005; 27(4): 245-53. [PMID: 16308474]

[49] Basílio-de-Oliveira CA, Aquino A, Simon EF, Eyer-Silva WA. Concomitant prostatic schistosomiasis and sdenocarcinoma: case report and review. Braz J Infect Dis 2002; 6(1): 45-9. [http://dx.doi.org/10.1590/S1413-86702002000100007] [PMID: 11980603]

[50] Hamid HKS. *Schistosoma japonicum*-associated colorectal cancer: a review. Am J Trop Med Hyg 2019; 100(3): 501-5. [http://dx.doi.org/10.4269/ajtmh.18-0807] [PMID: 30560774]

[51] Chen M. Assessment of morbidity due to *Schistosoma japonicum* infection in China. Infect Dis Poverty 2014; 3(1): 6. [http://dx.doi.org/10.1186/2049-9957-3-6] [PMID: 24529186]

[52] Zanger P, Habscheid W, Kremsner PG, Dahm HH. *Schistosoma japonicum* infection and rectal carcinoid tumour: underreported coincidence or neglected association? Epidemiol Infect 2010; 138(9): 1289-91. [http://dx.doi.org/10.1017/S095026880999152X] [PMID: 20056016]

[53] Qiu DC, Hubbard AE, Zhong B, Zhang Y, Spear RC. A matched, case–control study of the association between *Schistosoma japonicum* and liver and colon cancers, in rural China. Ann Trop Med Parasitol

2005; 99(1): 47-52.
[http://dx.doi.org/10.1179/136485905X19883] [PMID: 15701255]

[54] Ishii A, Matsuoka H, Aji T, *et al.* Parasite infection and cancer: with special emphasis on *Schistosoma japonicum* infections (Trematoda). A review. Mutat Res 1994; 305(2): 273-81.
[http://dx.doi.org/10.1016/0027-5107(94)90247-X] [PMID: 7510038]

[55] Zhang R, Takahashi S, Orita S, *et al.* p53 gene mutations in rectal cancer associated with schistosomiasis japonica in Chinese patients. Cancer Lett 1998; 131(2): 215-21.
[http://dx.doi.org/10.1016/S0304-3835(98)00154-2] [PMID: 9851256]

[56] Abdeen SH. Idiotype/anti-idiotype immunoregulatory network correlates with an improved clinical outcome of schistosomiasis mansoni in humans. Pak J Biol Sci 2011; 14(6): 375-84.
[http://dx.doi.org/10.3923/pjbs.2011.375.384] [PMID: 21902061]

[57] Cheever AW, Lenzi JA, Lenzi HL, Andrade ZA. Experimental models of *Schistosoma mansoni* infection. Mem Inst Oswaldo Cruz 2002; 97(7): 917-40.
[http://dx.doi.org/10.1590/S0074-02762002000700002] [PMID: 12471417]

[58] Zaghloul MS, Zaghloul TM, Bishr MK, Baumann BC. Urinary schistosomiasis and the associated bladder cancer: update. J Egypt Natl Canc Inst 2020; 32(1): 44.
[http://dx.doi.org/10.1186/s43046-020-00055-z] [PMID: 33252773]

[59] Ishida K, Hsieh MH. Understanding urogenital schistosomiasis-related bladder cancer: an update. Front Med (Lausanne) 2018; 5: 223.
[http://dx.doi.org/10.3389/fmed.2018.00223] [PMID: 30159314]

[60] Gouveia MJ, Santos J, Brindley PJ, *et al.* Estrogen-like metabolites and DNA-adducts in urogenital schistosomiasis-associated bladder cancer. Cancer Lett 2015; 359(2): 226-32.
[http://dx.doi.org/10.1016/j.canlet.2015.01.018] [PMID: 25615421]

[61] Khuntikeo N, Loilome W, Thinkhamrop B, Chamadol N, Yongvanit P. A comprehensive public health conceptual framework and strategy to effectively combat cholangiocarcinoma in Thailand. PLoS Negl Trop Dis 2016; 10(1): e0004293.
[http://dx.doi.org/10.1371/journal.pntd.0004293] [PMID: 26797527]

[62] Chaiyadet S, Smout M, Johnson M, *et al.* Excretory/secretory products of the carcinogenic liver fluke are endocytosed by human cholangiocytes and drive cell proliferation and IL6 production. Int J Parasitol 2015; 45(12): 773-81.
[http://dx.doi.org/10.1016/j.ijpara.2015.06.001] [PMID: 26187786]

[63] Chaiyadet S, Sotillo J, Smout M, *et al.* Carcinogenic liver fluke secretes extracellular vesicles that promote cholangiocytes to adopt a tumorigenic phenotype. J Infect Dis 2015; 212(10): 1636-45.
[http://dx.doi.org/10.1093/infdis/jiv291] [PMID: 25985904]

[64] Palmer WC, Patel T. Are common factors involved in the pathogenesis of primary liver cancers? A meta-analysis of risk factors for intrahepatic cholangiocarcinoma. J Hepatol 2012; 57(1): 69-76.
[http://dx.doi.org/10.1016/j.jhep.2012.02.022] [PMID: 22420979]

[65] Tyson GL, El-Serag HB. Risk factors for cholangiocarcinoma. Hepatology 2011; 54(1): 173-84.
[http://dx.doi.org/10.1002/hep.24351] [PMID: 21488076]

[66] Chng KR, Chan SH, Ng AHQ, *et al.* Tissue microbiome profiling identifies an enrichment of specific enteric bacteria in *Opisthorchis viverrini* associated cholangiocarcinoma. EBioMedicine 2016; 8: 195-202.
[http://dx.doi.org/10.1016/j.ebiom.2016.04.034] [PMID: 27428430]

[67] Plieskatt JL, Deenonpoe R, Mulvenna JP, *et al.* Infection with the carcinogenic liver fluke *Opisthorchis viverrini* modifies intestinal and biliary microbiome. FASEB J 2013; 27(11): 4572-84.
[http://dx.doi.org/10.1096/fj.13-232751] [PMID: 23925654]

[68] Kim EM, Bae YM, Choi MH, Hong ST. Cyst formation, increased anti-inflammatory cytokines and expression of chemokines support for *Clonorchis sinensis* infection in FVB mice. Parasitol Int 2012;

61(1): 124-9.
[http://dx.doi.org/10.1016/j.parint.2011.07.001] [PMID: 21820080]

[69] Matchimakul P, Rinaldi G, Suttiprapa S, *et al.* Apoptosis of cholangiocytes modulated by thioredoxin of carcinogenic liver fluke. Int J Biochem Cell Biol 2015; 65: 72-80.
[http://dx.doi.org/10.1016/j.biocel.2015.05.014] [PMID: 26007234]

[70] Smout MJ, Sotillo J, Laha T, *et al.* Carcinogenic parasite secretes growth factor that accelerates wound healing and potentially promotes neoplasia. PLoS Pathog 2015; 11(10): e1005209.
[http://dx.doi.org/10.1371/journal.ppat.1005209] [PMID: 26485648]

[71] Sripa B, Brindley PJ, Mulvenna J, *et al.* The tumorigenic liver fluke *Opisthorchis viverrini* – multiple pathways to cancer. Trends Parasitol 2012; 28(10): 395-407.
[http://dx.doi.org/10.1016/j.pt.2012.07.006] [PMID: 22947297]

[72] Boonmars T, Wu Z, Boonjaruspinyo S, *et al.* Alterations of gene expression of RB pathway in *Opisthorchis viverrini* infection-induced cholangiocarcinoma. Parasitol Res 2009; 105(5): 1273-81.
[http://dx.doi.org/10.1007/s00436-009-1548-0] [PMID: 19582476]

[73] Yothaisong S, Thanee M, Namwat N, *et al.* Opisthorchis viverrini infection activates the PI3K/AKT/PTEN and Wnt/β-catenin signaling pathways in a Cholangiocarcinogenesis model. Asian Pac J Cancer Prev 2015; 15(23): 10463-8.
[http://dx.doi.org/10.7314/APJCP.2014.15.23.10463] [PMID: 25556493]

[74] Haonon O, Rucksaken R, Pinlaor P, *et al.* Upregulation of 14-3-3 eta in chronic liver fluke infection is a potential diagnostic marker of cholangiocarcinoma. Proteomics Clin Appl 2016; 10(3): 248-56.
[http://dx.doi.org/10.1002/prca.201500019] [PMID: 26435198]

[75] Jusakul A, Kongpetch S, Teh BT. Genetics of *Opisthorchis viverrini*-related cholangiocarcinoma. Curr Opin Gastroenterol 2015; 31(3): 258-63.
[http://dx.doi.org/10.1097/MOG.0000000000000162] [PMID: 25693006]

[76] Chan-on W, Nairismägi ML, Ong CK, *et al.* Exome sequencing identifies distinct mutational patterns in liver fluke–related and non-infection-related bile duct cancers. Nat Genet 2013; 45(12): 1474-8.
[http://dx.doi.org/10.1038/ng.2806] [PMID: 24185513]

[77] Won J, Ju JW, Kim SM, Shin Y, Chung S, Pak JH. *Clonorchis sinensis* infestation promotes three-dimensional aggregation and invasion of cholangiocarcinoma cells. PLoS One 2014; 9(10): e110705.
[http://dx.doi.org/10.1371/journal.pone.0110705] [PMID: 25340585]

[78] Pak JH, Son WC, Seo SB, *et al.* Peroxiredoxin 6 expression is inversely correlated with nuclear factor-κB activation during Clonorchis sinensis infestation. Free Radic Biol Med 2016; 99: 273-85.
[http://dx.doi.org/10.1016/j.freeradbiomed.2016.08.016] [PMID: 27554973]

[79] Robbiani DF, Deroubaix S, Feldhahn N, *et al.* *Plasmodium* infection promotes genomic instability and AID-dependent B cell lymphoma. Cell 2015; 162(4): 727-37.
[http://dx.doi.org/10.1016/j.cell.2015.07.019] [PMID: 26276629]

[80] Thorley-Lawson D, Deitsch KW, Duca KA, Torgbor C. The Link between *Plasmodium falciparum* malaria and endemic Burkitt's lymphoma-new insight into a 50-year-old enigma. PLoS Pathog 2016; 12(1): e1005331.
[http://dx.doi.org/10.1371/journal.ppat.1005331] [PMID: 26794909]

[81] Bajnok J, Tarabulsi M, Carlin H, *et al.* High frequency of infection of lung cancer patients with the parasite *Toxoplasma gondii*. ERJ Open Res 2019; 5(2): 00143-2018.
[http://dx.doi.org/10.1183/23120541.00143-2018] [PMID: 31149623]

[82] Kalantari N, Ahangar Darabi Z, Siadati S, *et al.* Detection of *Toxoplasma gondii* DNA in Malignant breast tissues in breast cancer patients. Int J Mol Cell Med 2017; 6(3): 190-6.
[PMID: 29682491]

[83] Mostafa NES, Abdel Hamed EF, Rashed HES, Mohamed SY, Abdelgawad MS, Elasbali AM. The relationship between toxoplasmosis and different types of human tumors. J Infect Dev Ctries 2018;

12(2): 137-41.
[http://dx.doi.org/10.3855/jidc.9672] [PMID: 31825916]

[84] Jung BK, Song H, Kim MJ, Cho J, Shin EH, Chai JY. High *Toxoplasma gondii* seropositivity among brain tumor patients in Korea. Korean J Parasitol 2016; 54(2): 201-4.
[http://dx.doi.org/10.3347/kjp.2016.54.2.201] [PMID: 27180580]

[85] Shen DF, Herbort CP, Tuaillon N, Buggage RR, Egwuagu CE, Chan CC. Detection of *Toxoplasma gondii* DNA in primary intraocular B-cell lymphoma. Mod Pathol 2001; 14(10): 995-9.
[http://dx.doi.org/10.1038/modpathol.3880424] [PMID: 11598169]

[86] Uccelli F, Intelisano A, Piccinali D, *et al.* Ameboma *versus* colorectal cancer: a case report. Radiol Diagn Imaging 2018; 2(2): 1-3.

[87] Sengupta M, Mitra S, Ray S, Saha K. Amoeboma of colon mimicking colonic carcinoma. Trop Parasitol 2014; 4(2): 122-4.
[http://dx.doi.org/10.4103/2229-5070.138542] [PMID: 25250235]

[88] Sulżyc-Bielicka V, Kołodziejczyk L, Jaczewska S, *et al.* Colorectal cancer and *Cryptosporidium* spp. infection. PLoS One 2018; 13(4): e0195834.
[http://dx.doi.org/10.1371/journal.pone.0195834] [PMID: 29672572]

[89] Sawant M, Baydoun M, Creusy C, *et al. Cryptosporidium* and Colon Cancer: Cause or Consequence? Microorganisms 2020; 8(11): 1665.
[http://dx.doi.org/10.3390/microorganisms8111665] [PMID: 33121099]

[90] Certad G, Ngouanesavanh T, Guyot K, *et al.* Cryptosporidium parvum, a potential cause of colic adenocarcinoma. Infect Agent Cancer 2007; 2(1): 22.
[http://dx.doi.org/10.1186/1750-9378-2-22] [PMID: 18031572]

[91] Kopacz Ż, Kváč M, Karpiński P, *et al.* The first evidence of *Cryptosporidium meleagridis* infection in a colon adenocarcinoma from an immunocompetent patient. Front Cell Infect Microbiol 2019; 9: 35.
[http://dx.doi.org/10.3389/fcimb.2019.00035] [PMID: 30886833]

[92] Yang M, Li L, Jiang C, *et al.* Co-infection with *Trichomonas vaginalis* increases the risk of cervical intraepithelial neoplasia grade 2–3 among HPV16 positive female: a large population-based study. BMC Infect Dis 2020; 20(1): 642.
[http://dx.doi.org/10.1186/s12879-020-05349-0] [PMID: 32873233]

[93] Yang S, Zhao W, Wang H, Wang Y, Li J, Wu X. *Trichomonas vaginalis* infection-associated risk of cervical cancer: A meta-analysis. Eur J Obstet Gynecol Reprod Biol 2018; 228: 166-73.
[http://dx.doi.org/10.1016/j.ejogrb.2018.06.031] [PMID: 29980111]

[94] Saleh NE, Alhusseiny SM, El-Zayady WM, *et al. Trichomonas vaginalis* serostatus and prostate cancer risk in Egypt: a case-control study. Parasitol Res 2021; 120(4): 1379-88.
[http://dx.doi.org/10.1007/s00436-020-06942-7]

[95] Rai H, Dahoud W. *Trichomonas vaginalis* (TV) infection and its association with risk of cervical cancer and HPV status. Am J Clin Pathol 2019; 152 (Suppl. 1): S92-3.
[http://dx.doi.org/10.1093/ajcp/aqz118.002]

[96] Seo AN, Goo YK, Chung DI, Hong Y, Kwon O, Bae HI. Comorbid gastric adenocarcinoma and gastric and duodenal *Strongyloides stercoralis* infection: a case report. Korean J Parasitol 2015; 53(1): 95-9.
[http://dx.doi.org/10.3347/kjp.2015.53.1.95] [PMID: 25748714]

[97] Catalano C, Aron J, Bansal R, Leytin A. Colorectal cancer associated with *Strongyloides stercoralis* colitis. ACG Case Rep J 2017; 4(1): e104.
[http://dx.doi.org/10.14309/crj.2017.104] [PMID: 28879209]

[98] Sava M, Huynh T, Frugoli A, Kong L, Salehpour M, Barrows B. Colorectal cancer related to chronic *Strongyloides stercoralis* infection. Case Rep Gastrointest Med 2020; 2020: 1-5.
[http://dx.doi.org/10.1155/2020/8886460] [PMID: 32963848]

[99] Herrera LA, Ramirez T, Rodríguez U, *et al.* Possible association between *Taenia solium* cysticercosis and cancer: increased frequency of DNA damage in peripheral lymphocytes from neurocysticercosis patients. Trans R Soc Trop Med Hyg 2000; 94(1): 61-5. [http://dx.doi.org/10.1016/S0035-9203(00)90441-3] [PMID: 10748903]

[100] Cavellani CL, da Silva ACS, Ribeiro GKNA, Oliveira LF, Ferraz MLF, Teixeira VPA. Association between cysticercosis and neoplasia: a study based on autopsy findings. ScientificWorldJournal 2013; 2013: 1-4. [http://dx.doi.org/10.1155/2013/895942] [PMID: 24288510]

[101] Alberts B, Hopkin K, Johnson AD, *et al.* Essential Cell Biology: Vol. 5.5 (Fifth ed.). W. W. Norton & Company 2019.

[102] Akram N, Imran M, Noreen M, *et al.* Oncogenic Role of Tumor Viruses in Humans. Viral Immunol 2017; 30(1): 20-7. [http://dx.doi.org/10.1089/vim.2016.0109] [PMID: 27830995]

[103] McLaughlin-Drubin ME, Munger K. Viruses associated with human cancer. Biochim Biophys Acta Mol Basis Dis 2008; 1782(3): 127-50. [http://dx.doi.org/10.1016/j.bbadis.2007.12.005] [PMID: 18201576]

[104] Fontham ETH, Wolf AMD, Church TR, *et al.* Cervical cancer screening for individuals at average risk: 2020 guideline update from the American Cancer Society. CA Cancer J Clin 2020; 70(5): 321-46. [http://dx.doi.org/10.3322/caac.21628] [PMID: 32729638]

[105] White MK, Pagano JS, Khalili K. Viruses and human cancers: a long road of discovery of molecular paradigms. Clin Microbiol Rev 2014; 27(3): 463-81. [http://dx.doi.org/10.1128/CMR.00124-13] [PMID: 24982317]

[106] Wada N, Matsumura M, Ohba Y, Kobayashi N, Takizawa T, Nakanishi Y. Transcription stimulation of the Fas-encoding gene by nuclear factor for interleukin-6 expression upon influenza virus infection. J Biol Chem 1995; 270(30): 18007-12. [http://dx.doi.org/10.1074/jbc.270.30.18007] [PMID: 7543095]

[107] Colpani V, Soares Falcetta F, Bacelo Bidinotto A, *et al.* Prevalence of human papillomavirus (HPV) in Brazil: A systematic review and meta-analysis. PLoS One 2020; 15(2): e0229154. [http://dx.doi.org/10.1371/journal.pone.0229154] [PMID: 32084177]

[108] National Institute of allergy and Infectious Disease 2019. Https://Pave.Niaid.Nih.Gov/#explore/Proteins https://pave.niaid.nih.gov/#explore/proteins

[109] Liebowitz D. Epstein-Barr virus and a cellular signaling pathway in lymphomas from immunosuppressed patients. N Engl J Med 1998; 338(20): 1413-21. [http://dx.doi.org/10.1056/NEJM199805143382003] [PMID: 9580648]

[110] de Oliveira CM, Fregnani JHTG, Villa LL. HPV Vaccine: Updates and Highlights. Acta Cytol 2019; 63(2): 159-68. [http://dx.doi.org/10.1159/000497617] [PMID: 30870844]

[111] Reusser N, Downing C, Guidry J, Tyring S. HPV Carcinomas in Immunocompromised Patients. J Clin Med 2015; 4(2): 260-81. [http://dx.doi.org/10.3390/jcm4020260] [PMID: 26239127]

[112] Magalhães GM, Vieira ÉC, Garcia LC, De Carvalho-Leite MLR, Guedes ACM, Araújo MG. Update on human papilloma virus - part I: epidemiology, pathogenesis, and clinical spectrum. An Bras Dermatol 2021; 96(1): 1-16. [http://dx.doi.org/10.1016/j.abd.2020.11.003] [PMID: 33341319]

[113] Chang MH. Chronic viral hepatitis. Indian J Pediatr 1995; 62(6): 673-9. [http://dx.doi.org/10.1007/BF02825113] [PMID: 10829942]

[114] Gaglia MM, Munger K. More than just oncogenes: mechanisms of tumorigenesis by human viruses.

Curr Opin Virol 2018; 32: 48-59.
[http://dx.doi.org/10.1016/j.coviro.2018.09.003] [PMID: 30268926]

[115] Karayiannis P. Hepatitis B virus: virology, molecular biology, life cycle and intrahepatic spread. Hepatol Int 2017; 11(6): 500-8.
[http://dx.doi.org/10.1007/s12072-017-9829-7] [PMID: 29098564]

[116] Levrero M, Zucman-Rossi J. Mechanisms of HBV-induced hepatocellular carcinoma. J Hepatol 2016; 64(1) (Suppl.): S84-S101.
[http://dx.doi.org/10.1016/j.jhep.2016.02.021] [PMID: 27084040]

[117] Xiang WQ, Liu W. Role of HBx in hepatocellular carcinoma development. Zhejiang Da Xue Xue Bao Yi Xue Ban 2010; 39(3): 333-8.
[PMID: 20544999]

[118] Fischer R, Baumert T, Blum HE. Hepatitis C virus infection and apoptosis. World J Gastroenterol 2007; 13(36): 4865-72.
[http://dx.doi.org/10.3748/wjg.v13.i36.4865] [PMID: 17828818]

[119] Botlagunta M, Vesuna F, Mironchik Y, *et al.* Oncogenic role of DDX3 in breast cancer biogenesis. Oncogene 2008; 27(28): 3912-22.
[http://dx.doi.org/10.1038/onc.2008.33] [PMID: 18264132]

[120] Classon M, Harlow E. The retinoblastoma tumour suppressor in development and cancer. Nat Rev Cancer 2002; 2(12): 910-7.
[http://dx.doi.org/10.1038/nrc950] [PMID: 12459729]

[121] Sharp PM, Hahn BH. Origins of HIV and the AIDS Pandemic. Cold Spring Harb Perspect Med 2011; 1(1): a006841.
[http://dx.doi.org/10.1101/cshperspect.a006841] [PMID: 22229120]

[122] Peeters M, Sharp PM. Genetic diversity of HIV-1: the moving target. AIDS 2000; 14 (Suppl. 3): S129-40.
[PMID: 11086856]

[123] Lee CN, Wang WK, Fan WS, *et al.* Determination of human immunodeficiency virus type 1 subtypes in Taiwan by vpu gene analysis. J Clin Microbiol 2000; 38(7): 2468-74.

[124] Conley LJ, Ellerbrock TV, Bush TJ, Chiasson MA, Sawo D, Wright TC. HIV-1 infection and risk of vulvovaginal and perianal condylomata acuminata and intraepithelial neoplasia: a prospective cohort study. Lancet 2002; 359(9301): 108-13.
[http://dx.doi.org/10.1016/S0140-6736(02)07368-3] [PMID: 11809252]

[125] American Society of Clinical Oncology. HIV/AIDS-Related Cancer - Types of Treatment, (December 12, 2019). https://www.cancer.net/cancer-types/hivaids-related-cancer/types-treatment

[126] Ablashi DV, Chatlynne LG, Whitman JE Jr, Cesarman E. Spectrum of Kaposi's sarcoma-associated herpesvirus, or human herpesvirus 8, diseases. Clin Microbiol Rev 2002; 15(3): 439-64.
[http://dx.doi.org/10.1128/CMR.15.3.439-464.2002] [PMID: 12097251]

[127] Li S, Bai L, Dong J, Sun R, Lan K. Kaposi's Sarcoma-Associated Herpesvirus: Epidemiology and Molecular Biology. Adv Exp Med Biol 2017; 1018: 91-127.
[http://dx.doi.org/10.1007/978-981-10-5765-6_7] [PMID: 29052134]

[128] Alenzi FQ, Alotaibi AQ, Almotiri GM, *et al.* Role of Apoptosis in Microbial Infection. Open J Apoptosis 2014; 3(2): 32-8.
[http://dx.doi.org/10.4236/ojapo.2014.32004]

[129] Porto MAF, Alcântara LM, Carvalho EM, Castro N, Leal M. Atypical clinical presentation of strongyloidiasis in a patient co-infected with human T cell lymphotrophic virus type I. Am J Trop Med Hyg 2005; 72(2): 124-5.
[http://dx.doi.org/10.4269/ajtmh.2005.72.124] [PMID: 15741545]

[130] Juillard F, De León Vázquez E, Tan M, Li S, Kaye KM. Kaposi's Sarcoma-Associated Herpesvirus LANA-Adjacent Regions with Distinct Functions in Episome Segregation or Maintenance. J Virol 2019; 93(6): e02158-18.
[http://dx.doi.org/10.1128/JVI.02158-18] [PMID: 30626680]

[131] Kemp HI, Rice ASC, Adonis A, Davies NWS, Taylor GP. Human T-lymphotrophic virus—a neglected cause of chronic pain? Pain 2018; 159(8): 1433-7.
[http://dx.doi.org/10.1097/j.pain.0000000000001214] [PMID: 29554019]

[132] Eusebio-Ponce E, Anguita E, Paulino-Ramirez R, Candel FJ. HTLV-1 infection: An emerging risk. Pathogenesis, epidemiology, diagnosis and associated diseases. Rev Esp Quimioter 2019; 32(6): 485-96.
[PMID: 31648512]

[133] Beral V, Newton R. Overview of the epidemiology of immunodeficiency-associated cancers. J Natl Cancer Inst Monogr 1998; 1998(23): 1-6.
[http://dx.doi.org/10.1093/oxfordjournals.jncimonographs.a024164] [PMID: 9709294]

[134] Tello TL, Coggshall K, Yom SS, Yu SS. Merkel cell carcinoma: An update and review. J Am Acad Dermatol 2018; 78(3): 445-54.
[http://dx.doi.org/10.1016/j.jaad.2017.12.004] [PMID: 29229573]

[135] Pietropaolo V, Prezioso C, Moens U. Merkel Cell Polyomavirus and Merkel Cell Carcinoma. Cancers (Basel) 2020; 12(7): 1774.
[http://dx.doi.org/10.3390/cancers12071774] [PMID: 32635198]

[136] Dillon N, Grosveld F. Transcriptional regulation of multigene loci: multilevel control. Trends Genet 1993; 9(4): 134-7.
[http://dx.doi.org/10.1016/0168-9525(93)90208-Y] [PMID: 8516848]

[137] zur Hausen H, de Villiers EM. Cancer "causation" by infections-individual contributions and synergistic networks. Semin Oncol 2014; 41(6): 860-75.
[http://dx.doi.org/10.1053/j.seminoncol.2014.10.003] [PMID: 25499643]

[138] Krump NA, You J. Molecular mechanisms of viral oncogenesis in humans. Nat Rev Microbiol 2018; 16(11): 684-98.
[http://dx.doi.org/10.1038/s41579-018-0064-6] [PMID: 30143749]

[139] Purushothaman P, Uppal T, Verma SC. Human DNA tumor viruses and oncogenesis. Anim Biotechnol 2020; 131-51.
[http://dx.doi.org/10.1016/B978-0-12-811710-1.00007-0]

[140] Schiller JT, Lowy DR. An Introduction to Virus Infections and Human Cancer. Recent Results Cancer Res 2021; 217: 1-11.
[http://dx.doi.org/10.1007/978-3-030-57362-1_1] [PMID: 33200359]

[141] Choudhari SK, Chaudhary M, Gadbail AR, Sharma A, Tekade S. Oxidative and antioxidative mechanisms in oral cancer and precancer: A review. Oral Oncol 2014; 50(1): 10-8.
[http://dx.doi.org/10.1016/j.oraloncology.2013.09.011] [PMID: 24126222]

[142] Babior BM. NADPH oxidase: an update. Blood 1999; 93(5): 1464-76.
[http://dx.doi.org/10.1182/blood.V93.5.1464] [PMID: 10029572]

[143] Knight JA. Free radicals, antioxidants, aging and disease. Washington: AACC Press 1999.

[144] Zhu L, Gunn C, Beckman JS. Bactericidal activity of peroxynitrite. Arch Biochem Biophys 1992; 298(2): 452-7.
[http://dx.doi.org/10.1016/0003-9861(92)90434-X] [PMID: 1416976]

[145] Shahidi F, Zhong Y. Lipid oxidation and improving the oxidative stability. Chem Soc Rev 2010; 39(11): 4067-79.
[http://dx.doi.org/10.1039/b922183m] [PMID: 20617249]

[146] Finkel T, Holbrook NJ. Oxidants, oxidative stress and the biology of ageing. Nature 2000; 408(6809): 239-47.
[http://dx.doi.org/10.1038/35041687] [PMID: 11089981]

[147] Schrader M, Fahimi HD. Peroxisomes and oxidative stress. Biochim Biophys Acta Mol Cell Res 2006; 1763(12): 1755-66.
[http://dx.doi.org/10.1016/j.bbamcr.2006.09.006] [PMID: 17034877]

[148] Gross E, Sevier CS, Heldman N, *et al.* Generating disulfides enzymatically: Reaction products and electron acceptors of the endoplasmic reticulum thiol oxidase Ero1p. Proc Natl Acad Sci USA 2006; 103(2): 299-304.
[http://dx.doi.org/10.1073/pnas.0506448103] [PMID: 16407158]

[149] Cheeseman KH, Slater TF. An introduction to free radical biochemistry. Br Med Bull 1993; 49(3): 481-93.
[http://dx.doi.org/10.1093/oxfordjournals.bmb.a072625] [PMID: 8221017]

[150] Chiu YW, Chuang HY, Huang MC, Wu MT, Liu HW, Huang CT. Comparison of plasma antioxidant levels and related metabolic parameters between smokers and non-smokers. Kaohsiung J Med Sci 2009; 25(8): 423-30.
[http://dx.doi.org/10.1016/S1607-551X(09)70537-6] [PMID: 19605336]

[151] Nadiger HA, Marcus SR, Chandarkala MV. Lipid peroxidation and ethanol toxicity in rat brain – effect of vitamin E deficiency and supplementation. Med Sci Res 1988; 16: 1273-4.

[152] Aust SD, Chignell CF, Bray TM, Kalyanaraman B, Mason RP. Free radicals in toxicology. Toxicol Appl Pharmacol 1993; 120(2): 168-78.
[http://dx.doi.org/10.1006/taap.1993.1100] [PMID: 8511786]

[153] Vallyathan V, Shi X. The role of oxygen free radicals in occupational and environmental lung diseases. Environ Health Perspect 1997; 105(1) (Suppl. 1): 165-77.
[PMID: 9114285]

[154] Kojima C, Ramirez DC, Tokar EJ, *et al.* Requirement of arsenic biomethylation for oxidative DNA damage. J Natl Cancer Inst 2009; 101(24): 1670-81.
[http://dx.doi.org/10.1093/jnci/djp414] [PMID: 19933942]

[155] Obinaju BE. Mechanisms of arsenic toxicity and carcinogenesis. Afr J Biochem Res 2009; 3: 232-7.

[156] Weber LWD, Boll M, Stampfl A. Hepatotoxicity and mechanism of action of haloalkanes: carbon tetrachloride as a toxicological model. Crit Rev Toxicol 2003; 33(2): 105-36.
[http://dx.doi.org/10.1080/713611034] [PMID: 12708612]

[157] Kalyanaraman B, Sinha BK. Free radical-mediated activation of hydrazine derivatives. Environ Health Perspect 1985; 64: 179-84.
[http://dx.doi.org/10.1289/ehp.8564179] [PMID: 3007088]

[158] Ranguelova K, Rice AB, Khajo A, *et al.* Formation of reactive sulfite-derived free radicals by the activation of human neutrophils: An ESR study. Free Radic Biol Med 2012; 52(8): 1264-71.
[http://dx.doi.org/10.1016/j.freeradbiomed.2012.01.016] [PMID: 22326772]

[159] Kadiiska MB, Basu S, Brot N, *et al.* Biomarkers of oxidative stress study V: Ozone exposure of rats and its effect on lipids, proteins, and DNA in plasma and urine. Free Radic Biol Med 2013; 61: 408-15.
[http://dx.doi.org/10.1016/j.freeradbiomed.2013.04.023] [PMID: 23608465]

[160] Dreher D, Junod AF. Role of oxygen free radicals in cancer development. Eur J Cancer 1996; 32(1): 30-8.
[http://dx.doi.org/10.1016/0959-8049(95)00531-5] [PMID: 8695238]

[161] Acuña UM, Wittwer J, Ayers S, Pearce CJ, Oberlies NH, DE Blanco EJ. Effects of (5Z)-7-oxozeaenol on the oxidative pathway of cancer cells. Anticancer Res 2012; 32(7): 2665-71.

[PMID: 22753724]

[162] Cairns RA, Harris I, McCracken S, Mak TW. Cancer cell metabolism. Cold Spring Harb Symp Quant Biol 2011; 76(0): 299-311.
[http://dx.doi.org/10.1101/sqb.2011.76.012856] [PMID: 22156302]

[163] Valko M, Leibfritz D, Moncol J, Cronin MTD, Mazur M, Telser J. Free radicals and antioxidants in normal physiological functions and human disease. Int J Biochem Cell Biol 2007; 39(1): 44-84.
[http://dx.doi.org/10.1016/j.biocel.2006.07.001] [PMID: 16978905]

[164] Valko M, Izakovic M, Mazur M, Rhodes CJ, Telser J. Role of oxygen radicals in DNA damage and cancer incidence. Mol Cell Biochem 2004; 266(1/2): 37-56.
[http://dx.doi.org/10.1023/B:MCBI.0000049134.69131.89] [PMID: 15646026]

[165] Blau S, Rubinstein A, Bass P, Singaram C, Kohen R. Differences in the reducing power along the rat GI tract: lower antioxidant capacity of the colon. Mol Cell Biochem 1999; 194(1/2): 185-91.
[http://dx.doi.org/10.1023/A:1006994800272] [PMID: 10391139]

[166] Guz J, Foksinski M, Siomek A, *et al.* The relationship between 8-oxo-7,8-dihydro-2′-deoxyguanosine level and extent of cytosine methylation in leukocytes DNA of healthy subjects and in patients with colon adenomas and carcinomas. Mutat Res 2008; 640(1-2): 170-3.
[http://dx.doi.org/10.1016/j.mrfmmm.2007.12.013] [PMID: 18281064]

[167] Haklar G, Sayin-Özveri E, Yüksel M, Aktan AÖ, Yalçin AS. Different kinds of reactive oxygen and nitrogen species were detected in colon and breast tumors. Cancer Lett 2001; 165(2): 219-24.
[http://dx.doi.org/10.1016/S0304-3835(01)00421-9] [PMID: 11275372]

[168] Rainis T, Maor I, Lanir A, Shnizer S, Lavy A. Enhanced oxidative stress and leucocyte activation in neoplastic tissues of the colon. Dig Dis Sci 2007; 52(2): 526-30.
[http://dx.doi.org/10.1007/s10620-006-9177-2] [PMID: 17195121]

[169] Murrell TGC. Epidemiological and biochemical support for a theory on the cause and prevention of breast cancer. Med Hypotheses 1991; 36(4): 389-96.
[http://dx.doi.org/10.1016/0306-9877(91)90018-T] [PMID: 1809862]

[170] Brown NS, Jones A, Fujiyama C, Harris AL, Bicknell R. Thymidine phosphorylase induces carcinoma cell oxidative stress and promotes secretion of angiogenic factors. Cancer Res 2000; 60(22): 6298-302.
[PMID: 11103787]

[171] Lim SD, Sun C, Lambeth JD, *et al.* Increased Nox1 and hydrogen peroxide in prostate cancer. Prostate 2005; 62(2): 200-7.
[http://dx.doi.org/10.1002/pros.20137] [PMID: 15389790]

[172] Brar SS, Corbin Z, Kennedy TP, *et al.* NOX5 NAD(P)H oxidase regulates growth and apoptosis in DU 145 prostate cancer cells. Am J Physiol Cell Physiol 2003; 285(2): C353-69.
[http://dx.doi.org/10.1152/ajpcell.00525.2002] [PMID: 12686516]

[173] Hoagland LFM IV, Campa MJ, Gottlin EB, Herndon JE II, Patz EF Jr. Haptoglobin and posttranslational glycan-modified derivatives as serum biomarkers for the diagnosis of nonsmall cell lung cancer. Cancer 2007; 110(10): 2260-8.
[http://dx.doi.org/10.1002/cncr.23049] [PMID: 17918261]

[174] Opanuraks J, Boonla C, Saelim C, *et al.* Elevated urinary total sialic acid and increased oxidative stress in patients with bladder cancer. Asian Biomed 2010; 4(5): 703-10.
[http://dx.doi.org/10.2478/abm-2010-0092]

[175] Gecit I, Aslan M, Gunes M, *et al.* Serum prolidase activity, oxidative stress, and nitric oxide levels in patients with bladder cancer. J Cancer Res Clin Oncol 2012; 138(5): 739-43.
[http://dx.doi.org/10.1007/s00432-011-1136-4] [PMID: 22258852]

[176] Sabharwal SS, Schumacker PT. Mitochondrial ROS in cancer: initiators, amplifiers or an Achilles' heel? Nat Rev Cancer 2014; 14(11): 709-21.
[http://dx.doi.org/10.1038/nrc3803] [PMID: 25342630]

[177] Helfinger V, Schröder K. Redox control in cancer development and progression. Mol Aspects Med 2018; 63: 88-98.
[http://dx.doi.org/10.1016/j.mam.2018.02.003] [PMID: 29501614]

[178] Lee SR, Yang KS, Kwon J, Lee C, Jeong W, Rhee SG. Reversible inactivation of the tumor suppressor PTEN by H_2O_2. J Biol Chem 2002; 277(23): 20336-42.
[http://dx.doi.org/10.1074/jbc.M111899200] [PMID: 11916965]

[179] Salmeen A, Andersen JN, Myers MP, *et al.* Redox regulation of protein tyrosine phosphatase 1B involves a sulphenyl-amide intermediate. Nature 2003; 423(6941): 769-73.
[http://dx.doi.org/10.1038/nature01680] [PMID: 12802338]

[180] Son Y, Cheong Y K, Kim N H, Chung H T, Kang D G. Pae HO. Mitogen-activated protein kinases and reactive oxygen species: how can ROS activate MAPK pathways?,J Signal Transduc 2011, Article ID 792639.

[181] Klaunig JE, Wang Z, Pu X, Zhou S. Oxidative stress and oxidative damage in chemical carcinogenesis. Toxicol Appl Pharmacol 2011; 254(2): 86-99.
[http://dx.doi.org/10.1016/j.taap.2009.11.028] [PMID: 21296097]

[182] Peshavariya H, Dusting GJ, Jiang F, *et al.* NADPH oxidase isoform selective regulation of endothelial cell proliferation and survival. Naunyn Schmiedebergs Arch Pharmacol 2009; 380(2): 193-204.
[http://dx.doi.org/10.1007/s00210-009-0413-0] [PMID: 19337723]

[183] Monaghan-Benson E, Burridge K. The regulation of vascular endothelial growth factor-induced microvascular permeability requires Rac and reactive oxygen species. J Biol Chem 2009; 284(38): 25602-11.
[http://dx.doi.org/10.1074/jbc.M109.009894] [PMID: 19633358]

[184] Hwang AB, Lee SJ. Regulation of life span by mitochondrial respiration: the HIF-1 and ROS connection. Aging (Albany NY) 2011; 3(3): 304-10.
[http://dx.doi.org/10.18632/aging.100292] [PMID: 21389351]

[185] Sibenaller ZA, Welsh JL, du C, *et al.* "Extracellular superoxide dismutase suppresses hypoxia-inducible factor-1α in pancreatic cancer." Free Radic Biol Med 2014; 69: 357-66.

[186] Chio IIC, Tuveson DA. ROS in cancer: the burning question. Trends Mol Med 2017; 23(5): 411-29.
[http://dx.doi.org/10.1016/j.molmed.2017.03.004] [PMID: 28427863]

[187] Basuroy S, Dunagan M, Sheth P, Seth A, Rao RK. Hydrogen peroxide activates focal adhesion kinase and c-Src by a phosphatidylinositol 3 kinase-dependent mechanism and promotes cell migration in Caco-2 cell monolayers. Am J Physiol Gastrointest Liver Physiol 2010; 299(1): G186-95.
[http://dx.doi.org/10.1152/ajpgi.00368.2009] [PMID: 20378826]

[188] Tochhawng L, Deng S, Pervaiz S, Yap CT. Redox regulation of cancer cell migration and invasion. Mitochondrion 2013; 13(3): 246-53.
[http://dx.doi.org/10.1016/j.mito.2012.08.002] [PMID: 22960576]

[189] Cannito S, Novo E, Compagnone A, *et al.* Redox mechanisms switch on hypoxia-dependent epithelial–mesenchymal transition in cancer cells. Carcinogenesis 2008; 29(12): 2267-78.
[http://dx.doi.org/10.1093/carcin/bgn216] [PMID: 18791199]

[190] Lamouille S, Xu J, Derynck R. Molecular mechanisms of epithelial–mesenchymal transition. Nat Rev Mol Cell Biol 2014; 15(3): 178-96.
[http://dx.doi.org/10.1038/nrm3758] [PMID: 24556840]

[191] Anand P, Kunnumakara AB, Sundaram C, *et al.* Cancer is a preventable disease that requires major lifestyle changes. Pharm Res 2008; 25(9): 2097-116.
[http://dx.doi.org/10.1007/s11095-008-9661-9] [PMID: 18626751]

[192] Boffetta P, Donaldson K, Moolgavkar S, Mandel JS. A systematic review of occupational exposure to synthetic vitreous fibers and mesothelioma. Crit Rev Toxicol 2014; 44(5): 436-49.

[http://dx.doi.org/10.3109/10408444.2014.899558] [PMID: 24766058]

[193] Nakamura N. A hypothesis: radiation carcinogenesis may result from tissue injuries and subsequent recovery processes which can act as tumor promoters and lead to an earlier onset of cancer. Br J Radiol 2020; 93(1115): 20190843.
[http://dx.doi.org/10.1259/bjr.20190843] [PMID: 31860335]

[194] Moon JH. Health effects of electromagnetic fields on children. Clinical and Experimental Pediatrics 2020; 63(11): 422-8.
[http://dx.doi.org/10.3345/cep.2019.01494] [PMID: 32683815]

[195] Belpomme D, Irigaray P, Hardell L, *et al.* The multitude and diversity of environmental carcinogens. Environ Res 2007; 105(3): 414-29.
[http://dx.doi.org/10.1016/j.envres.2007.07.002] [PMID: 17692309]

[196] Nasca PC, Pastides H. Fundamentals of Cancer Epidemiology. Aspen Publishers 2001.

[197] Mechanisms of Carcinogenesis. Springer Publishing 2012; pp. 43-61.
[http://dx.doi.org/10.1007/978-90-481-3725-1_3]

[198] Bernardes N, Seruca R, Chakrabarty AM, Fialho AM. Microbial-based therapy of cancer: Current progress and future prospects. Bioeng Bugs 2010; 1(3): 178-90.
[http://dx.doi.org/10.4161/bbug.1.3.10903] [PMID: 21326924]

[199] Khan MI, Bouyahya A, Hachlafi NEL, *et al.* Anticancer properties of medicinal plants and their bioactive compounds against breast cancer: a review on recent investigations. Environ Sci Pollut Res Int 2022; 29(17): 24411-44.
[http://dx.doi.org/10.1007/s11356-021-17795-7] [PMID: 35064485]

CHAPTER 4

Biology of Cancer

Rawiah A. Alsiary[1,*], **Hanadi A. Katouah**[2], **Hiba S. Al-Amodi**[3] and **Mashael Al-Toub**[4]

[1] *King Abdullah International Medical Research Center (KAIMRC), WR King Saud Bin Abdulaziz University for Health Sciences (KSAU-HS), P.O. Box 9515, Jeddah, Saudi Arabia*

[2] *Chemistry Department, Faculty of Applied Sciences, Umm Al-Qura University, Makkah, Saudi Arabia*

[3] *Department of Biochemistry, Faculty of Medicine, Umm Al-Qura University, P.O. Box 715, Makkah, Saudi Arabia*

[4] *Department of Clinical Laboratory Sciences, College of Applied Medical Sciences, King Saud University, Riyadh, Saudi Arabia*

Abstract: Loss of genomic stability in the cell due to defects in the checkpoint of DNA damage, mitotic checkpoint, and telomere maintenance led to increased incidences of base pair alterations. Therefore, that genomic instability plays a critical role in tumor initiation and progression. Tumor progression requires a dynamic tumor/normal exchange in their microenvironment to support tumor growth. The histological alteration seen in the tumor at early stages confirms that the surface between the epithelium and the stroma undergoes progressive disturbance. Tumor progression is also affected by the immune system in which chronic inflammations promote the growth of tumor. Tumor cells experience altered metabolic profiling to support their growth. Cancer cells are characterized by uncontrolled cell division. For that, they utilize glucose as a source of energy to help them grow faster than normal cells. Hence, Glycolysis is a key metabolomics pathway consumed at a high rate during carcinogenesis.

Keywords: Cancer Biology, Cancer Cell Metabolism, Cell Cycle, Pericytes, TME.

INTRODUCTION

Stem cells are distinguished by their ability to continue to grow and differentiate into various cell types. In this chapter, we'll glance at the most common types of cells in the human body. The body's cells go through a constant cycle of renewal,

* **Corresponding author Rawiah A. Alsiary:** King Abdullah International Medical Research Center (KAIMRC), WR King Saud Bin Abdulaziz University for Health Sciences (KSAU-HS), P.O. Box 9515, Jeddah, Saudi Arabia; E-mail: alsiaryra@ngha.med.sa

aging, and eventually death. Endothelial cells, for example, are renewed every 150 days in adults. Mutations disturb this cycle in some cases, causing an abnormal accumulation of defects in the tissues, which finally leads to the formation of cancer cells. The cancer spreads uncontrollably and is linked to cell mass, which is influenced by a variety of factors, including blood supply, extracellular matrix, and cell-cell interactions, as well as changes in oncogenes and tumor suppressor genes. Endothelial cells are important in the function of blood vessels, including angiogenesis. As a result, endothelial cell defects may contribute to tumor development. As endothelial cells line the inside of the vessel wall, pericytes cover the surface of the vascular tube and sustenance the tumor microenvironment and cross-talk with cancer cells.

CANCER CELLS AND CANCER STEM CELLS

INTRODUCTION

In the human body, stem cells can differentiate into different cell types. They are characterized by a continuation of development, differentiation and tissue repair. There is a relationship between stem cells and cancer cells; they share the self-renewal property, which is a highly essential characteristic. Indeed, stem cells are affected by mutations that cause the accumulation of cancer and produce cancer cells [1].

Several studies have reported that the cells in the body are in a continuous cycle of renewal, aging and then dying. In fact, this cycle is disrupted in some conditions by mutations to the deoxyribonucleic acid (DNA)and causes abnormal accumulation of tissues and different types of cancer cells, including cancer stem cells (CSCs), which are generated from stem cells. Therefore, both stem cells and cancer stem cells show a critical role in the initiation and progression of cancer (Fig. **4.1**) [2]. Furthermore, there are always changes in the mechanism of cancer due to cancer proliferation. In fact, cancer development is uncontrolled and has a relationship with cell mass, which depends on many factors such as blood supply, extracellular matrix, cell contacts, differentiation, immune attack and cell death. In addition, cancer development is dependent on any changes to the cancer regulatory systems, which are oncogenes and tumor suppressor genes [3].

Cancer and Tumor

There is a misunderstanding between the definition of cancer, tumor and neoplasm. The following explanation is to clarify the meaning and the difference between them. Cancer is an abnormal progression of cells, which divide uncontrollably anywhere in the body tissues and invade neighboring tissues [4, 5].

Indeed, the actions of cancer are changeable during cancer development. Thus, the process involved in the formation of cancer is the multi-pathway mechanism called carcinogenesis [6].

However, cancer is illustrated by oncogenic mutations in a target cell or appears after several years [1]. In fact, the breast, lung, bone marrow, gut and prostate tissues contain stem cells that play an important role in cancer development [1]. Moreover, there are different types of cancers, such as carcinoma, leukemia, lymphoma, melanoma and sarcoma. The main diagnosed type is carcinoma, which is a cancer of many organs and glands, such as the breast, lungs, pancreas and skin. Furthermore, the cancer of the blood is called leukemia. In addition, the cancer of lymphocytes is lymphomas, and the cancer of melanocytes is melanoma. However, the rarest type of cancer is sarcoma, which starts in the bones and in the soft connective tissues, such as tendons of the arms or legs [4].

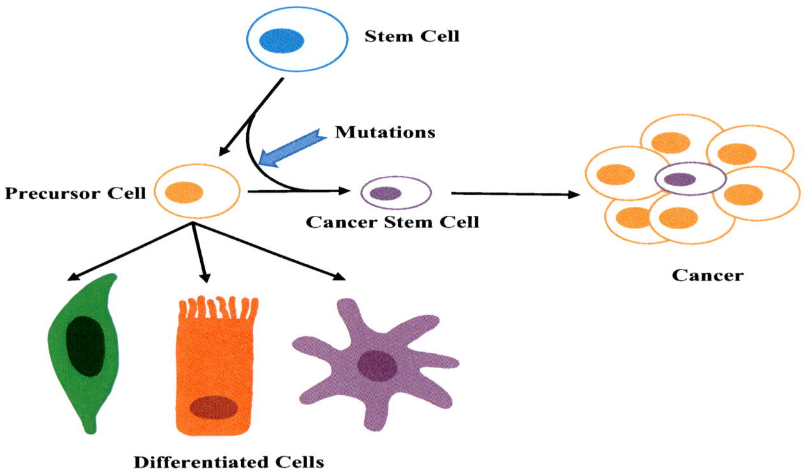

Fig. (4.1). Generation of cancer stem cells (CSCs) from stem cells and progenitor cells and formation of cancer [4].

A tumor is not certainly cancer. Moreover, a tumor is an uncontrolled development of cells without inflammation in the body tissues. In addition, the body does not need them, and they don't die [5]. However, the origination of the tumor is from the transformation of normal stem cells [7]. Furthermore, a tumor can be benign or malignant. Also, a collection of pus can be a tumor [5]. Indeed, tumors heterogeneity plays an important role in cancer cell types [8].

On the other hand, neoplasms are defined as the innovative growth independent from the nature of that growth [6].

Cancer Cells

Cancer cells are abnormal cells which are divided permanently and distributed in the body by blood and lymph systems. Actually, the classification of cancer cells is dependent on the site of the cells origin. The cancer cells in a carcinoma originate from epithelial cells. While, cancer cells in leukemia are derived from bone marrow. Though, lymphomas and melanomas come from cells of the immune system. However, sarcoma originates from cells of the connective tissue of muscle, bone and fat [9]. Furthermore, there is a difference between cancer cells; they are not identical. Whereas, the stem cell principle suggests that some cancer cells act as stem cells that replicate and maintain cancer [7].

A recent study showed therapeutic approaches for different types of cancer cells by protein arginine *N*-methyltransferase 5(PRMT5) selective inhibitor and (S)-*N*-(3, 4-dihydroisoquinolin-2(1H)-yl)-2-hydroxypropyl)-6-(oxetan-3-ylamino)pyrimidine-4-carboxamide (EPZ015666) [10]. Another recent study showed cancer cells inhibiting resistance to drugs *via* flap endonuclease 1 (FEN1) stability. It also showed that the response of DNA can be regulated by protein arginine *N*-methyltransferase 1 (PRMT1)-mediated arginine methylation [11].

Cancer Stem Cells

Cancer stem cells (CSCs) or tumorigenic cells are rare cancer cells that originated from stem cells. Also, these malignant cells are termed leukemic stem cells (LSCs). They grow and replicate rapidly to influence initiation, development, spread, tumorigenesis and metastasis of cancer. However, the main cause of cancer-related deaths is metastasis [8]. In addition, cancer stem cells are described by having the capability of self-renewal from a portion of malignant cells, proliferation, tumorigenic growth and differentiation for tumor growth (Fig. **4.2**) [12]. Differentiation of cancer stem cells will be by a similar pathway of differentiation of stem cells and cancer cells [13]. On the other hand, the differentiation of cancer stem cells for tumor growth will form non-tumorigenic cancer cells, which are the tumor bulk cells. In contrast, non-tumorigenic cancer cells are incapable of giving rise to more cells or maintaining tumorigenesis [14].

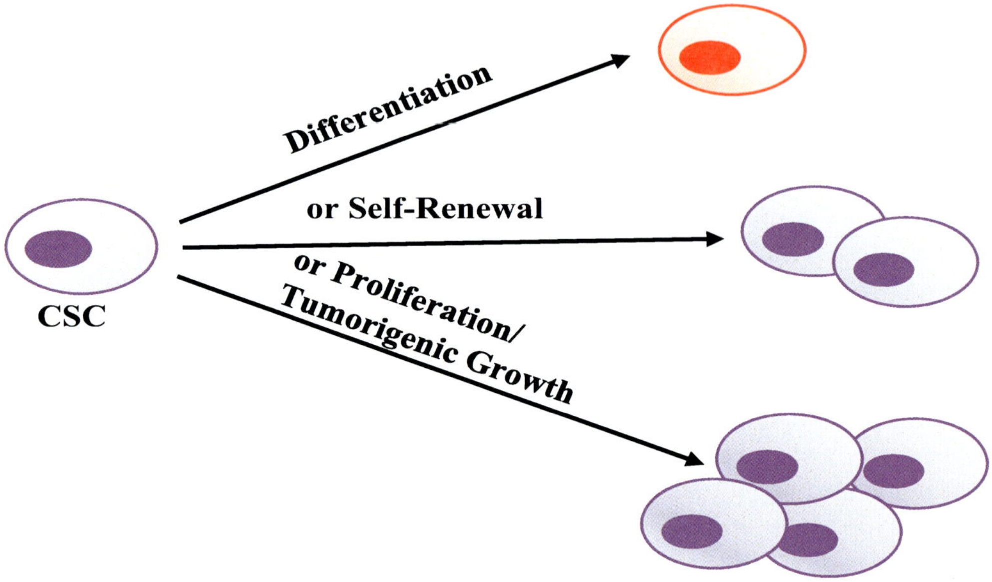

Fig. (4.2). Properties of cancer stem cells (CSCs) [12].

In fact, mesenchymal stem cells (MSCs) are essential in cancer management, where they improve tumor angiogenesis and antagonisms. They are also a precursor to a specific individual cancer stem cell, but the mechanism of initiation of cancer stem cells is still unclear [8]. Furthermore, there are several theories about the origin of cancer stem cells that include: i) cell synthesis [15], ii) microenvironment [16], iii) gene transmission [17], and iv) genomic renovation [18]. Moreover, cancer stem cells are resistant to treatments [19]. Also, they are characterized by disrupting the regulation of self-renewal pathways, possessing of cell surface markers and are involved in tumor formation [8]. In contrast, non-tumorigenic cancer cells, which form the bulk of the tumor, have superficial biomarkers as well, but they are unable to maintain tumorigenesis and self-renewal [1]. In all malignancies and solid tumors, there is an increase in CD47 cell surface marker [20, 21]. However, the antibody blockade of CD47 increases phagocytosis and elimination of cancerous cells [22].

ENDOTHELIAL CELLS

INTRODUCTION

Endothelial cells (ECs) are the cells found on the inner surface of the lumen of blood vessels and lymphatic vessels. Precisely, they are mesodermal in origin. In adults, endothelial cells are renewed once every 150 days. Moreover, endothelial cells represent the intracellular structure and the extracellular adhesions. The mechanical state of the structure depends on the actin fibers, cortex and cell membrane [23].

Endothelial cells resemble a pyramid shape. Furthermore, in large vessels, endothelial cells are surrounded by smooth muscle cells (SMCs), which give vessels stability and provide proteins that control the vessel's diameter. Whereas, the small capillaries are wrapped by perivascular cells called pericytes that also provide the capillaries with stability [24]. In addition, blood vessel stability is provided by the extracellular matrix (ECM), which is defined as the basement membrane. The extracellular matrix consists of proteins such as collagen, laminin and fibronectin [25].

However, endothelial cells play an important role in the vessel's function, such as angiogenesis, vasoconstriction, vasodilation, blood clotting, and regulation of nutrition movement into tissues, sustaining the flow of blood, and during inflammations, they contribute to sending the signals to white blood cells (WBCs) [23, 26].

Angiosarcomas

Any defect in the function of the normal endothelial cells will lead to the formation of malignant endothelial cells, also called tumor endothelial cells (TECs) [24]. In fact, these malignancies are rare and have a high degree of resistance to the treatment. Moreover, these malignancies depend on vascular endothelial growth factor stimulation, angiopoietin, hypoxia and Notch pathways. Therefore, angiosarcomas are produced by an increased number of malignancies. Whereas, the high potential of angiosarcomas causes metastasis [23, 26]. In particular, there are two types of angiosarcomas, primary angiosarcomas, that are able to take place all over the body; the most popular positions are breast, liver, spleen, heart, bone and scalp [27]. However, secondary angiosarcomas occur when there is peripheral lymphedema or after breast cancer treatment due to exposure to radiation [28].

Tumor Endothelial Cells (TECs)

Tumor endothelial cells (TECs), derived from normal endothelial cells, are involved in the initiation and progression of tumor endothelium leading tometastasis [29]. Thus, the morphological modifications in the blood vessels will participate in the formation of tumor blood vessels with an unregulated angiogenesis process [30]. Moreover, blood vessel tumors are characterized by abnormalities such as irregularity in the diameters, weakness of the wall and intercellular gaps, which release blood, fluid and fibrin into the neighboring spaces (Fig. **4.3**) [23, 24]. The abnormal phenotypes of tumor endothelial cells are dependent on the tumor microenvironment [31]. Indeed, tumor blood vessels contribute to supplying the tumor with nutrition and oxygen. In addition, tumor blood vessels consider the major effective goal of antiangiogenic therapies with the same mechanism as in the normal blood vessels [30, 31].

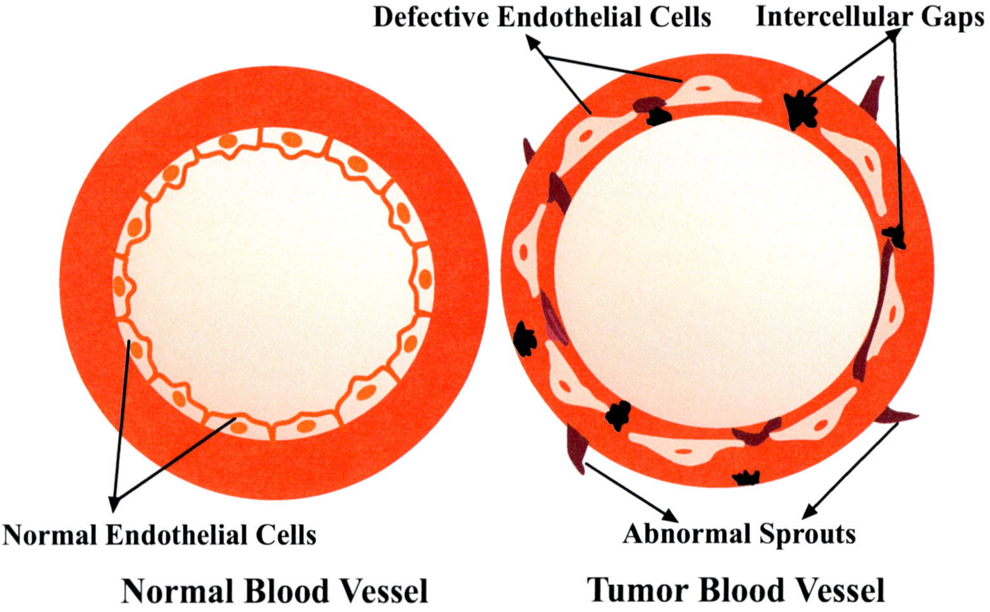

Fig. (4.3). Morphology of endothelial cells in cross-section of normal blood vessels and tumor blood vessels [24].

Tumor Endothelial Markers (TEMs)

During angiogenesis, large portions of tumor endothelial markers (TEMs) are detected in tumor vessels, specially TEM1, TEM5 and TEM8 [24]. The TEM5 is a G-protein-coupled receptor (GPCR) and contains seven transmembrane domains with an amino terminal [32]. While TEM8 is an anthrax toxin receptor (ANTXR1) and contains one transmembrane domain [33]. Furthermore, TEM1 is an endosialin or CD248 that also contains a single transmembrane glycoprotein with a lectin-like domain at the carboxyl-terminal [34]. It was demonstrated that the potential treatment of tumor growth is dependent on these genes' expression [24].

Metastasis

Metastasis is the single form of metastases, which is described as the distribution of cancer cells from one part of the body to different parts of the body by breaking away from the original site of cancer and passing through the bloodstream or lymph system. Therefore, metastasis depends on many factors, such as cancer type, progression speed and behavior [3].

Cancer Regulatory Systems

There are two regulatory systems involved in the growth of cancer. They are oncogenes and tumor suppressor genes. Oncogenes are responsible for the normal regulation of cell progression. On the other hand, tumor suppressor genes are genes that are responsible for controlling replication and result in cancer if mutated [3].

Angiogenesis

Angiogenesis is a reversible and self-controlled process that is involved in the formation of new blood vessels with new vascular structures from pre-existing blood vessels. These new blood vessels become stable with their basement membrane matrix protein and pericytes. This stability is provided by extracellular matrix (ECM), endothelial cell (EC) mitoses and spreading [35, 36]. Though, the reconfiguration of the extracellular matrix is involved in the reduced spreading of endothelial cells (ECs) by materials released from new blood vessels [35]. The nascent vascular tree is controlled by angiogenic factors such as the vascular endothelial growth factor VEGF/Dll4/notch axis with communication of neuronal and vascular systems [37, 38].

Any dysregulation in angiogenesis is called tumor angiogenesis which makes changes in the morphology of the nascent blood vessels and forms tumor blood vessels [24, 35]. The uncontrolled regulation is due to mutation in angiogenesis-related genes, viral infection and chromosomal translocations [24]. However, tumor angiogenesis depends on angiogenic stimulators and inhibitors formed by the tumor [31].

However, this mutation leads to the migration of endothelial cells by breaking down the basement membrane and stopping pericytes. Therefore, this migration depends on vascular endothelial growth factor (VEGF)/VEGF receptor (VEGFR) signaling, which is enhanced by VEGFR-1, VEGFR-2 and VEGFR-3, the tyrosine kinase vascular endothelial growth factor receptors. However, in cancer cells, the upregulation of vascular endothelial growth factor depends on molecules stimulated by hypoxia as well as oncogenes and tumor suppressor genes. Vascular endothelial growth factor motivates endothelial cells to spread for angiogenesis production. VEGFR-1 and VEGFR-2 are specific for blood endothelial cells, and VEGFR-3 is specific for lymphatic endothelial cells [31, 39].

On the other hand, there is abnormal VEGF/VEGFR pathway signaling at endothelial cell neoplasms [26]. The mechanism of this mutation is still under exploration, but it can activate angiosarcomas [40]. Furthermore, the role of spreading endothelial cells in tumor angiogenesis is still not understood [24].

In contrast, vasculogenesis is characterized as the differentiation of progenitor cells (angioblasts) into endothelial cells and the formation of a new immature vascular network [41].

On the other hand, intussusceptive angiogenesis (IA) is also defined as the formation of new vessels but in an unusual and fast way, while providing normal circulation [42]. Actually, intussusceptive angiogenesis is still considered as an unknown process for the development of new tumor blood vessels or inhibition tumor progression [24].

PERICYTES

INTRODUCTION

Pericytes (PCs) (*peri*, around; *cyte*, cell) are one of the two types of blood vessel-mural cells. The *vascular smooth muscle cells* (vSMCs) are the other blood vessel-mural cells. Collectively, they are called mural cells, since the endothelial cell tube is associated and covered with them. In contrast, the inner side of any blood vessel wall is formed by endothelial cells. In order to differentiate between PCs and vSMCs, a collection of parameters, including; cell density, morphology, location, and the pattern of specific markers (genes or proteins) expression, are used [43 - 45]. For instance, regarding the morphology and the micro-anatomical position of these cells, vSMCs, which are short, ring-shaped, and thickly lined, surround the arteries and arterioles. In comparison, the capillaries are surrounded by PCs with sporadic, protruding cell bodies and thin processes that extend longitudinally around and cover the capillaries and are implanted within the vascular basement membrane (BM) [46].

Before 1923, PCs were known as "Rouget cells", since, their finding is generally credited to the French scientist Charles-Marie Benjamin Rouget, who described a group of contractile cells circling the endothelial cells of the blood micro-vessels and occupying the perivascular compartment [47]. However, the existence of PCs was reported earlier, in 1871, by Eberth [46]. Subsequently, Zimmermann re-named these cells and introduced the term "pericytes". Also, he categorized them into three subtypes according to the morphology of their processes. As such, PCs at the arteriolar end of the capillary bed exhibited peripheral processes, but PCs at the mid and the venular end of the capillaries, shows longitudinal and stellate shape processes, respectively [48, 49]. This morphological heterogeneity may reveal a functional diversity of these cells [50].

In practice, PCs recognition in standard histological slides is challenging. It is feasible, however, to identify them, at the ultrastructural level and in semi-thin sections, where it is possible to reveal their position within the vascular basement membrane, and so distinguish them from the other perivascular compartments cells. In tandem with immunological staining approaches, the use of these procedures helps their distinctive morphology and position to be demarcated [48]. PCs show specific characteristics by expressing a variety of surface markers, in response to certain growth factors. Therefore, PCs expression pattern of these specific receptors for the growth factor can be employed for their recognition. However, and analogous to CAFs, there is no known single molecular marker that can be used to classify PCs unambiguously and separate them from vSMCs or other stromal cells. Instead, it is a pattern of inclusion and exclusion markers that may expand with the advancement of researches. For instance, PCs should be positive for; the tyrosine-kinase receptor, beta-type platelet-derived growth factor receptor (PDGFR-β) and it's co-receptor, the chondroitin sulfate proteoglycan, Neuron-glial 2 (NG2) - which also known as high-molecular-weight melanoma-associated antigen, or (HMWMAA) [51]. Although, PDGFR-β can be expressed by other types of cells, such as, astrocytes, particular tumor cell types, andmyofibroblasts [52]. Besides, they should be negative for the endothelial cells specific markers (*e.g.,* CD31), the other stromal specific markers (*e.g.,* fibroblast-specific protein 1 (FSP1), and the hematopoietic cells specific markers (*e.g.,* CD45, and CD11b) [50, 53, 54].

PCs Origins and Activation

Tumor cells have the ability to recruit stromal cells from distant sites, for the purpose of supporting their microenvironment and vasculature. These recruited stromal cells considered to be a precursor of some other TME-stromal cells, such as pericytes. PCs have been documented to be a part of stem cell niches and MSCs [55]. Recruited stromal cells that are derived from the bone marrow (*e.g.,* BM-MSCs) can contribute more strongly to pericytes and/or endothelial populations when local cells are unable to meet the tumor vasculature growth requirement [56]. Furthermore, the homing of MSCs to the TME and their differentiation into PCs can be induced by soluble factors released by the neoplastic cells, in response to some radio-therapeutic strategies. This facilitates the recurrence of the tumor, by supporting its vasculature through these newly formed PCs [57]. Moreover, there is extensive evidence of cellular transdifferentiation within the tumor microenvironment, both from stromal cell to stromal cell and from tumor cell to stromal cell [58]. The example most commonly quoted is that PCs can be originated from *cancer stem cells* (CSCs) in some tumor types. CSCs can be recruited through the SDF-1/CXCR4 axis against endothelial cells and induced by TGF-β primarily to become PCs. As a result, CSCs lead to vascular PCs that can actively reshape perivascular niches [59]. Pericytes are a type of mesenchymal cell (similar to smooth muscle cells) with finger-like projections that wrap around blood vessel endothelial tubing. Pericytes are known to secrete paracrine support signals to the normally quiet endothelium in normal tissues. For instance, Ang-1 secreted by pericytes transmits anti-proliferative stabilizing signals that are recognized by Tie2 receptors expressed on the surface of endothelial cells; some pericytes also produce low levels of VEGF, which serves an alimentary function in endothelial homeostasis [45]. Pericytes as well collaborate with endothelial cells to create the vascular basement membrane, which protects both pericytes and endothelial cells while also allowing vessel walls to withstand the hydrostatic pressure of blood flow. In contrast, normal vessel pericytes are not prone to such pharmacological interruption, providing an alternate illustration of the differences in regulation of normal quiescent and tumor vasculature. The RIP-tag2 transgenic mouse has recently become a popular model for studying pericyte biology. Pericytes express a variable profile of markers, including populations of cells expressing a subset of SMA, NG2, desmin, and PDGFR, according to these studies [60]. Confocal microscopy revealed SMA+/desmin+ cells as both abnormal mural cells (pericytes) connected to blood vessels and interstitial cells (myofibroblasts) free within the stroma, with no obvious cooperation with blood vessels. Tumor pericytes form an abnormally loose alliance with microvessels, tending to lift off endothelium and cytoplasmic processes extending deep into the tumor parenchyma [61]. Pericyte coverage is present in 97 percent of vessels in larger pancreatic Islet cell cancers; however, in other cancer models, pericyte density has been shown to be quite variable. Some cancers, such as human glioblastoma (which has 10–20% microvessel coverage) [62]. Despite endothelial synthesis of PDGF-B ligand, recruitment of PDGFR+ expressing cells to endothelium was relatively inadequate in two transplantable tumors, T241 fibrosarcoma and KRIB osteosarcoma. T241 tumor cells were co-injected with embryonic stem cells from mice bred to express the pericyte marker protein lacZ, demonstrating that these cells could be efficiently selected to a periendothelial site [63]. It's uncertain what function pericytes play in cancer. *via* heterotypic contacts and soluble factors, pericytes may be able to stabilize blood vessels, inhibit endothelial proliferation, support capillary diameter, control blood flow, and provide endothelial survival signals.

PCs Contribution to Tumor Microenvironment and Cross-Talk with Cancer Cells

PCs play essential roles in both physiological and pathological conditions. In the physiological contexts, for example, they have been concerned predominantly with blood flow stability and hemodynamic processes. Their roles are far more diverse, though. They can detect angiogenic factors, direct sprouting channels, induce functions of endothelial survival, and also demonstrate behaviors that are similar to macrophages [54].

Equally important, in pathological contexts, PCs are considered one of the essential cellular features in the tumor microenvironment. Hence, they are frequently associated with tumor vasculature. PCs have the capability to participate in and enhance cancer invasion and metastasis through the trans-differentiation program, the *pericyte–fibroblast transition* (PFT). As they have the ability to revamp tumor vessels into a mature phenotype. So that, when PCs disengage from tumor micro-vasculatures, they will undergo trans-differentiation to become stromal fibroblasts in response to *Platelet-Derived Growth Factor-BB* (PDGF-BB), secreted by the tumor cells itself [64]. This also shows the reciprocal manner by which the pericytes interact with the tumor cells within the TME. This mutual cross-talk can also be seen when the neoplastic cells are stimulated by *stereotactic body radiation therapy* (SBRT). As and upon this stimulation, the neoplastic cells will increase their release of two soluble factors; *stromal cell-derived factor-1α* (SDF-1α) and *platelet-derived growth factor-B* (PDGF-B). Subsequently, these factors will be bound to the receptors ((chemokine (C-X-C motif) receptor 4 (CXCR4) and PDGFR-β) on the circulating bone marrow-derived MSCs and recruit them to the tumor parenchyma. So, this newly engrafted can be differentiated to give rise PCs, which in turn will support tumor angiogenesis [56].

IMMUNE INFLAMMATORY CELLS

INTRODUCTION

The first link between cancer and inflammation was seen in the 19th century, when Rudolf Virchow observed the presence of leukocytes infiltrating tumors tissues, which led him to hypothesize that cancer originates from chronically inflamed reactions [65]. However, concrete evidence confirming the critical role of inflammation as one of the main causes of tumorigenesis was obtained only during the last decade. Therefore, it is important to eliminate the inflammation to inhibit tumorigenesis even before its initiation in the microenvironment [66].

Research shows that the inflammatory cell component always exists in all tumors microenvironments (TME) [67]. TME is a complex system containing a diverse group of cells that act in autocrine and paracrine manners and communication through direct contact, cytokine, and chemokine production [68]. High levels of inflammatory chemokines and cytokines have been linked to the aggravation of tissue damage and cancer progression. These chemokines and cytokines include the tumor necrosis factor (TNF)-a, interleukin family (*i.e.,* IL-1, IL-6, and IL-10), and *inducible nitric oxide synthase* (*iNOS*) and *cyclooxygenase-2* (COX-2) [69 - 71].

TME includes the following cells:

1. Cancer cells (fibroblasts, endothelial cells, pericytes, and mesenchymal cells).

2. Several inflammatory cells.

- Adaptive immune cells (T lymphocytes and B lymphocytes).
- Innate cells (mast cells, neutrophils, myeloid-derived suppressor cells, dendritic cells, macrophages, natural killer cells, and dendritic cells.

Hence, let's discuss the most frequently found immune cells in the TME: Tumor-associated macrophages (TAMs), B lymphocytes and T lymphocytes. B and T lymphocytes are the two primary types of lymphocytes present in the tumor microenvironment.

TAMs

Present in abundance in TME, and in contrast to normal macrophages, they are regulated by several microenvironmental cytokines, epigenetic regulators, and growth factors. They may also be regulated *via* other signals derived from the tumor itself or stromal cells in the surroundings. Evidence suggests that TAMs promote tumor growth by producing proteolytic enzymes, growth factors, and inhibitory immune checkpoint proteins in T cells [72 - 74]. Hence, TAMs play an important role in the relationship between chronic inflammation and cancer and play a crucial role in angiogenesis, invasion, and metastasis [75]. *In vitro*, TAMs were triggered by exposing them to various immune regulatory cytokines [76].

TAMs congregate in necrotic areas of tumors, and cover cancerous cells from normal immune cells by secreting IL-10 [77], then, Nitric oxide synthase (NOS) and vascular endothelial growth factor (VEGF) are released, which aid angiogenesis (VEGF) and promote tumor growth by the secretion of epidermal growth factor (EGF) [77, 78].

Excessive TAM expression was linked to poor prognosis. Therefore, in recent years, researchers' focused their interest and attention worldwide to target TAMs as a therapeutic strategy to prevent tumor development [79, 80]. TAMs have been linked to the delivery of invasion-potentiating microRNA into tumor cells, *via* exosomes (organelles used to secrete intracellular contents) [81].

B Lymphocytes

B lymphocytes are also known as B cells; it is express clonally diverse cell surface immunoglobulin (Ig) receptors recognizing specific antigenic epitopes. Based on their cell surface phenotype, location, activation routes, and Ag specificity, mature B lymphocytes can be categorized into multiple subsets [82].

T Lymphocytes

T lymphocytes, aka T cells, are a type of leukocyte that originates in the bone marrow and mature in the thymus. As T cells mature, they either become memory T cells or multiply and differentiate into regulatory, helper, or cytotoxic T cells. They undergo further differentiation into specialized cells that perform varying functions in the periphery. Initially, subsets of T cells were categorized by function. However, they also have distinct protein expression patterns and associated genes [83]. Based on the T cell receptors (TCR), T cells are divided into two main groups, namely γδ and αβ. αβ T cells use CD8 or CD4 co-receptors. That further classifies T cells into groups of effector T cells based on their effector function. T cells using CD8 become cytotoxic (CTLs), while T cells with CD4 become T helper (Th) cells. Different T cells specialize in different tasks. Together, CD4+/Th cells can differentiate further into multiple subtypes that perform different roles based on the type of cytokines they secrete. These subtypes include Th1, Th2, Th3, Th9, Th17, Th22, and follicular helper T cells, commonly known as Tfh (Table **4.1**). These subsets can promote several inflammatory responses, depending on their interaction with other cells, respective cytokine profiles, and responses to chemokines [84].

Regulatory T cells (Tregs) are a type of T lymphocytes that maintain the host's homeostasis. They inhibit the initiation of the self-immune system. It is hypothesized that the accumulation of Tregs is triggered to repress anti-tumor activity in response to chemokines and cytokines released in thc TME by tumor stroma infiltrating cells and dysplastic cells [85]. Based on their localization in the tumor, Tregs work to suppress multiple immune responses. Tregs may suppress the anti-tumor response of the immune system against tumor-associated antigens at the invasive margin, where cytotoxic CD8+ and IFN-producing Th1 cells are predominant [86]. The opposite is reported when the tumor is located in the stroma; regulatory T cells may negatively control the inflammatory response that stimulates the tumor progression [87].

It is essential to establish memory CD8+ T cell responses to attain lasting immunity against tumors [88, 89]. The circulating memory compartment typically consists of the following:

1. Central Memory (Tcm): These cells circulate between blood and secondary lymphoid organs.

2. Effector Memory (Tem) CD8+ T cells: These cells circulate between blood and non-lymphoid tissues [90].

Unlike the circulating subsets, many T cells reside in the peripheral tissue. These $CD8^+$ memory T cells are retained in lymphoid and non-lymphoid tissues. They offer local and powerful innate and adaptive immune responses [91, 92]. Memory T cells are heterogeneous cells that develop at different stages during the immune response with varying life spans, different migration patterns, and distinct functions, not just an ordinary cells that escape activation-induced cell death following infection [93 - 96].

Table 4.1. CD4+ helper T cell subsets.

Cell Type	Transcription Factor	Cytokines	Function
Th1	STAT4 and T-bet.	IFNγ, IL-2, IL-10, and TNF-α/β	• Increase the killing efficacy of the macrophages. • Provide defense against intracellular bacteria and viruses. • Help in tumor rejection by enhancing the proliferation of cytotoxic T lymphocytes (CTLs). • Promote the production of IgG.

(Table 4.1) cont.....

Cell Type	Transcription Factor	Cytokines	Function
Th2	STAT6 and GATA3	IL-4, IL-5, IL-6, IL9 Il10 and IL-13	• Help the differentiation and antibody production by B cells. • Play a crucial role in responses against intracellular parasites. • Enhance the production of neutralizing antibodies, including IgG, IgM, IgA, and IgE antibodies.
Th9	IRF4, STAT6, IRF, GATA3	IL-9 IL-10 and IL-21	• Provide defense against parasitic worms (helminths). • Play a crucial role in pro- and anti-tumorigenic activity (depending on cancer type).
Th17	RORγt STAT3	IL-17A and IL-17F, IFNγ, TNF-α, IL-10, IL-21, IL-22 and IL-26	• Offer defense at mucosal barriers and against gut pathogens. • Help in the activation of CTLs. • Help in the production and recruitment of neutrophils. • Promote tumor formation induced by inflammation of the colon.
Th22	aryl hydrocarbon receptor (AhR)	IL-22, IL-13, and TNF-α	• Promote gastrointestinal tumors. • Induce innate immune responses. • Play a significant role in the regulation of skin homeostasis and inflammation. • Aid in wound healing and promote barrier function at mucosal sites against enteropathogenic bacteria and *Candida albicans*. • Play a crucial role in the pathogenesis of psoriasis and keratinocytes.
Tfh	B cell lymphoma 6 (Bcl6)	IL-21, IL-4 IL-17, IL-22, and IL-10	• Present in B cell follicles and germinal centers of B cells and help them in the production of antibodies.

CD41 T cells can be further classified into Th1, Th2, Th9, Th17, Th22, or follicular helper T cells (Tfh). Each type can secret different cytokine profiles that promote different inflammatory responses. They respond differently to chemokines, and interactions with other cells also vary in Interleukin (IL), Interferon-gamma (IFNγ), Lymphotoxin (TNF) [97 - 107].

Infiltrating Cells

Immune system infiltrating cells are being more widely recognized as general components of tumors. These inflammatory cells have opposing functions: in most, if not all, neoplastic lesions, both tumor-antagonizing and tumor-promoting leukocytes can be present in varying proportions.

For the last century, researchers have discovered that genes involved in the effector activities of different immune cell types, as well as pharmacological inhibitors of these cells or their functions, play a variety of important roles in tumorigenesis [108]. Investigations of that kind havc proposed an increasing number of signaling molecules produced by inflammatory cells as effectors of their tumor-promoting behavior. That includes the angiogenic growth factor VEGF, and proangiogenic factors like FGF2. Proangiogenic and/or proinvasive matrix-degrading enzymes, such as MMP-9 and other matrix metalloproteinases, heparanase, and cysteine cathepsin proteases, may be generated by these cells [79, 109].

A number of partially differentiated myeloid progenitors have been identified in tumors, in addition to completely differentiated immune cells found in the stroma [79].

Tumor-Infiltrating Lymphocytes (TILs)

They are lymphocytes that get into cancer cells and share the same origin with myelogenous cells at the Hematopoietic stem cells (HSCs) [77]. Cancer cells have the ability to induce apoptosis in activated T cells *via* secreting exosomes with death ligands (TRAIL and FasL), or *via* switching off the normal cytotoxic response of natural killer cells by the same mechanism (NK cells) [110]. This suggests that tumor cells define the roles and responsibilities of TILs.

Myeloid-Derived Suppressor Cells (MDSCs)

They are a diverse population of myelogenous cells with the potential to inhibit T-cell responses. They are rapidly spread in tumors, implying that symptoms of inflammation can be seen in the majority of cancer sites. They also regulate wound healing in cancer [67]. Tumor-associated macrophages (TAMs) are included in this community of cells.

CANCER-ASSOCIATED FIBROBLAST (CAF)

INTRODUCTION

In healthy stromal tissue, *Fibroblasts*, which are elongated, fusiform cells with tapering ends, and oval or round central nuclei, exhibited heterogeneity and reside in few numbers. However, the metabolically active fibroblasts will appear stellated in shape, and they render *myofibroblast* phenotype [111, 112]. The concept of myofibroblast was first introduced for granulation tissue in wound healing [113, 114]. The phenotype of myofibroblast includes the formation of stress fiber, consisting of *alpha-smooth muscle actin* (α-SMA/*smooth muscle aortic alpha-actin* (ACTA2),), an actin isoform, and the secretion of *Extracellular matrix* (ECM) components such as collagen type-1 [115]. The activation of Fibroblasts plays a critical role in wound healing [116], and since "tumors are wounds that never heal" [117], they reside in abundance number in the cancerous tissues [118, 119], and so they are called *cancer-associated fibroblasts* (CAFs) or *tumor-associated fibroblasts* (TAFs) [120].

CAF was defined for the first time in 1979 by Gilles Tremblay as a stromal population of mesenchymal cells with myofibroblast characteristics. These cells exhibited prominent rough endoplasmic reticulum, well-developed Golgi zones, and longitudinal microfilament bundles with dense bodies. The nucleus often had irregular contours with nuclear membrane indentations, by Electron microscopic study [121]. CAFs can be recognized based on their spindle appearance and elongated cytoplasmic processes in light-microscopic studies of tissue slides [119, 122].

In addition to the phenotypic appearance, and in order to identify and isolate CAFs, the differentially expressed markers can be used. However, there is no single specific marker that may use to identify CAFs, instead, a group of inclusion and exclusion criteria may use [123]. CAFs should be negative for the non-mesenchymal tumor-microenvironment stromal cell markers. As such as epithelial cell adhesion molecule (EPCAM/CD326 or Tacstdl) and cytokeratin, an epithelial cells surface marker [124, 125]; high molecular weight caldesmon (CALD1), a pericytes marker; smoothelin (SMTN), a smooth muscle cells surface marker;protein tyrosine phosphatase receptor type C (PTPRC), a leukocytes surface marker;platelet and endothelial cell adhesion molecule 1 (PECAM1/CD31), an endothelial cell surface marker [126, 127, 128]. Besides and on the basis of inclusion criteria, CAFs can be identified by the expression of a number of postulated mesenchymal markers. However, Different forms of tumors can be present with varying occurrence and overlap in a given range of CAF markers. The availability of a given CAF marker in a tumor form may reflect the activation characteristics of the dominant type of resident fibroblasts in the affected tissue [123]. CAFs may possess myofibroblastic (activated fibroblast)and fibroblastic markers. Thus, the most commonly used markers for CAFs are α-SMA and *fibroblast activation protein* (FAP) [129]. In addition, there are other markers have also been identified in previous research, such as *platelet-derived growth factor receptor alpha/beta* (PDGFRα/β); *fibroblast-specific protein-1* (FSP-1//S100A4); *tenascin-C* (TNC); *microfibrillar-associated protein 5* (MFAP5); *collagen type XI alpha 1 chain* (COL11A1); *podoplanin* (PDPN);

integrin α11β1 (ITGA11); *neural/glial antigen 2* (NG2); *vimentin* (VIM); and *periostin* (POSTN) [128].

Similar to the normal stromal fibroblast, CAF within the tumor microenvironment exhibited heterogeneity among the different cancer types [130]. In general, the heterogeneity of the cancer-associated stromal cells arose from the various origin of the tumor-microenvironment stromal components, however, there are some factors that may alter the microenvironment composition like differing tumor types, modes of tumor establishment, age of the host and time of evaluation [56]. In the case of CAFs, the heterogeneity which gives rise to the different CAFs subpopulations among various cancer types may be explained by two main factors: (I) the broad spectrum of precursor cells of origin, and (II) the variation of stimuli that trigger the activation of CAFs [131].

CAFs Origins and Activation

Tumors have an ability to use numerous sources of structural cells in an orderly and discriminatory manner [56]. *Mesenchymal stem cells* (MSCs) have a probable tumor tropism; they are capable of migrating and infiltrating into the microenvironment of the tumor [132]. In several tumor microenvironments, MSCs may differentiate into α-SMA + myofibroblast cells that are abundant [120]. This, at least 20% of CAFs that express α-SMA and lead to cancer progression emerge from bone marrow (BM) and originate from MSCs in a mouse model of inflammation-induced gastric cancer [133]. MSCs-originated CAFs subpopulations may be recruited from two distinct sources. For instance, within ovarian and breast murine tumors stromal populations, the majority of FSP-positive and FAP-positive TAFs originate from MSCs located in bone marrow sources. However, most fibrovascular (pericytes, α-SMA+ myofibroblasts, and endothelial cells) and vascular stroma originate from neighboring adipose tissue [56].

Besides, CAFs may originate from the resident fibroblasts in the vicinity of neoplastic cells. The activation of these fibroblasts is partly due to the damage stemming from the neoplasm that is forming [119]. In addition to that, and through transdifferentiation programs; the epithelial-to-mesenchymal transition (EMT) and the endothelial-to-mesenchymal transition (EndMT), CAFs may arise from epithelial and endothelial cells, respectively [134].

CAFs activation can be motivated by a number of stimuli, including soluble factors that are secreted by tumor cells and immune cells. These soluble stimuli may comprise; growth factors such as *platelet-derived growth factor* (PDGF) (PDGFα and PDGFβ), *Transforming growth factor beta 1* (TGF- β1), *fibroblast growth factor* (basic FGF/bFGF/FGF2), and *Hepatocyte growth factor* (HGF); in addition to interleukins like IL-6, metalloproteinases, and reactive oxygen species [135]. Furthermore, it has become evident that some other factors rather than tumor-secreted factors may play an important role in CAFs activation, such as the stiffness of the matrix in the tumor microenvironment [136]. Both of these stimuli can collaborate to decide different CAF phenotypes that further add another dimension to their heterogeneity [136].

CAFs Contribution to the Tumor Microenvironment and Cross-Talk with Cancer Cells

The theory of 'seed and soil' (Paget, 1989) introduced the crucial role of the microenvironment in controlling tumor growth [137]. In a mutual communication way, tumor cells interact with stromal cells, within the tumor microenvironment [138]. CAFs considered one of the most significant players in the field of cancer progression, as they facilitate the development of tumor cells, both *in vitro* and *in vivo* [139, 140]. Precisely, CAFs develop a close association with cancer cells. This provides benefits for both types of cells; while cancer cells activate and maintain CAF activation, cancer cell formation, motility and invasion are assisted by CAFs. The reciprocal dynamic interaction between CAFs and cancer cells may lead to tumor growth, chemo-resistance and metastasis [135]. For example, this can be seen in the role of CAFs in enhancing cancer invasion, as they are the principal source of MMP13, a stromal mediator of cancer cell invasion [120]. Furthermore, by inducing tissue fibrosis, they also encourage the possibility of cancer growth [141, 142]. Also, CAFs can help tumor cell development and survival by the secretion of chemokines, like CXCL12, enhancing neovascularization, and the recruitment of immune cells to the tumor microenvironments [143].

Additionally, CAFs able to remodel and increase the extracellular matrix (ECM) deposition in tumors, which may boost the matrix stiffening, cancer cell invasion and angiogenesis, through activation of (*yes-associated protein*) YAP transcription factor, which is a signature feature of CAFs [136].

Moreover, CAFs-secreted growth factors, chemokines and ECM enables endothelial cells and pericytes to be recruited angiogenically. Therefore, activated tumor-fibroblasts or CAFs are a central determinant of cancer malignancy development and provide a significant focus for cancer therapies [119].

TUMOR MICROENVIRONMENT (TME)

INTRODUCTION

Malignant tumors are considered to be disarrayed masses of several living tissues, where typical and cancerous constituents are intermixed. The environment around the tumor is known as tumor microenvironment (TME), and it is generated from the tumor and controlled by tumor-induced interactions. Therefore, TME is influenced by cancers cells but through the release of bioactive molecules (chemokines, cytokines, lipid mediators, *etc.*) [144 - 146], stroma cells with signaling molecules, immune cells (lymphocytes, microglia, macrophages, *etc.*), neighboring blood vessels, and non-cellular components of extracellular matrix (ECM) (such as interstitial fluid, laminin, fibronectin, hyaluronan [147, 148]. The functions related to cellular and non-cellular constituents in the tumor microenvironment are controlled by tumor cells *via* complex signaling networks. As a result, they utilize the non-malignant cells to their advantage by building an environment that encourages tumor escape; that is, to grow and progress. The immunosuppressive environment is generated by Tumor cells in two different ways: 1) by a congregation of immunosuppressive cells around the tumor, and 2) by activation of immunosuppressive molecules, which contain several immune checkpoints, resulting in immune escape. Non-malignant cells in the tumor microenvironment release bioactive molecules [149, 150], contributing to cancer progression by inducing uncontrolled cell proliferation and metastasis [67, 76, 98, 151, 152].

Tumor microenvironment involves all the processes associated with the initiation and development of tumor, including all genetic and epigenetic alterations [153]; it also involves all the complex structures as well as functional modifications that are believed to be at the interface existing between putative tumors cells and the neighboring non-neoplastic host cells during tumor progression [154, 155]. This fact has been ignored for decades, and researchers believed that these nuclear changes in the tumor cells were significant causes for tumor initiation and progression. On the other hand, the researchers also regarded the neighboring tissues' changes as random bystander effects during tumor development. Nevertheless, this was disapproved by Judah Folkman and other experts studying the formation of new blood vessels for tumor growth, after determining the advancing mass of tumor cells also required some extrinsic support from the host [156]. Furthermore, scientists reported distinctly visible alterations at the tumor-host interface in tumors from diverse organs in their microscopic studies on tumor development [157, 158]. Carcinogenic agents, which can either be chemicals (such as asbestos, kepone, benzene, EDB), radiant energy, víruses, (such as human papillomavirus (HPV), hepatitis viruses' B and C), can induce these constant changes in various animal species at the tumor-host interface. These changes turn out to be more unhinged as the tumor continues to expand into the host. Another evidence is the hormonal and metabolic influence of the tumor on the host, occasionally evidently disrupting the function of other separate organs located far away [159, 160].

All this evidence has made researchers conclude that carcinogenesis in the target tissue is functionally influenced by physical changes and significant disturbances in the regulatory interactions of adjacent normal tissues, regardless of the causative a gentnature, such as excess hormonal stimulation, viruses, and/or chemicals [161]. Thus, the host surrounding tumor environment is imperative as it influences the tumor initiation, growth, invasion and metastasis. Consequently, understanding the cancer-non-cancer cell interactions in the tumor microenvironment is vital to comprehending the mechanisms attributing to cancer progression and patients' survival. Subsequently, this may introduce new opportunities for developing therapeutics.

Cancer-Non-Cancer Cell Interactions Mechanism

For the development of the tumor in microenvironments and for tumor cells to grow, invade, and metastasize, cancer cells often communicate with their complex and dynamic neighboring microenvironments. This cancer-non-cancer cell communication is bidirectional and occurs through several signaling networks. This interaction includes:

1. Cell-free contacts.

2. Juxtacrine interactions such as desmosomes and cell-cell junctions.

3. Interaction through facilitating mediators.

The mediators initiate the interactions between cancer and non-cancer cells *via* a complex network secreted by TME constituents, including chemokines, cytokines, growth factors, matrix remodeling enzymes, and inflammatory mediators. Additionally, the tumor cells and host surface communication also involve cell-free DNA (cfDNA), exospores, circulating tumor cells (CTCs), and apoptotic bodies [162 - 164].

Cytokines and chemokines are the most investigated mediators in the TME that facilitate intracellular interaction. Cytokines are an extensive group of small extracellular proteins or peptides secreted by different types of cells, such as fibroblasts, endothelial cells and immune cells. Also, some types of stromal cells produce cytokines. Cytokines are believed to be involved with cell signaling mediation *via* cell surface receptors to control the tumors development, since they cannot pass through the cell membrane into the cytoplasm [165, 166].

On the other hand, chemokines are small peptides and described as a subtype of cytokines. Chemokines are similar to growth factors in structure and function in that they stimulate chemoattraction by binding to G-protein-coupled receptors to direct angiogenesis and the migration of cells.

Unlike cytokines and chemokines, Exosomes and fatty acid mediators are still under study. Exosomes are small extracellular vesicles containing proteins, lipids, and genetic materials. They act as mediators to facilitate cell interaction and potent signalling molecules between cancer cells and the adjacent non-cancer in the TME. Also, exosomes have been associated with cancer progression stages and play a significant role in response to treatment. Fatty acid mediators have less attention due to a deficiency in the quantification and localization of lipids techniques [167, 168]. Nevertheless, recent lipidomics advancements have shown promising impacts in the field of carcinogenesis [169 - 171].

Surface stress-induced ligands (ULBP, MICA, and MICB) are processed by metalloproteases released in the TME, allowing cancer cells to avoid recognition in a procedure called shedding [172, 173]. Shedding facilitates immune evasion in a variety of ways.

1. The ligands do not stimulate receptor binding sites since they don't attach to cells and remain free in the bloodstream.

2. Binding to NK cells or CTLs leads to ligands internalization, allowing immune escape [174].

3. As ligands bind consistently to the NKG2D receptor, other NK receptors and T-cell activation are suppressed [175].

Heat Shock Proteins (HSPs)

Heat shock proteins (HSPs) exist intracellularly. In response to stressors in the microenvironment, they are discharged into the extracellular matrix *via* extracellular vehicles (EVs) such as oncosomes and exosomes [175]. HSP receptors are found on both immune and cancer cells. HSP90, is an example of the heat shock protein, which is implicated in cancer development by facilitating the maturation of different proteins involved in the process. HSP90 carries out its role with the help of around ten co-chaperones [176]. HSP90 upregulation has been linked to a poor prognosis in a variety of cancers, including lung cancer, breast cancer, colon cancer and others [177 - 181].

In response to heat shock factor 1 (HSF 1) and hypoxia-inducible factor-1 (HIF-1), tumor cells produce alarmins *via* oncosomes. Alarmins are extracellular heat shock proteins (ex-HSPs), and they are linked to resistance-associated secretory phenotype (RASP) that foster immune escape by granting resistance to stressful environmental factors like hypoxia, radiation, immune factors, and therapeutic medications [182]. TIGIT-A, which stands for T cell receptor immunoglobulin and ITIM domain, functions as an inhibitory receptor that interacts with CD155 on APCs or tumor cells to suppress NK and T cell functions. CD155, CD112, and CD113 have been identified as TIGIT ligands [183]. CD155 and CD112 have been shown to be overexpressed in a variety of human cancers and up-regulated by IFN [184 - 188]. ECM plays a significant role in tumor formation and progression and is considered a major barrier to metastasis [189]. In solid tumors, fibroblast/myofibroblast involved in initial invasion is accompanied by desmoplasia, which is an immense buildup of collagenous ECM. This is linked to a bad prognosis and resistance to treatment [190, 191].

Tumor Microenvironment Alterations at the Histological Level During Carcinogenesis

The two-dimensional cell culture cannot be used to evaluate the disorientation of systematic cellular interactions during tumor development. This disorientation can only be assessed by examining samples removed from intact tumors developing within an entire living organism. David Tarin reviewed the histological changes at the tumor-host surface during tumor progression [192].

TME at the Early Human Carcinogenesis Stage

Dysplasia is a disorder that results in the development of tumor. Studying this kind of disorder delivers substantial information regarding the involvement of the TME in the initiation of tumors. These disorders also offer helpful insignias regarding to comprehend the series of reactions occurring at the surface between the pre-tumor unsteady epithelial cells and the stroma of the host in the initial stages of tumor development. Observations have indicated that this surface remains undamaged, but in the affected regions, the cell alignment gets increasingly disturbed, which increases the epithelium's thickness. The steady increase in rarefaction and density of stromal cells underneath the affected area then follows [155].

TME at the Advanced Human Carcinogenesis Stage

At the advanced stage, it's difficult to outline the surface separating the epithelium from the stroma, soon afterwards, it disappears, and the interpretation becomes complicated. Eventually, the tumors expand, and the cancer cells keep dividing and start to invade the neighboring stroma. As a result, the number of stromal cells increases with an increase in capillary vessel quantity in the stromal-epithelial junction, which shows the ability of tumor cells to support its development through the recruitment of the host tissue constituents [192].

CONCLUSION

To sum up, the histological features observed at a microscopic level in biopsies obtained during the early stages of tumor progression from different organs confirm that the boundary between the epithelium and the stroma undergoes progressing disturbance. Pre-cancerous cells interact with their non-neoplastic neighbors during neoplastic transformation, which are vital indicators for pathologists to ascertain whether the suspect lesions are malignant. Also, to determine whether it is a need for treatment or not. Thus, the histological change observed under the microscope microscopic in tumors can be used to validate that considerable and progressive alterations happen in the TME during carcinogenesis.

GENOMIC INSTABILITY AND MUTATION

INTRODUCTION

Genome instability (GIN) is a hallmark of most human cancers. It includes small structure alterations like increased frequencies of base pair mutation, which is also known as nucleotide instability (NIN) and microsatellite instability (MSI), in addition to significant structural alterations like changes in the number or structure of chromosome that is also called chromosome instability (CIN) [193, 194]. The genetic changes accumulation ranging from mutations of single nucleotide to rearrangements of chromosomes can derive cells to be predisposed towards malignancy. Moreover, the sustentation of GIN enables cancer cells to be survived under selective pressure and adapt to their microenvironments by promoting mechanisms to resist various therapies [195].

Genomic stability is frequently challenged by exogenous and endogenous factors, which can persuade a diversity of lesions in DNA, causing alterations and impairment within chromosomes [196]. All species need to conserve genome stability to warrant a correct transmission of their genetic content to the following generations. In order to maintain genome integrity, diverse protection mechanisms have been established through development. Imperfections in these protection mechanisms can initiate the buildup of mutations named GIN. The GIN existence eventually influences gene overexpression, and the synthesis and activity of many proteins, leading to alterations of phenotype, which disturb cellular suitability and develop diseases such as cancer [197].

In fact, damages and mutations of DNA are quite different. DNA damages involve physical anomalies, such as breaks of single and double strands, remnants of 8-hydroxydeoxyguanosine, and abducts of polycyclic aromatic hydrocarbon. Moreover, enzymes can recognize DNA damages, and subsequently, they might be efficiently mended if redundant information, for instance, the undamaged sequence in the complementary DNA strand or in a homologous chromosome, is accessible for replication. Therefore, within the cell keeps DNA damage, it is possible to counteract the transcription of a gene, and in this way, a protein produced by gene translation will be blocked as well. Copying could additionally be blocked, or the cell could pass by and die. Contrary to DNA damage, a DNA mutation involves an alteration in the DNA base sequence. An alteration can't be predictable by enzymes when the base mutation is presented in both DNA strands; consequently, a mutation can't be restored. At the cellular level, DNA alterations can lead to modifying protein functions and regulation. Moreover, Mutations are copied in cell proliferation.

The current topic displays the life cycle of cells and its regulation as it is the major driving force for GIN tumorigenesis in genomic mutations. Various levels of GIN, as well as global trends in GIN across several tumor types, are discussed. Ultimately, caretaker genes as well as mechanisms are explained, which are responsible for maintenance against GIN and then protection from tumorigenesis.

Cell Cycle

One of the greatest significant traits in cell biology is the cell cycle, which supports development and progression, and is principal to preserve the homeostatic system throughout the grownup lifespan of multicellular creatures. It is an intricate series of proceedings over which each cell copies its contents and splits, causing the production of two genetically indistinguishable daughter cells.

The cell-division cycle consists of an interphase that comprises two gap phases; gape 1 and gap 2 (G1 and G2), the synthesis (S) phase, and the mitosis (M) phase (Fig. **4.4**) [198]. Throughout interphase, a cell gets ready to divide by means of

DNA development and replication. The G1 phase is the gap between the cytokinesis termination of a former division and the starting of S phase. It is the first progressive phase within that the cell develops in preparation for DNA replication; in addition, it is the phase in which the cell decides whether it will split again or go into a quiescent state (G0) [199, 200]. A deletion of growth factors in initial G1 forces the cell to enter G0; however, their deletion later on; next the G1 phase restriction checkpoint, permits the cell to endure into S phase [201]. Throughout S phase, DNA duplication happens, and each chromosome is replicated into two identical chromatids. The G2 phase happens directly next DNA replication and prior to the mitotic phase. At this time, each cell creates constituents required for cell division, like proteins and RNA [202]. The M phase initiates with mitosis that involves five stages; starting with prophase, then pro-metaphase, metaphase, anaphase, and ending up by telophase, which finishes with the form of two separate daughter cells through the process known as cytokinesis [198]. Cell division and imitation over the cell cycle produce two genetically identical daughter cells.

Regulation of the Cell Cycle

Each cell-division cycle phase is accomplished by the activity of cyclin-dependent kinases (CDKs), which are self-stimulated or activated by cyclins. They are crucial regulators of the cell-division cycle development by controlling substrates essential in that phase [203, 204]. In the initial G1 phase, cells motivated with signaling pathways of mitogen, like through mitogen-activated protein kinase (MAPK), by growth stimulating factors leading to up-regulation of the family of cyclin D (cyclin D1, D2, and D3) that stimulates CDK 4/6 [205]. However, During the late stage of the G1 phase, the cyclin D, and CDK 4 and 6 expression levels start to reduce, whereas the family of cyclin E (cyclin E1 and E2) of nucleus proteins and CDK2 is stimulated using cyclin E [206, 207]. The stimulation of cyclin E-CDK2 triggers hyperphosphorylation and inhibition of retinoblastoma (Rb) components of protein (Rb/p107 and Rb/p130) [208]. Additionally, the inactivation of Cdh1, one of the component adaptor proteins of cyclosome, also known as anaphase-promoting complex (APC/C), persuades permanent obligation to cell division [209, 210]. Cdh1 inactivation by activated cyclin E/CDK2 at the late stage of G1 phase inhibits the cyclosome activity. This permits E2F1 in S phase gene transcription as well as prompts the cells development and entrance into the S phase [211]. During the synthesis (S) phase, cyclin E could be broken, causing the cyclin A-CDK1and 2 complex activation that supports S-phase development. Through the G2/M moving, cyclin B, the significant controller of entrance into the mitotic phase, directly transfers into the nucleus in a companion with CDK1 and phosphorylates many targeted proteins implicated separation of chromosome-sister chromatids and cytokinesis on the spindle fibers of mitosis phase. The cyclin B-CDK2 complex degradation after the mitotic phase indicates the starting of the following G1 phase [212].

Generally, four major mechanisms are mainly involved in normal mammalian cells to preserve their genomic integrity for the period of the cell-division cycle (Fig. **4.4**):

1. high-fidelity during DNA replication (S-phase).
2. precise segregation of chromosomes between the two new daughter cells throughout mitosis (M phase).
3. precise repair mechanism of DNA damage during the cell division.
4. control of cell cycle checkpoints.

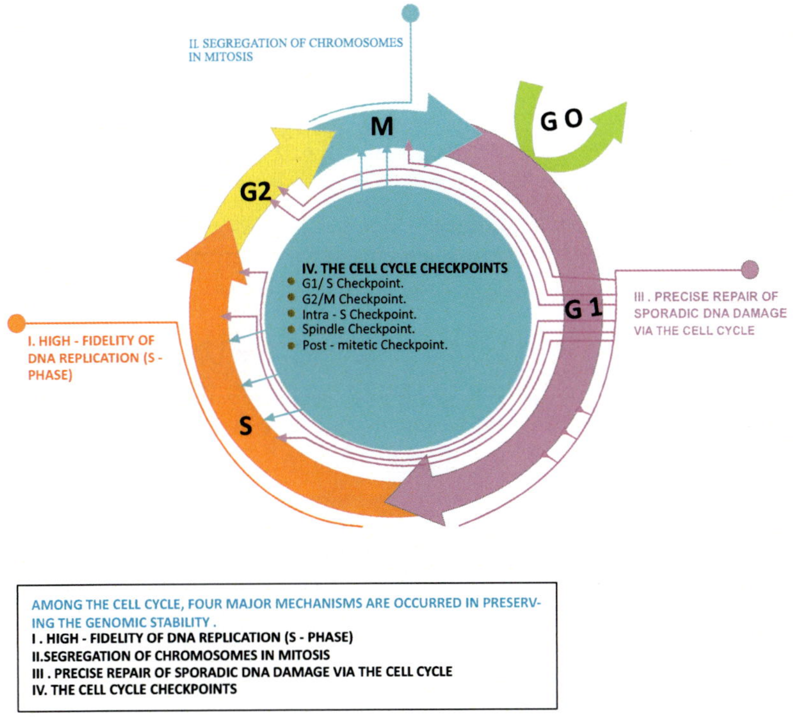

Fig. (4.4). Summary of the four main mechanisms used to preserve the integrity of the genome through the cell-division cycle.

In addition, further mechanism(s), like control of abnormal regulation of cell fate, involving apoptosis (programmed cell death) and senescence, can be considered as a result of GIN and can do additional participation to the progression benefit of tumorous cells. Moreover, four major mechanisms restore manifold molecular pathways [199].

Genomic Instability Levels

Nucleotide Instability (NIN)

Nucleotide instability (NIN) generally develops as a result of replication errors, as well as defects in repair tracks like base- or nucleotide-excision repair (BER and NER, respectively), causing alterations in nucleotides sequences either by substitutions, deletions, or insertions, that is able to affect the structure of the gene and/or its expression. In fact, NIN has been reported to occur in hereditary cancers, in which losing the function of DNA repair genes leads to increased occurrences of base pair alteration. For instance, inherited MUTYH-associated polyposis that is bi-allelic germline alterations (BER; *MUTYH* results in an increased incidence of G•C to T•A transmission, leading to carcinogenesis [213]. Even though NIN exists, single nucleotide alterations can lead to great phenotypes changes. For instance, hereditary impairments in these repair signaling paths (germline alterations in *ERCC2, DDB2, XPC,* and *MUTYH*) cause ailments like MUTYH-associated polyposis and xeroderma pigmentosum that result in GIN and the buildup of DNA alterations, accordingly prompting these entities to be affected by colon and skin cancers, respectively [214].

Like the genomic nucleus, the mitochondrial genomic DNA also shows NIN, and the link of the high-level generation of reactive oxygen free radicals with a failure or inadequacy of DNA repair pathways leads to an increase in the rate of mitochondria DNA alterations, which is a substantially greater than that of DNA of the nucleus [215].

The evidence of NIN laterally with MSI existed in other inherited cases of DNA impairment repair gene alteration might be a reason for GIN and the onset of cancer. It has been suggested that an initial step in the development of cellular alteration is the expression of mutant genes, which normally function in the maintenance of genetic integrity [216].

Microsatellite Instability (MSI)

Microsatellites (MSs), also known as Tandem Repeats (TRs) or Simple-Sequence Repeat (SSRs), are defined as repetitive DNA sequences containing 1–6 bps located within the genome, in both exons and introns [217, 218]. The spreading features range from 15 to 65 nucleotide sequences tandem repeats recurrence of tandemly repeated DNA commonly situated close to the terminals of chromosomes [219]. MS size is variable; nevertheless, the sole MS of a set of length are existent in the human genome of each individual. Errors of replication are occurred frequently within MS, assuming their repetitive nature, which can be corrected through DNA mismatch repair (MMR) [217].

MSI generation mechanism is mostly supposed to be DNA slippage in the replication processes, or slippage basic group mismatch as well as complementary strands in the DNA replication process and repair, leading to missing or insert of one or more of the nucleotide units. Normally, MMR can repair the errors in the process of DNA replication. However, as a result of the shortage of mismatch repair genes within tumorous cells or failure in the replication DNA repair, the chance of gene mutation is raised [220]. Every MS definite location contains two parts; the peripheral flanks the dominant core, and the specificity of MS is mainly a result of the variation in the number of core repeating units [221].

Microsatellite instability (MSI) is produced from disorders in DNA (MMR) during the replication process that leads to multiple mutations at microsatellites, particularly mutations of the *PMS2, MLH1, MSH2*, and *MSH6* genes, which leads to random insertion or deletions, microsatellites expansion, and a hypermutable phenotype. It is a distinctive feature of numerous cancers, such as endometrial, stomach, lung, ovarian, and colon cancer, wherever and it has been comprehensively diagnosed and described [222, 223]. MSI occurs in about 15% of colorectal cancer that naturally arises in the proximal colon and is linked with more effective prediction compared to non-MSI cancers.

MSI arises in either sporadic forms of colon cancer or hereditary "Lynch syndrome", even though through different mechanisms [224]. Sporadic forms of CRC with MSI are related to hypermethylation and expression loss of *MLH1*; however, hereditary non-polyposis CRC (Lynch syndrome) is described by deactivating germline alterations to *PMS2, MLH1, MSH2*, or *MSH6* [225]. The bulk of sporadic CRC forms with MSI develops in an extensive abnormal promoter methylation background, stated as the "CpG island methylator phenotype (CIMP)" [226, 227]. The progression and development of CIMP tumors occur through methylation of the promoters of tumor-suppressor genes (*e.g., MLH1, p16* and *IGF-2*), and have clinical characteristics distinctive from non-CIMP tumors [228 - 230].

Microsatellites (MSs) are extremely polymorphic and mutated, are biomarkers represented in forensic medicines and molecular genetics and have predictive value in several cancers. The prevalence and profile of MIS within lung cancer (LC) is still debatable; however, it is allied with carcinogenesis in the early stages

[231]. MSs can assist in stratifying patients with LC for immunotherapeutic, providing their neoantigen expression, develop tumor mutational burden [232] and Deficiency of MMR is measured through MSI and is associated with tumor mutational burden levels. However, the MSI frequency in non-small cell lung cancer (NSCLC) in a comprehensive study, including 480 adenocarcinomas cases of lung cancer using staining of mononucleotide immunohistochemistry and marker panel of MMR proteins, was only 0.8%, mostly in smoking patients and initially diagnosed stage [233, 234]; however, an additional study demonstrated only 1 case of 341 adenocarcinomas of patients with LC (0.3%) [234, 235].

Chromosomal Instability (CIN)

Genomic cancers are characterized by frequent chromosomal abnormalities, known as chromosomal instability (CIN), which is characterized by the elevation in the gain or loss level of entire and segment of chromosomes in the cellular division. In solid tumors, CIN is the utmost notable GIN form, with approximately 90% of humanoid tumors showing chromosomal aberrations and aneuploid chromosomes [236, 237].

Translocations, amplifications, global aneuploidy, deletions, homozygous deletions, loss of heterozygosity (LOH), and inversions are considered as main characteristic features of CIN tumors [238]. However, the main importance of CIN is the production of cells with disturbing content of chromosomes, a state recognized as aneuploidy [239], which is a state of an unequal separation of newly replicated chromosomes to daughter cells *via* mitosis [240]. These mutations cause karyotypic instability and the diverse tumor subpopulations simultaneous growth, leading to genomic intra- and inter-tumor heterogeneity [236].

Extensive CIN leads to genome disorders in several cancer styles undergoing complex and high genomic changes. High missegregation of chromosomes takes place in cancerous cells; 1 in 5 cell divisions in comparison to normal cells, which involve 1 in 100 cell divisions. The CIN mechanisms at the molecular level include repair and duplication defects in DNA as well as failure in spindle assembly, kinetochore-microtubule attachment, telomeres dysfunction, and sister chromatid interconnection [238]. In addition, CIN progresses early in tumors, is noticeable in premalignant lesions, is linked to inherent multiple drug resistance, and has a very unfortunate prognosis, thence creating its detection clinically relevant [241, 242].

Even though the fundamental and prominent significance of CIN to cancer biology, the mechanisms at the molecular level originating CIN in periodic cancers are still unclear. This is because the countless genes disturbance can lead to CIN, however not restricted to those implicated in segregation and chromosome condensation (STAG2) [243], DNA damage (ATM) [244], as well as telomeres dysfunction (TRF1 and Tankyrase) [245] and spindle checkpoint genes (BUB1, Mad2) [246], emphasizing the CIN heterogeneous nature in periodic cancers. In attempting to elucidate the CIN existence and molecular basis in periodic cancers have directed to three prevailing theories development: the oncogene-induced DNA damage model, the mutator hypothesis, and instability as a result of telomere erosion that is revised in [197, 216, 247].

Numerical chromosomal instability (nCIN) generates from the missegregation of whole chromosomes within anaphase, leading to the formation of two daughter cells with a karyotype distinguishing from the species natural karyotype, also known as aneuploidy. However, errors of segregation can also lead to structural chromosomal instability (sCIN), displaying structural variations of chromosomes. Even though both types of CIN originated from different mitotic [248, 249], as well as pre-mitotic alterations [250], they overwhelmingly co-exist and are interrelated [251, 252].

Even though, CIN has been identified as a hallmark of a common cancers, it is still unconvincing if CIN is a final stage or an early detection of cancer development. Accurate of chromosome segregation during mitosis is essential for maintenance the genomic integrity. Failure of accurate segregation of chromosomes unavoidably leads to cell death or malignant transformation. Equal segregation of chromosome in cell division process is controlled and protected by numerous closely related processes that until now particularly considered as diverse molecular machineries [195].

Maintenance of genomic integrity by caretaker genes and pathways implicated in the maintenance of genomic integrity.

Checkpoints of DNA Damage

Conventionally, malignancy is known as a set of diseases, which are characterized by gradual genetic anomalies that contain mutations in tumor-suppressor genes, oncogenes, and chromosomal aberrations. Even so, it has ended up obvious that cancer is also determined by epigenetic modifications [253]. Even though considerable amounts of epigenetic modifications are discovered in tumors, the epigenetic changes in DNA repair genes, causing diminished expression of DNA repair proteins, seem by all accounts to be especially important. Though considerable amounts of epigenetic alterations are revealed in tumorigenesis, the epigenetic modifications in DNA repair genes, producing reduced expression of

DNA repair proteins, appear by all accounts to be specifically significant. Moreover, diminished expression of DNA repair genes leads to deficient DNA repair. Furthermore, when DNA repair is inadequate, DNA damages remain within cells at a higher level than an ordinary one and these excess damages cause extended incidences of mutation. Additionally, lacking expression of DNA repair proteins due to an inherited mutation can expand the risk of cancer. Furthermore, an inherited debilitation in any of the 34 DNA repair genes can cause a prolonged risk of cancer. A few deformities bring up to a 100% lifetime risk of malignancy, such as p53 transformations [254].

The p53 tumor suppressor gene functions as a key component in a complicated network of signal transduction termed the p53 pathway, which is considered a key protection mechanism against tumor. The p53 signaling pathway identifies different forms of cellular oncogenic stress and transforms them into suitable cellular responses to diminish carcinogenic development. Cell survival is a response to stress by inhibiting the DNA damage and/or directly supporting DNA repair. Activated p53 stimulates programmed cell death (apoptosis) or senescence and finally prevents the potential malignancy transformation, when the damaged DNA is away from repair or too severe [195, 255].

One of the most common cellular serine/threonine kinase is the ataxia-telangiectasia mutated (ATM) protein which has an essential role in the modulation of cellular response to DNA damage [256]. ATM becomes activated by its phosphorylation at Ser-1981, in response to DNA damage. The stimulated ATM phosphorylates several molecules, including γH2AX, p53, and Chk2 [257]. ATM-mediated p53 phosphorylation on serine 15 play a crucial role in the stimulation of p53 pathway in response to DNA damage [255].

The expression of p19Arf as a response to oncogenic stress does not usually occur in normal tissues; however, it is expressed by elevated and sustained proliferation signals [258]. For instance, Myc and Ras signaling physiologic thresholds do not stimulate Arf gene expression; however, upregulation of Myc and oncogenic Ras lead to induction of Arf [259, 260]. Then, Induced Arf inhibits the Mdm2 activity that requires stabilizing p53 that, gives rise to cell cycle arrest or apoptosis. This process counteracts signaling of oncogenic proliferation by activating cell cycle arrest or apoptosis in cells, which may lead to tumors as an alternative mechanism.

Mitotic Checkpoints

Several surveillance mechanisms or checkpoints occur in eukaryotic cells to preserve chromosomal stability throughout cell division; these checkpoints control the success of important molecular and cellular processes of one stage before getting into the next one. The checkpoints in G1 and G2 prevent DNA repair of the cells; however, the spindle assembly checkpoint (SAC) is an advanced preserved surveillance mechanism, which drives the correct distribution of chromosomes to daughter cells. SAC holds cells within metaphase until the assembly and attachment of mitotic spindle are completed to the sister chromosomes through bi-orientation of the chromosome. This takes place prior to the nuclear division in the mitosis process. Several regulatory proteins involved in this process have been identified, including mitotic arrest-deficient members such as benzimidazole and components of the mitotic spindle checkpoint, which inhibit aneuploidy.

The ubiquitin ligase is inhabited by forming the mitotic checkpoint complex that targets *securin* and *cyclin B* for ubiquitination and degradation, leading to change from metaphase to anaphase and finally inhibiting chromosome segregation. Several MCC proteins have been recognized as characterized as requirements for checkpoint functions, such as *Bub1, Bub3, Mad1, Mad2, Mad3 (BubR1), MPS1/Mph1*, and *Cdc20* [261 - 263]. A number of further gene products comprising Aurora B, Shugoshin, PP2A, and Plk1 as well as play an essential role in the regulation of spindle checkpoint [264 - 266].

The *Mad2* protein acts together with *Mad1* to attach the kinetochore; then *Mad2* binds to *Mad3-Bub3-Cdc20,* resulting in conformational changes for MCC assembly. When chromosomes are correctly binding to the mitotic spindle, MCC no longer needs to block APC/C, and then the anaphase will start [267].

Telomere Maintenance

Human telomeres consist of hexanucleotides of TTAGGG tandem DNA copies with connected proteins. The chromosome fusion is protected by telomeres caps, which prevent the double-strand breaks and inhibit the recognition of chromosomes ends [268]. Telomeres within humans are kept in germ cells, and shortened in cell division of somatic cells that minimize cell proliferation. This is accomplished by telomerase down expression. It's no wonder to find that the highly proliferative tumor cells can effectively preserve the length of their telomeres, mostly by the telomerase expression; while only some human cancer (10%) as an alternative mechanism hold telomeres [269]. Nevertheless, simultaneously tumor cells with high levels of telomerase display a high rate of telomere loss. A critical feature occurs in tumor cells with low frequency through the spontaneous loss of telomere. Therefore, the cancer cells acquire fundamentally infinite proliferative capacity. Loss of telomere participates in chromosome instability as well as cancer cell progression [270, 271]. One of the essential mechanisms of chromosome instability is the excessive shortening of telomeres before the telomerase expression, which can trigger chromosome fusion [272].

The absence of mice RNA component of telomerase (mTERC) exhibits progressive shortening of telomere as well as eventually chromosomal instability (end-to-end fusions) due to ageing and successive generational mating [273]. Telomere shortening within ageing mTERC−/− mice is related to the increase in cancer occurrence, proposing that the genetic integrity loss related to telomere dysfunction can expedite transformation *in vivo* [274]. Furthermore, in cultured human cells, telomerase high-level expression expedites malignant transformation [195, 275].

DNA Repair Pathways

DNA replication in normal cells is achieved with extreme fidelity (alteration rate of 10^{-10}/base pair/cell-division). Damage of cellular DNA characteristically happens over the three processes: (1) exposing to agents: like genotoxic chemicals, ionizing radiation, and ultraviolet irradiation; (2) spontaneous events of DNA damage like forming a basic site; and (3) events of cellular DNA treating and replication failure like stalling of replication forks. These lead to enhancement, alkylation, cross-linking, oxidation, dimerization, and strand breaks in DNA that should be repaired.

Damage to DNA could predispose individuals to raised tumorigenesis when left without correction. Therefore, a system responds to such errors by engaging DNA repair or induction of apoptosis. Repairing DNA damage is essential to maintain genome stability and prevent cancerogenesis.

The excision repair system is multiple evolutionarily conserved pathways that involve three excision repair pathways, which are able to repair a single strand of DNA damage: (NER); nucleotide-excision repair, (BER); base-excision repair, and (MMR); DNA-mismatch repair [276].

Nucleotide-Excision Repair (NER)

Nucleotide-excision repair (NER) is a predominant DNA repair process that removes large DNA lesions created by UV radiation, oxidizing and alkylating agents or chemotherapy drugs, which shape huge, helix-deforming adducts. NER works over numerous steps involving damage site recognition, the damaged DNA-strand incision, the synthesis of DNA, and lastly, the ligation of uncoupled edges by particular ligase enzymes [277]. Three different NER mechanisms; differentiation-associated repair (DAR), transcription-coupled repair (TCR), and global genomic repair (GGR), have been recognized [278]. TCR is exclusively involved in lesion removal, which blocks the transcription of constitutively expressed genes. Whereas GGR works by restoring nearly all impaired sites within the whole DNA genome irrespective of the status of active transcription of genes [279 - 281].

All components of the NER mechanisms are essential in completing the fruitful repair of the damaged sites. There is an association between several human diseases and functional genetic impairments within the genes of NER-related proteins; these diseases, such as Cockayne's syndrome, Trichothiodystrophy, xeroderma pigmentosum that can lead to severe skin cancer, and many cancers [282, 283].

Base-Excision Repair (BER)

The BER system repairs damaged bases DNA, produced *via* deamination, methylation, and oxidation [284, 285]. These damages are detected and eliminated by glycosidase enzymes that cut out the glycosidic bond between the impaired nucleotide base and the sugar molecules on the DNA backbone, and create an apurinic/apyrimidinic (AP) site. For short-patch BER, AP endonuclease (APE1) detects the AP lesion and BER enzymes set (DNA polymerase β (Pol β), DNA ligase III (Lig III), and X-ray repair cross-complementing 1 (XRCC1)) repair this lesion. For long-patch BER, APE1 recognizes single-strand breaks (SSBs) that are usually fixed by DNA Polδ/ε-dependent recruitment of BER-associated proteins [284]. However, in extra complex damages, proliferating cell nuclear antigen (PCNA), flap endonuclease 1 (FEN1), and Pol β, with/without POL δ/ε, act to repair the lesion. BER events are assisted by poly ADP-ribose polymerase 1 (PARP1) that recruits proteins that participate in the response of DNA repair, like DNA ligase, DNA polymerase, and X-ray repair cross-complementing protein 1 (XRCC1) [286].

Since cells are continuously exposed to harmful environments of DNA damage, the BER pathway is essential to preserve genome stability, as observed in mice embryonic lethality, which deactivates key molecules of this pathway [287]. The somatic mutation in the adenomatous polyposis coli gene in certain families results in an increased incidence of colorectal tumors within these families because of a defect of biallelic germline in a DNA glycosylase (mutY Homology (MUTYH)) [213]. This type of mutation increases colon cancer risk by 93- folds in old age (60 years) [288]. In addition, it may confer raised risk for endometrial cancer [289]. Other glycosylase mutations, 8 Oxoguanine (OGG1), have been related to laryngeal cancer patients [290], whereas the inactivation of glycosylase endonuclease VIII-like 1 (NEIL1) is related to gastric cancer [291]. Finally, all these studies affirm the BER importance in the suppression of tumorigenesis.

DNA-Mismatch Repair (MMR)

Many findings propose that the activity of DNA-mismatch repair (MMR) mechanisms and replicative DNA polymerase proofreading act within series in mammalian cells [292, 293]. MMR system particularly removes the base mismatches created either by endogenous or exogenous agents, which lead to changes in the chemical nature of nucleotide bases by oxidation, deamination, or methylation. Mostly, MMR targets base mismatches and large deletion-insertion loops [276]. MMR systems consist of several steps; the DNA lesion recognition, discrimination of strand, excision, and repair. MutS and MutL proteins contribute to identifying the base mismatches. In addition, the homologues of MutS, *e.g.,* MSH1–6, MLH1 and MLH3 and homologues of MutL *e.g.,* PMS1 and PMS2 are described to be accountable for distinguishing the sites of mismatched base. The heterotetrametric complex generated by the interaction of MutS and MutL recognizes the mismatched bases [294]. Subsequently, exonuclease I enzyme (EXO1) removes the base pair mismatches, and then polymerase δ/ε enzyme (POLδ/ε) resynthesizes the missing base, then ligation takes place by ligase [295, 296].

Double-Strand Repair (DSR) & Cancer-Predisposition

Double strand break (DSB) is the greatest fatal type of DNA impairment, as it can cause substantial damage to DNA by numerous genomic alterations, including deletions, amplifications, and translocation formation, leading to heritable cellular genomic damage/ instability, which can cause malignancy [297, 298]. DSBs are fixed by non-homologues end joining (NHEJ) and homolog repair (HR) pathways.

NHEJ pathway is an important DNA repair, which directly glues damaged DSB ends of DNA. Therefore, NHEJ ligates the ends of damaged DNA without detecting the sequence homology of DNA, so it is highly error-prone. However, the repair of HR depends upon the DNA sequence homology; so, it is moderately free of error [298, 299]. NHEJ is not limited to a particular phase of the cell cycle, whereas HR prevails within the S and G2 phases of the cell cycle [298, 300].

NHEJ pathway began with the Ku heterodimer, which is comprised of two subunits; KU70 and KU80, which identifies and links to DSBs trimmings [301].

The catalytic polypeptide, known as DNA-PKcs is directly recruited by the KU heterodimer, and directed towards the DNA ends to produce an active DNA-PK complex [302].

HR repair has multiple-gene products, some of that are recruited in the repair of stalled replication forks [299]. MRN complex (NBS, RAD50 and MRE11, known as Nibrin) started HR of damaged DNA ends and eliminated the damaged base in direction 5′ to 3′ end. Endonucleases or exonucleases (EXO1and retinoblastoma binding protein 8 (RBBP8) create the two short strands of ssDNA at DSBs, leading to ssDNA overhangs, which are covered by RPA to avert the formation of DNA secondary structure. Then, RAD52 substitutes RPA with RAD51in ssDNA, forming a "synaptic complex", the recombination mediator. Eventually, the synaptic complex allows homologues ssDNA to attach and anneal to matching DNA strand. ssDNA gap is then filled by DNA polymerase and the synaptic complex is committed and created crossover and non-crossover products [297, 300]. The Repair process that-associated with DNA biosynthesis is ended by numerous networks of DSB repair, including the creation of a double-Holliday junction (dHJ) [303, 304].

BRCA1 and *BRCA2* are important molecules within the HR repair mechanisms, as well as, acting as tumor suppressors by preserving genome integrity. Early onset breast cancer was observed in families that have *BRCA1* susceptibility genes [305]. Consequently, early-onset breast and ovary cancer have been reported to be associated with *BRCA1* mutation [306]. In addition, a new locus (encoding *BRCA2)* has been detected and related to breast cancer susceptibility [307]. Furthermore, in one meta-analysis, accumulative risks for *BRCA1* mutation carriers to the development of ovarian (40%) and breast cancer (57%) have been reported [308]. Moreover, hereditary mutations of *BRCA* have also been linked to prostate, colon, and pancreatic cancers [309].

Fanconi anemia (FA) is an autosomal recessive disorder that cause congenital deficiencies, bone marrow failure, and cancer predisposition (ovarian, breast, and oral cancers) [310]. FA/BRCA pathway involved the FA genes (15 genes) and coordinated to complete the DNA repair process. Excitingly, two of these genes *BRCA2* (*FANCD1*) and *PALB2* (*FANCN*), play a modulatory role in FA and HR [311]. Significantly, there are differences between BRCA-associated cancers, and FA-associated cancers that FA defects lead to develop of hypersensitive to cross-linking agents (*e.g.,* cisplatin and mitomycin C, and radiation) [312]. Lastly, biallelic damage of ataxia telangiectasia mutated (ATM) leads to ataxia telangiectasia disorder which increases the incidence of lymphoma (roughly 1000-folds) [313].

Conclusion Remarks

GIN shows an essential role in cancer origination and progression. The genome fidelity is safeguarded at each phase of the cell-division cycle. GIN involves small structure differences like increased base pair alteration frequencies, resulting from defects in pathways of (BER and NER), MSI, and CIN. As well as, it is recognized that genomic stability is thoroughly monitored by numerous observation mechanisms, checkpoint of DNA damage, mitotic checkpoint, telomere maintenance, and machinery of DNA repair. The regulation defect of any of these mechanisms frequently leads to the loss of genomic stability that predisposes the cell to malignancies.

TUMOR-PROMOTING INFLAMMATION

INTRODUCTION

A small number of tumors have been noticed to be thickly filled by cells of both arms of the innate and adaptive immune system and accordingly reflect cases of inflammatory responses developing in non-neoplastic tissues [314]. It is presently clear that principally each neoplastic lesion grips immune cells existing at densities ranging from small infiltrations discernable merely with cell type-specific antibodies to gross inflammatory responses, which are obvious even by procedures of standard histochemical staining [315].

Inflammation is an ancient advanced process that includes stimulation, recruitment, and action of innate and adaptive immune cells. It is a biological protective response of immune system within a vascular organism that can be triggered by a variety of internal and external harmful stimuli, including infection by pathogens; viruses, bacteria, parasites, and fungi, injured ischemic tissues; initiated by an insufficient blood supply to an organ, exposure to toxic compounds, and other types of trauma. These stimuli may motivate acute and/or chronic inflammatory responses to invade these factors, remove damaged cells, and ultimately maintain tissue homeostasis [316, 317].

Acute inflammatory response aims to overhaul damaged cells and eradicate or neutralize undesirable elements. It's ideal outcome thorough and well-timed resolve through back-to-tissue stability that is dynamically programmed using specific pro-resolving anti-inflammatory intermediaries, comprising lipoxins (LXs), protectins (PDs), resolvins (Rvs), and maresins (MaRs) [317, 318]. SPMs effectively prevent neutrophil infiltration as well as stimulate macrophage efferocytosis of apoptotic neutrophils within the inflammatory loci [319, 320]. On the other hand, when the inflammation-causing agent within the body persists for a long time of period, the response to it develops into a prolonged inflammatory response, 'chronic inflammation' that is described as either non- or delayed-resolving and may cause disease. The signs and symptoms of the chronic inflammatory response are not considered as severe as those of acute inflammatory response; however, chronic or persistent inflammatory response is classically quite dangerous as it can mediate more damages, such as organ dysfunction, necrosis, fibrosis, and gene mutation; as well as, a huge proportion of refractory diseases, like Alzheimer's disease (AD) [321], cardiovascular diseases, diabetes, arthritis [322], and cancer [320, 323].

In the 19th century, the leukocytes presence in neoplastic tissues was observed for the first time by Dr. Virchow. He proposed the first indication of a potential association between inflammatory response and cancer [66]. Virchow's hypothesis "lympho-reticular infiltrate" reflected the cancer origin at locations of chronic inflammation within several cancer patients as *Helicobacter pylori*, hepatitis pancreatitis, colitis, cholangitis esophagitis, and other chronic inflammatory diseases that are established risk factors for tumor in these tissues [324 - 327]. Through the past decade, the understanding of the inflammatory microenvironment of malignant tumor has supported the hypothesis of Virchow; as well as, the connections between tumor and inflammation have started to have prevention and therapeutic implications [328].

Cancer is considered a key reason for deaths worldwide; as well as, through an ageing population, 8 million cancer is annually reported, which is anticipated to rise [329]. In this regard, carcinogenesis can be broadly split into two groups: non-metastasis and metastasis which is the primary cause of cancer-associated deaths [330]. Conventionally, metastatic cancer has been considered to take place in the later stages of tumor development; on the other hand, collecting evidence has also characterized metastasis dissemination through early tumor progression [331, 332]. In metastatic cancer, disseminating cancer cells get away from the origin site of tumors and obtain cellular features, which let them travel as well as colonize distant tissues and organs [333, 334].

During "tumor-promoting inflammation", which is referred to cancer initiation, promotion, and progression, the immune system shows a different role. Tumor-related inflammation exists through various carcinogenesis stages; it participates in epigenetic modification, genomic mutation, tumor anti-apoptotic pathway enhancement, stimulation of tumor cell proliferation, induction of angiogenesis, and, eventually, cancer dissemination [335]. During the past few decades, several studies have established that immune cells of inflammation function as important actors in cancer-associated inflammation [332].

The current review focuses on the cancer-promoting role of the immune system and inflammation. We reviewed diverse types of inflammation and general mechanisms. Then, we explained how tumor cells corrupt the immune system using tumor immunoediting, a dynamic process for tumor initiation and progression, and how inflammation stimulates tumor. Finally, we described the mediation of inflammatory mediators in genetic instability as paving the way for tumorigenesis.

"Normal" Inflammation & Inflammatory Response in Tumor and General Mechanisms

An inflammatory response is a protective mechanism started in responding to damaged tissues triggered by exposure to infectious agents, chemicals, or concurrent trauma [316, 336]. At an early stage of inflammation, neutrophils are the first responders, infiltrating toward mediators of inflammation produced at the inflammatory loci [337]. As the inflammatory process proceeds, numerous other inflammatory players like macrophages and lymphocytes are induced and employed to the location of the inflammation. Infiltration of immune mediators is assisted by the high expression levels of growth factors, chemokines, and cytokines. These cells aim to enhance the defense process of the body; as well as, to neutralize the offending agents [338, 339].

On the other hand, when the acute inflammation is not resolved within the body, this results in a persistent and chronic inflammatory response [340]. Today, clear evidence has been achieved that chronic and persistent inflammatory response is a critical hallmark of carcinogenesis, with up to 25% of cancers linked to it [337, 341, 342]; as well as, potential underlying sources, including microbial infections, immune deregulation, and autoimmunity. For instance, persistent infection with *Helicobacter pylori* (*H. pylori*) is closely related to gastric adenocarcinoma and MALT lymphoma [343], hepatocellular carcinoma (HCC) triggered by chronic hepatitis B and C virus infection [344], infection with human papillomavirus (HPV) increases the incidence of cervical cancer [345], Epstein–Barr virus infection is thoroughly linked to nasopharyngeal carcinoma [346], and infections with *Bacteroides* or *Schistosoma* species are highly associated with colon and bladder cancer, respectively [347]. The inflammation activated by infection leads to tumor progression; it is also a part of natural host protection, which aims to remove pathogens. On the other hand, carcinogenic pathetical agents disrupt host immune response and create stubborn infections related to low grade but persistent inflammatory response.

Whereas persistent inflammation plays a crucial protagonist in cancerogenesis, fewer is obvious about the acute inflammatory response influence on tumor development. For instance, triggering acute inflammation of the urinary bladder with a vaccine having a weakened strain of *Mycobacterium bovis* effectively cures squamous cell carcinoma of the urinary bladder [348 - 350]. Therefore, with the leukocyte infiltration and consequent inflammation, the influence of inflammatory mediators can sometimes recruit and eradicate cancer cells and avoid tumor progression [351]. In addition, this twin role of inflammation becomes clinically more obvious, where diagnosed HIV patients are more frequently diagnosed with tumor [352]. Excitingly, long-lasting usage of NSAIDs, suppressing the immune system, is associated with a decrease in tumor risk [353]. Although tumor carcinoma is stimulated by chronic inflammation, what makes it exclusively sensitive to acute inflammatory response is currently not clear. This is an essential issue, and its resolution ought to disclose how to effectively deploy inflammation in the treatment of cancers [336, 344]. An additional type of chronic inflammatory response that leads to tumor progression is triggered by the deregulation of the immune system and autoimmunity. Ulcerative colitis and Crohn's disease, also recognized as inflammatory bowel disease (IBD), are greatly related to the high jeopardy of colon cancer [354, 355].

Nevertheless, not all chronic inflammations increase tumor risk; some of them, like psoriasis, may even decline the tumor risk [340]. It is unclear what makes IBD or chronic hepatitis cancer stimulating, in contrast to conditions like psoriasis or rheumatoid arthritis that do not considerably promote carcinogenesis. One possible cause could be associated with the liver and gastrointestinal tract exposure to environmental and dietary carcinogens, which do not make their way into the skin or joints. In addition, chronic or persistent inflammation is triggered by exposure to environmental agents [344]. Tobacco smoke and other irritants are able to participate in chronic obstructive pulmonary disease (COPD), a condition related to the increase in the incidence of lung cancer risk [356]. Inhalation of airborne pollutants, such as asbestos or silica particles, increases the incidence of lung cancer, but no obvious mutagenic activity occurs. However, these particles can initiate inflammation by affecting the processing of leukocytic endogenous mediators [357] and this could facilitate their carcinogenic performance. Even chronic inflammation related to obesity increases tumor risk by 1.6 times [358, 359], which promotes hepatocellular carcinoma progression [360]. Adding fuel to the fire, Persistent DNA damage, and age-associated cellular senescence can also induce tumor-promoting chronic inflammation by triggering several inflammatory programs [361, 362].

Most solid tumors activate intrinsic inflammation, promoting pro-tumorigenic microenvironments [316, 344, 363]. Additional to cell-autonomous proliferation, certain oncogenes, like MYC and RAS family members, trigger a transcriptional program, leading to the tumor microenvironment remodeling through lymphocytes and leukocytes recruitment, tumor-promoting chemokines and cytokines expression, and angiogenic induction [364, 365]. At some point, all solid malignancies outstrip their supplied blood and come to be under nutrient and oxygen deprivation. This leads to necrotic death of cancer cells, and pro-inflammatory mediators release IL-1 family and High Mobility Group-box1 (HMGB1) superfamily [366]. The resultant inflammation stimulates neo-angiogenesis and supplies survived cancerous cells with further growth factors, created through the recent recruitment of immune and inflammatory cells [66].

Lung cancer, and other tumor promotes inflammatory response out of vigorous secretion of molecules, like the extra-cellular matrix component (EMC) versican, which triggers macrophages over Toll-like receptor-2 (TLR-2) [367]. According to the endless cell regeneration and propagation prompted by tumor-related inflammatory response, tumors are described as "chronic wounds that don't heal" [368, 369]. This inflammation type is mostly a disrupted wound healing as well as regenerative tissue response.

Last but not least, cancer treatment can originate a strong cancer-associated inflammation. In fact, chemotherapy and radiation treatment lead to enormous necrosis of tumor cells as well as adjacent tissues, which consecutively activate inflammatory reactions similar to a response of healing the wounds [370, 371]. In addition, the therapy-stimulated inflammation outcome is debatable because; although, it has cancer-promoting functions exactly similar to necrosis, which causes rapid growth of tumor [344, 372], it can also increase the production of cancer antigens and consequently initiate an anti-cancer immune response [355, 373].

Inflammation & Tumor Initiation and Progression

The inflammatory response can take part in various properties of tumors by affording bioactive molecules to the tumor microenvironment (TME), integrating pro-angiogenic growth factors and extracellular matrix (ECM)-modifying enzymes, which promote angiogenesis, metastasis, and invasion; growth factors, which progress proliferative signaling; survival factors, which limit cell death; and inductive signals, which prompt stimulation of EMT and other hallmark accelerating programs [374].

A marginal number of cancers are produced by germline alterations; however, most malignant tumors (95%) have been associated to somatic mutations in genes encoding proteins controlling progression of cell cycle and/or death [375, 376]. Etiologic insight into numerous of these alterations has been provided by previous epidemiological studies, consequently revealing that 35% of human malignancies are linked to dietary factors, 30% to tobacco use and inhaled pollutants, 18% to infectious agents, 14-20% to obesity, and 7% to environmental and radiation pollutants [377]. Besides "initiating" the cancerous cell formation, these factors may likewise act as cancer promoters by activating acute stimulation of immune effector programs resulting in infiltration of "initiated" tissue by cells of the immune system [378]. When these cells persist for long periods without resolution, these assaults of tissue become chronic then, by several mechanisms, provide the underpinnings for cancer progression [379, 380].

Several questions ascend as to which immune cell subsets directly or indirectly stimulate malignant tumors, which of these subsets can be reprogrammed centered on their functional plasticity to instead fight tumor, and to what degree these possessions are generic or tissue-specific. Even though the majority of adult solid tumors comprise infiltrates of different subsets of leukocytes and other phagocytic cells, data from Flow cytometric (FACS analysis) of solid tumors within different genetic abnormalities; *e.g.,* lung, mesothelioma, and breast display that complexity of leukocytes diverges according to the location of organ or tissue as well as malignant stage, proposing that immune-based treatments will require to reflect these small differences and be more tailored [381, 382].

Tumor cells capture inflammatory mechanisms to support their own evolution and survival. By the innate and adaptive immune system 'through a typical inflammatory/immune response', immune cells perform their particular job of devastating or sweeping over any foreign intruders. In the heterogeneous microenvironment of the cancerous cells, these cells corrupt the fighting cycle of the immune system. Consequently, rather than devastating the altered cells, the antitumor cells are disrupted into cancer-promoting cells of the immune system, which secrete pro-migration, pro-survival, and anti-recognition factors that permit the tumor to progress, invade and metastasize [335]. Significant biomolecules and signaling pathways mediators that facilitate this immune response to the microenvironment of cancer comprise NF-κB, inflammatory signaling biomarkers, tumor-infiltration biomarkers of the immune cell and the checkpoints of the immune system [383].

Within cancer biology, cells and biomolecules that form the essential components of the complex tumor microenvironment play a central role in tumor initiation, progression, and resistance to therapeutic approaches. Through the process known as immunoediting, tumor initiation and progression are marvelously altered in their immunogenicity as a result of the anti-tumor response of the immune system. The Immunoediting concept of tumor broadly consists of 3 sequential phases: elimination, equilibrium, and escape phase [384 - 386]. The tumor elimination stage, also identified as immunosurveillance, comprises the response of innate and adaptive immunity to tumor cells. Elimination of tumor cells is achieved by effective immunogenicity within the immune system prior to they being clinically detectable. Through innate immunity, numerous cellular effectors, including natural killer (NK) cells and T-cells, are stimulated by cytokines produced by cancerous cells, macrophages, and mesenchymal stem cells (MSCs) neighboring tumor cells. Enrolled NK cells and macrophages produce interleukin 12 (IL-12) and interferon-gamma (IFN-γ), which get rid of tumor cells by stimulating the response of cytotoxic factors, like ROS, interferon alpha (TNF-α), and perforin [384, 387]. Antigen-presenting cells (APCs) like macrophages, dendritic cells (DCs), and B-cells adopt and display tumor-specific antigens to cytotoxic T-lymphocytes and trigger T-cells through costimulatory biomolecules [388, 389]. Hence, in comparison with pro-tumor IM, anti-tumor inflammatory mediators (IM) mainly contribute through this phase. Tumor cells escape the elimination phase and progress into the equilibrium stage, the next step in tumor immunoediting when anti- and pro-tumor IM are balanced. During this stage, tumor cell variants that escaped the immune recognition breach the defense of the immune system of the host organism, and several genetic alterations are produced that further increase overall resistance to immune attack [384]; however, they have a nonimmunogenic phenotype that is designated for growing, such as loss expression of major histocompatibility complex (MHC) components and antigenic tumor peptides (ATPs) [390]. Remarkably, this stage is the longest of the three stages may last over a period of many years until other variants of immune resistance appear that are expected to run away from immune surveillance [387, 391]. During this situation, the balanced IM is twisted in the direction of the pro-tumor IM production as the immune system loses the ability to limit tumor outgrowth and expansion, which may lead to malignancies. Ultimately, the immune-resistant variants lead to the formation of clinically detectable solid tumors [387, 392, 393]. There are numerous mechanisms, which help tumor cells to escape the immune system, for instance, loss or down-regulation of expression of classical MHC class-I that is important for functional T-cell mediated-immune response [394], improvement of tumor microenvironments that repress innate and adaptive immune systems and functions as a defensive line of tumor cells [138, 390]. In addition, cells involved in tumor microenvironments can create several cytokines that lead to apoptosis of stimulated T-cells [395, 396]. The further cellular machinery of cancer to evade the immune system is the up-regulation of non-classical MHC-I that inhibits the immune response mediated by NK cells [397]. Consequently, it is worth saying that during the escape stage, tumor escape from immune system control. Indeed, during this phase, pro-tumor immune cells, comprising of tumor-associated dendritic cells (TADCs), myeloid-derived suppressor cells (MDSCs), Th17, tumor-associated macrophages (TAMs), and regulatory T (Tregs) lymphocyte, together with cancerous tissues as well as stem cells (CSCs) trigger the immunosuppressive effect through cytokines and biomolecules secretion. Moreover, T-lymphocytes overexpress inhibitory receptors, acting as immune checkpoints that are stimulated by expression of ligands on pro-tumor immune cells [398 - 400]. Totally, these immunosuppressive mechanisms collaboratively counteract antitumor immune effect, as well as, speed up tumor progression.

The classical mechanisms thru which inflammation stimulates tumors include (1) genetic alterations: DNA damage/ mutation, loss of genomic integrity, epigenetic dys-regulation of gene expression, and loss of DNA repair [401, 402]. Mutated DNA sequentially motivates inflammatory response, creating a malicious circle, which cooperatively initiates oncogenesis [402]; (2) angiogenesis: it is critical for the invasion and growth of sarcomas, carcinomas, and lymphomas [335]. Pro-inflammatory cytokines, like TNF-α and IL-1 trigger the signaling of chemokine receptor-4 and chemokine ligand 12 (CXCR4/CXCL12) that up-regulates expression of vascular permeability factor (VPF) through the phosphatidylinositol 3-kinase (PI3K)/protein kinase B pathway. Besides chemokine and cytokine proteins,prostaglandin-endoperoxide synthase (PTGS2) and part of its metabolic products are also involved in vascular synthesis [403, 404]; (3) metastases and invasion: inflammatory response similarly participates to hypoxic processes that further stimulates glycolytic pathway, invasion, and angiogenesis [320, 404]. Moreover, cytokine-mediated inflammation produced by immunosuppressive cells contributes to cancer progress. For instance, suppressor cells derived from bone stimulate epithelial-mesenchymal transition (EMT) by triggering epidermal growth factor (EGF), hepatocyte growth factor (HGF), and transforming growth factor β (TGF-β) pathways and change ant-inflammatory (M2) macrophages into pro-inflammatory (M1) macrophages; tumor-associated macrophages (TAMs) [405, 406]. TAMs lack tumoricidal action and subsidize immune suppression over the up-regulation of several inflammatory mediators, such as TGF-β, IL-10, and CC motif chemokine ligand 22 (CCL22) that trigger Treg recruitment and T-cell anergy [407].

Involvement of Inflammatory Mediators in Genetic Mutations; Paving the Way for Carcinogenesis

Several epidemiological studies have stated that chronic inflammation and infections contribute to about 25% of all human cancer cases, including various cancer types such as bladder, hepatocellular, and prostate cancer are associated with [408, 409]. In the period of inflammation, the generation of reactive nitrogen oxygen species (RNOS) is linked to the increase of immune cells such as eosinophils, neutrophils, and macrophages. These RNOS, such as nitric oxide (·NO), peroxynitrite (ONOO−), superoxide ($\bullet O^-_2$), hydroxyl radical (·OH), hydrogen per-oxide (H_2O_2), and hydrochlorous acid (HOCl·) eliminate the pathological and biological insults [410]. However, the predominant macrophages and other white blood cells in inflammatory immune tissues, as a result of the persistent presence of injurious stimuli, lead to continuous expression of RNOS to cope with the microbial invasion [336]. These RNOS tends to be linked to the genomic DNA, causing frameshift mutation or point mutation. In addition, RNOS interacts with lipids causing lipid peroxidation and damage of cell membranes, interacting with proteins causing protein denaturation or loss of protein functions, and interacting with DNA nucleotide bases. All these events lead to chronic inflammation and malignancy development [339, 411]. In gastric and esophageal carcinoma, for example, chronic inflammations are responsible about the DNA damage and development of cancer [412]. Therefore, in respect of the above-mentioned context, it is proposed that excessive DNA damage is associated with increases in the generation of RNOS in a microenvironment of chronic inflammation [339]. Moreover, increasing cellular proliferation, angiogenesis, and genomic instability are the triggers of chronic inflammation to develop cancer (Fig. **4.5**) [413].

Chronic IBD patients, including ulcerative colitis and Crohn's disease, have displayed increased tumor progression, and it has been reported that the opportunity of CRC development increased from 2% to 8% and to 18% after 10, 20, and 30 years of diagnosis with IBD, respectively [414]. An environment of chronic inflammation can drive cancer progression, since such an environmental hostility is related to increased secretion of growth factors by inflammation, and such proliferating cells are more predisposed to acquire genetic alteration and DNA damage, with subsequent tumorigenesis development of cells [415]. Furthermore, migration inhibitory factors and tumor necrosis factor-α (TNF-α) synthesized by inflammatory immune cells aggravate DNA damage [336, 339].

Tumor progression is a multifactorial described as uncontrolled proliferation and cell growth, escape from the immune system and inhibition of apoptosis, unresponsiveness to the anti-growth signals effect, increased angiogenesis, and the ability to metastasize from the primary site to distinct organ sites [336]. Similarly, the immune cells and cytokines impact different metastasis stages, especially the epithelial-mesenchymal transition stage, that affected by numerous cytokines and transcription factors, including TNF-α, IL-1β, IL-6, and transforming growth factor-β (TGF-β), NF-κB and signal transducer and activator of transcription 3 transcriptions (STAT3). Correspondingly, these inflammatory mediators increase the production and activity of a number of protease enzymes, which support the destruction of tissue and extracellular matrix (ECM) and cancer invasion. Chemokines and TNF-α enhance vascular permeability and stimulate the migration and extravasation of tumor cells (Fig. **4.5**) [416].

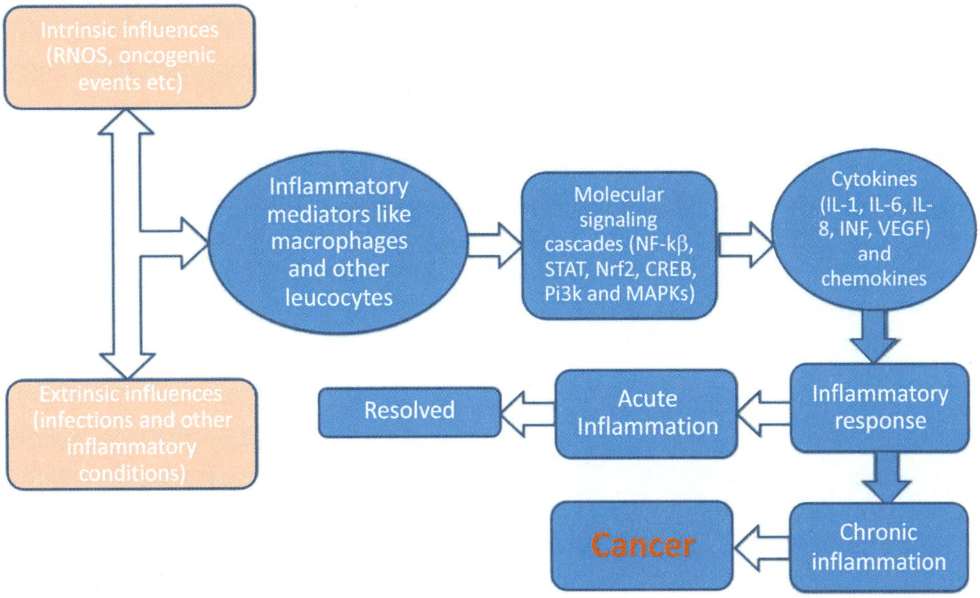

Fig. (4.5). Effect of intrinsic and extrinsic factors on tumor progression.
Abbreviations:NF-kβ, Inhibition of nuclear factor kappa beta; **STST**, signal transducer and activator of transcription; **Nrf2**, nuclear factor erythroid 2-related factor 2; CREB, cyclic AMP response element binding protein; **Pi3K**, phosphoinositide-3-kinase; **MPKs**, mitogen-activated protein kinases; **IL-1**, **IL-6**, **IL-8**; interleukin-1, 6, 8; INF, interferon; VEGF, vascular endothelial growth factor.

The pathway of Ras-Raf signaling has been shown to cooperate with a chronic inflammatory response to support cellular transformation. Both chronic pancreatitis and mutated K-ras 'through a murine model' are required to prompt pancreatic intra-epithelial neoplasia and invasive ductal carcinoma. Whereas different Ras-Raf signaling can lead to tumor-promoting inflammatory response to a large degree, an extrinsic condition of inflammation, such as pancreatitis, is required to cause oncogenesis [417].

A key organizer of innate immune response and inflammation is NFκB signaling pathway. It assumes vigorous roles in a precancerous chronic inflammatory response and tumor-stimulated inflammation. Frequent activation by cancer gene alteration, NFκB is a significant regulator of tumor initiation and progression. Origination of this pathway triggers cytokines expression of inflammation, enzymes, and adhesion molecules in the prostaglandin-synthesis pathway, like COX2, inducible nitric oxide synthase (iNOS) angiogenic factors and genes of anti-apoptosis, like Bcl-2 [418].

Stimulation of Myc oncogene has been associated with the remodeling of the extracellular microenvironment, a procedure requiring chemokines, cytokines, and enrolled mast cells. The current procedure stimulates tumor angiogenesis and metastasis [419]. Tumor suppressor genes, such as PTEN, p53, p16 and VHL, have similarly been connected in the initiation of inflammatory mediators, which might help tumor progression [420].

Similar to NFκB, the STAT3, as well as TGFβ signaling pathways, are involved in numerous carcinogenic signaling pathways [421]. These transcription factors are constitutively triggered in cancerous cells and are involved in carcinogenesis and prevention of the apoptotic pathway. The stimulation of STAT3 in cancer cells has correspondingly been entangled in immune evasion over suppression of dendritic cell maturation and the consequent immunity.

Different intrinsic and extrinsic factors activate the inflammatory/immune cell recruitment to the location of the inflammatory offense, with the resultant stimulation of numerous molecular signaling cascades. These signaling cascades are linked to the augmented creation of inflammatory cytokines and chemokines, and, therefore establishment of inflammation. This inflammation is either of acute nature that can be resolved or is of chronic nature that leads to cancer initiation.

CONCLUSION

Chronic inflammation predisposes the growth of the tumor and stimulates all stages of tumorigenesis. Tumor initiation progression is thoroughly associated with prolonged inflammation. The immune system shows a significant, albeit changeable, role during carcinogenesis. On the one hand and on the other hand, it fights cancer, and conversely, it facilitates tumor growth and metastasis through typical mechanisms such as genetic alterations, angiogenesis, and metastasis and invasion. As well as, the twin immune system action in malignancies has exposed the modern concept of tumor immunoediting that comprises three Es sequential phases of elimination, equilibrium, and escape. Tumor immunoediting is a dynamic process wherein the immune system is not just defending against tumor growth, it supports outgrowth of tumor capable of evading immune system control.

REPROGRAMMING ENERGY METABOLISM

INTRODUCTION

Reprogramming energy metabolism or metabolic alteration is the 9th hallmark of cancer that involves uncontrolled growth and division [422]. Metabolism is cellular life's fundamental architecture. Normally, either directly or indirectly, each cell in the body undergoes metabolic reactions. It is a summation of natural biochemical reactions that harvest energy for life-supporting processes and biological large molecule biosyntheses, such as carbohydrates, lipids, proteins, and nucleic acids. Overgrowth of cancer cells requires a replication of the whole of their cellular components; their sugars, proteins, lipids, DNA and RNA must all be duplicated to distribute into daughter cells, with a view to meet the rapidly dividing cells. Undoubtedly, this process needs energy. Cancer cells should modify their metabolism accordingly to allow this frenzied growth [423].

Naturally, mitochondria are considered the powerhouses or power generators of cells. They play a vital role in energy metabolism, both by their direct influence and their important role in signal transduction pathways. They are hearts for reprogramming and alterations of metabolism. Moreover, mitochondria are the producers of adenosine triphosphate (ATP) and play fundamental roles in oxidation/reduction hemostasis, cell signaling, Ca regulation, cellular death, and various intermediates synthesis, which are essential for macromolecule synthesis [424, 425].

The complex association between metabolic reactions and carcinogenesis is an encouraging part of carcinoma research. Therefore, aggregate consideration has been provided to the metabolism role within mitochondria in cancer cell biology. Growing indication has confirmed that targeting the metabolism of mitochondria within cancerous cells can be existent as a new strategy for cancer treatment [426 - 428].

To sum up the existing knowledge, there is an intercrossing association between the biology of mitochondria and tumorigenesis through various levels as follows: i) tumorigenesis is promoted by mitochondria direct signals; ii) functions of mitochondria can be changed by signaling pathways mediated by oncogenes; iii) functional perturbations of mitochondria have been exhibited as a key role in controlling bioenergetics and metabolic reactions; iv) alterations of DNA, proteins, and enzymes within mitochondria lead to changed levels of metabolites that support tumor progression and development [429, 430]. Metabolic alterations and/or metabolic pathways dysregulation characterize tumor cells [431]. This review highlights the significance of numerous classical changes in the metabolism of cancer cells. Therefore, biological cancer will be superior understood as well as new anti-cancer treatments will be established by realizing this metabolic aspect.

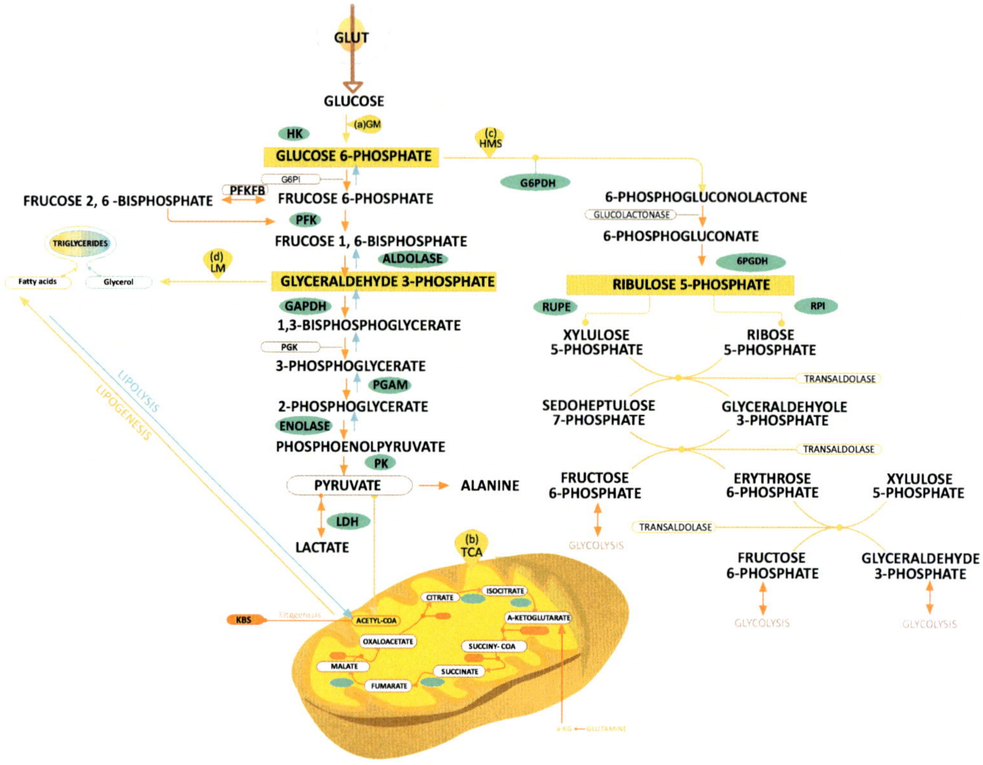

Fig. (4.6). Important reactions of intermediary metabolism. **(a) GM**: Glucose metabolism (glycolysis) is the catabolic process in that glucose is broken down to pyruvate through 10 enzymatic steps. Various glycolytic enzymes are changed in tumor cells (green ovals). GLUT, glucose transporter; HK, hexokinase; GAPDH, glyceraldehyde-3-phosphate dehydrogenase; PGAM, phosphoglycerate mutase; PK, pyruvate kinase; LDH, lactate dehydrogenase; PFKFB, 6-phosphofructo-2-kinase/fructose 2,6-bisphosphatase. **(b) TCA**: Tricarboxylic acid cycle consists of a series of enzyme-catalyzed reactions, situated in the mitochondrial matrix. Numerous enzymes (green ovals) of the TCA cycle are mutated and/or changed in several types of cancer. IDH, isocitrate dehydrogenase; OGDC, oxoglutarate dehydrogenase complex; SCS, succinyl-CoA synthetase; SDH, succinate dehydrogenase; FH, fumarate hydratase; MDH, malate dehydrogenase; CS, citrate synthase. **(c) HMS**: Hexose monophosphate shunt that branches out from glycolysis at the first committed step of glycolysis, is essential for nucleotide synthesis in tumor cells. Various enzymes of the HMS are related to numerous types of cancer (green ovals). G6PDH, glucose 6-phosphate dehydrogenase; 6PGDH, 6-phosphogluconate dehydrogenase; RuPE, ribulose-5-phosphate-3-epimerase; RPI, ribose-5-phosphate isomerase. **(d) LM (Lipid Metabolism)**: The interactions between GM, TCA cycle, and LM. Lipolysis is the breakdown of lipids, while Lipogenesis is the biosynthesis of lipids. TGAs, Triglycerides are made up of glycerol and fatty acids. Fatty acids undergo ß-oxidation generating acetyl CoA, which enters the TCA cycle. α-KG, α-ketoglutarate is generated from the deamination of glutamine. KBS, ketogenesis is the biosynthesis of ketone bodies from acetyl C.

Glycolysis

Energy is required by all tissues in the body to do their work. Food consumption is used to derive this type of energy. Naturally, breaking down foodstuff into small molecules creates energy, known as ATP. ATP is an organic molecule created through the regulated oxidation of glucose as well as other molecules. Glycolysis is the cytoplasmic catabolic pathway of glucose in all cells. Under aerobic conditions, the transportation of dietary glucose into cells occurs by a wide group of glucose-transporter proteins on the cell membrane, and then it is broken down to pyruvic acid through a chain of enzymatic reactions (Fig. **4.6a**). Pyruvic acid is the glycolysis end-product that can be later transformed into acetyl-CoA, a fuel of the tri-carboxylic acid (TCA) cycle known as Krebs cycle. NADH and $FADH_2$ are created by Krebs cycle to supply a series of chemical reactions within mitochondria, known as a respiratory chain (RC), with electrons for ATP creation. This is an energy creation effective mode as up to 36 ATP can be produced by each glucose molecule. However, in the lack of oxygen supply, pyruvate is converted into lactate, through the pathway termed anaerobic glycolysis. Theoretically, one glucose molecule produces 2 pyruvate molecules and 2 ATP molecules through glycolysis [429].

Anomalies of glycolysis in cancerous tissues have been detected since the beginning of the 20th century. Otto Warburg, a Nobel laureate and a German physiologist, has observed that cancer 'proliferating' cells need exclusively glycolytic pathways for energy synthesis, even in the existence of an adequate amount of O_2. This observed phenomenon is later termed 'aerobic glycolysis' (Warburg effect) of cancer cells in order to differentiate from anaerobic glycolytic pathway of normal 'non-proliferating' cells [432, 433]. Indeed, energy metabolism reprogramming is obviously significant, in that proliferating cells do so to some extent by culminating glucose transporters, conspicuously GLUT1, which fundamentally enhances glucose import into the cytoplasm [434]. Moreover, dependence on glycolytic pathways might be additional featured under the lack of oxygen (hypoxia) cases, which work inside several tumor cells. The reaction system of hypoxia performs pleiotropically to construct glucose transporters and numerous proteins of the glycolysis [434, 435]. Moreover, aerobic glycolysis increases the query as to why cancerous cells change their metabolic pathway to aerobic glycolysis, contrasting healthy cells that are contingent on classical cellular respiration to produce energy [436, 437]. Even though the exact causes remain unclear, the up-to-date explanations comprise: i) a quick production of ATP by aerobic glycolysis; even though it is less efficient than classical cellular respiration; ii) intermediates of glycolysis deliver adequate building blocks for the synthesis of macromolecules necessary for the cell proliferation enhancement [438, 439]. As a result of these features of malignant cells, several research works have been devoted to new approaches to selectively inactivate metabolic pathways and/or glucose transportation in cancerous cells [440, 441].

In fact, 2 molecules of ATP are made by one molecule of glucose through glycolysis, whereas the mitochondrial respiratory chain can harvest up to 36 ATP/consumption of glucose. Therefore, cancerous cells ought to recompense for the 18-fold lower efficiency of energy synthesis. Part to solve this issue is to up-regulate glucose transporters, particularly Glut1-4, to uptake more glucose [442 - 444]. Therefore, the elevation in glucose uptake is a main characteristic differentiating cancer-proliferating cells from healthy non-proliferating cells.

Remarkably, two subpopulations of tumorigenesis have been identified within a few cancerous cells, which differ in their energy-generating pathways. One subpopulation involves glucose-dependent ("Warburg-effect") cells that release lactate, even though cells of the second subpopulation particularly import and utilize the lactate created by their neighbors as their major energy source [445]. Amusingly, a few numbers of cancerous transformations have been exposed to hold both subpopulations of cancer cells that differ in their energy-generating pathways. One subpopulation contains glucose-dependent ("Warburg-effect") cells, which release lactate, though cells of the second subpopulation particularly import and utilize the lactate produced by their neighboring cells as their major energy source [445].

Previous research work has indicated that glycolytic fueling is related to stimulated oncogenes, such as RAS, MYC and mutated tumor suppressors, such as Tp53 [434], whose changes within tumorigenesis have been selected essentially for their interests in providing the abilities of cell proliferation, evasion of cytostatic controls, and minimizing of apoptosis [435, 444]. Additionally, tumors abnormally increase the production of most enzymes of glycolysis. Most important oncogenes like Ras, Myc, and HIF-1α are documented to be the main stimulators of glycolysis in cancerous cells [444]. Numerous glycolytic enzymes are up-regulated in tumor cells, resulting from raised transcriptional activity of c-Myc and HIF-1α and deficient control by p53. In fact, c-Myc and HIF-1α transcription factors are known as two principal glycolytic promoters over direct or indirect increased expression of glycolytic genes in cancerous cells. Both these transcriptional factors directly stimulate the expression of key glycolytic enzymes like HK2,PFK1, TPI1, and LDHA, among others, in tumor cells [446, 447]. Indeed, most promoter areas of glycolytic genes have unanimity binding motifs of Myc and HIF-1α. C-Myc is quite recognized to stimulate the expression of its target glycolysis genes in normoxic conditions, whereas HIF-1α is primarily functional in a hypoxic condition. This organization permits metastasis to constantly drive glycolysis in order to support their accelerated biosynthesis and quick proliferation [447, 448].

Noticeable development has been gained in recognizing the cancerous molecular mechanisms causing constitutive up-regulation of glycolytic pathways within cancers [449]. Several glycolytic enzymes are known as multi-functional proteins involving high levels of gene expression in cancerous cells. For instance, hexokinase (HK), the glycolytic enzyme that catalyzes the irreversible phosphorylation of glucose, the first reaction of the glycolytic pathway, and is implicated in transcriptional regulation; as well as, its expression in cancerous cells is frequently up-regulated [450]. Most malignant tissues show higher levels of type II isoform (HK-II) expression that could increase the glycolytic rate [449, 451]. Phosphofructokinase (PFK), the regulatory enzyme of glycolysis, has been documented to be up-regulated in some breast cancers [449, 452]. Another critical key regulatory glycolytic enzyme is 6-phosphofructo-2-kinase/fructose 2,6-bisphosphatase (Pfkfb), which is a family of bi-functional enzymes that regulate fructose 2,6-bisphosphate levels, and that in turn is a dominant allosteric effector of PFK1 activation. Both isoforms of Pfkfb; Pfkfb-2 and Pfkfb-3, are linked to carcinogenesis [453, 454]. Subsequently, aldolase, the enzyme catalyzing the reversible conversion of fructose-1,6-bisphosphate to dihydroxyacetone phosphate and glyceraldehyde-3-phosphate, has been confirmed to overexpress in epidermoid carcinoma lung [449, 455]. In addition, glyceraldehyde-3-phosphate dehydrogenase (GAPDH), the well-known classic glycolytic enzyme, is also involved in cancers. Its overexpression is considered a significant feature of numerous types of carcinoma, which has been proposed to be a promising target for carcinoma therapy [456, 457]. Pyruvate kinase (PK) is the enzyme involved in the final rate-limiting step in glycolysis, catalyzing the transferring of a phosphate group from phosphoenolpyruvate to ADP and thereby producing pyruvate and ATP. Many earlier studies have confirmed that tumor cells have high expression of the type M2 isoform of PK (PKM2); therefore, PK seems to be implicated in cancer [458, 459]. Due to the dependence of most cancerous cells on the aerobic glycolytic pathway for the creation of ATP, the lactate dehydrogenase (LDH) enzyme, catalyzing the reduction of pyruvate to lactate, is important to define the phenotype of glycolysis in cancerous cells. Therefore, LDH is considered an encouraging target for anticancer treatment. The inhibited LDH suppresses tumor development of pancreatic cancer xenografts and cancer of the lymphatic system [449, 460]. These outcomes show that selective targeting of glycolysis and/or its enzymes in tumor tissues might be existed as nominal approaches to manage various cancer types.

Krebs Cycle

Krebs cycle, also known as the tricarboxylic acid cycle (TCA), is a chain of chemical reactions employed by most aerobic living organisms for creating energy through the oxidation of acetate derived from carbohydrates, proteins, and fats into CO_2 (Fig. **4.6b**). TCA cycle provides different precursors for the synthesis of metabolites like amino acids, and nicotinamide adenine dinucleotide (NADH) and flavin adenine nucleotide ($FADH_2$), which are later used to produce energy by transferring electrons from NADH or $FADH_2$ to the oxygen molecule through the electron-transport chain (ETC). The Krebs cycle is the central metabolic axis of cells, which happens mainly in the matrix of mitochondria in comparison to cytoplasmic glycolysis. While mutations within mitochondrial DNA have been estimated for over twenty years [461 - 463], lots of care has been concentrated on the documentation of genetic alterations in numerous enzymes of TCA cycle [464]. Eight steps catalyzed by eight different enzymes are involved in the cycle. Alterations in genes, encoding fumarate hydratase (FH), succinate dehydrogenase (SDH), isocitrate dehydrogenase (IDH), and aconitase enzymes may drive to cancer [465].

FH is the enzyme catalyzing the reduction of fumarate to malate. Mutations of FH gene are related to aggressive forms of uterine, cutaneous, and renal cancer [466, 467]. Cancerous tissues which harbor FH mutations harvest up to a hundred-fold more fumarate, and 7-fold more succinate, but reduced levels of citrate and malate [468]. In tumor cells, FH deficiency changes redox homeostasis, leading to tumorigenesis promotion [467]. SDH is the enzyme, responsible for converting succinate to fumarate, and SDH mutations are involved in paraganglioma, pheochromocytoma, papillary thyroid cancers, and renal cell carcinoma [469, 470]. Reduction of expression and Loss of heterozygosity in the SDH gene are detected in the colon and gastric carcinoma [471]. Down-regulation of SDH leads to succinate accumulation, resulting in oncogenic signal transmission from the mitochondrial matrix to the cytoplasm [472]. IDH catalyzes the conversion of isocitrate to α-ketoglutarate (α-KG). Glioblastoma multiforme, which is one of the greatest common and fatal types of brain cancer, is characterized by a mutated

IDH1 gene [473]. Similar studies have exposed mutated genes of IDH1 and IDH2 in the pathogenesis of malignant gliomas and other human tumors [474, 475].

Mutations that take place within the single amino acid residue of active sites of IDH1 not only lead to the novel ability for the mutated enzyme to convert α-KG to 2-hydroxyglutarate that is suggested to participate in the gliomas formation and malignant progression [476]. Aconitase isomerizes citrate to isocitrate by the action of the cis-aconitase enzyme. Changed expression levels of aconitase are involved in human cancer of the prostate, in which the normal citrate-producing glandular secretory epithelial cells undergo a metabolic transformation to malignant citrate-oxidizing cells, causing abnormal citrate metabolism and prostatic malignancy [477].

Hexose Monophosphate Shunt (HMS)

Hexose monophosphate shunt (HMS) that branches out from the glycolytic pathway at the first committed step comprises 2 twigs. Through the oxidative branch, HMS catalyzes the irreversible conversion of glucose-6-phosphate (G6P), an intermediate of the glycolysis pathway, producing ribulose-5-phosphate (Ru5P) and NADPH, a cofactor utilized by anabolic reactions (Fig. **4.6c**). Then, NADPH is used to create antioxidant glutathione and synthesize macromolecules such as lipids. The non-oxidative HMS arm encompasses a series of reversible reactions, which are followed by the production of fructose-6-phosphate (F6P) and glyceraldehyde-3-phosphate (G3P). These metabolic products are able to contribute to the glycolytic pathway, as well as downstream metabolic pathways [478, 479]. HMS is generally seen as a route of protection against oxidative stress through NADPH production as well as producing ribose-5-phosphate (R5P), a precursor for nucleotide synthesis. On the other hand, several studies propose that numerous aspects of tumors are influenced by HMS, such as invasion, metastasis, proliferation, apoptosis and drug resistance [479]. These thrilling findings uncover HMS as a probable target for anti-cancer metabolism treatments.

HMS goes parallel to the glycolytic pathway, and stimulation of these metabolic pathways is a mutual stamp of tumor cells [480]. Cancer cells need a continuous supply of nucleotides to meet the rapid dividing of them; therefore, most of the pentose phosphates are produced by the HMS to meet this demand [442]. Hence, by providing pentose phosphate and NAPDH for nucleic acid synthesis, HMS is essential and commonly up-regulated in various types of tumors [442, 479, 481].

In fact, the glucose-6- phosphate dehydrogenase (G6PD), catalyzing the first step in the HMS, is extremely overexpressed in proliferating tumor cells [482, 483]. Raised G6PD levels are accountable for clear cell renal cell carcinoma (ccRCC)

[484]. In the human bone osteosarcoma-derived U2OS cell line, the overexpressed G6PD increases HNADPH production by HMS [485, 486]. Additionally, it has been established that oxidative stress can be prompted, and malignant human tumor cell lines are sensitized to radiation treatment through simultaneous inhibition of HMS and glycolysis, seemingly through the stimulation of numerous modalities of cell death, comprising mitotic catastrophe, necrosis, and apoptosis [487]. Numerous cancer types and accelerated tumor proliferation elevate several HMS enzymes, such as G6PD and transketolase (TK) [488, 489]. Moreover, cancer survival is stimulated by G-6PD, through NADPH, which is an important tool for tumor cells for protecting against chemotherapy-stimulated cytotoxic damage, oxidative stress, and stimulating biosynthesis [478, 479]. Therefore, the function of G-6PD is strongly regulated by the tumor suppressor p53 by preventing the formation of active G-6PD dimer complexes [490]. It is remarkable that G-6PD is a direct transactivated target of HIF-1α [491]. The function of G-6PD is firmly controlled within healthy cells, however, extremely stimulated within cancer cells, causing G-6PD to be a robust oncogene candidate [479]. Excitingly, the functions of G-6PD and TK are both inhibited by a plant antioxidant compound, "resveratrol" [492], proposing the expenditure of this natural remedy to treat and prevent cancerogenesis [478].

6-phosphogluconate dehydrogenase (6PGDH) is the next enzyme, which has a part in tumor. 6PGDH catalyzes ribulose 5-phosphate production *via* the oxidative decarboxylation of 6-phosphogluconate plus NADPH production. It has been publicized to be critical for malignant lung tumor; therefore, its suppression could be a new treatment approach for glycolytic lung tumorigenesis [481]. Another critical enzyme in the HMS is ribulose-5 phosphate isomerase, converting Ru5P to R5P and xylulose-5 phosphate (Xu5P), which is likewise linked with carcinogenesis [481]. R5P is significant due to its role as a precursor for nucleotide biosynthesis in quickly dividing cancer cells. In addition, Xu5P elevates 6-phosphofructose-2-kinase/fructose-2,6-biphosphatase (PFKFB) levels that activate phosphofructokinase 1 (PFK1) and raise the flux through the glycolysis [493]. Consequently, all of these studies involve vigorous HMS regulation for cancer cell survival and spread. Moreover, HMS may control directly or indirectly amplified glycolytic flux in cancerous cells, therefore, this may signify an encouraging strategy for cancer cell therapy [429].

In addition, HMS defends tumor cells from apoptosis by facilitating DNA damage repair and counteracting oxidative stress. Indeed, NSAIDs prompt apoptosis and reduction of polyps and colon carcinoma by HMS regulation [482]. Furthermore, inhibitors of G-6PD, such as dehydroepiandrosterone (DHEA) or 6-aminonicotinamide (6-AN), stimulate cellular apoptotic pathways in mouse PC-12 neural cells and fibroblasts whereas overexpression of G-6PD defends cells against H_2O_2-induced cell death [494]. As well as, G-6PD knocking down enhances toxicity mediated by oxidative stress in malignant melanoma [495]. Moreover, the HMS vital role is proven in cell protection against apoptotic cell death *in vivo,* like in stem cells as well as mononuclear cells of peripheral blood in patients with G-6PD deficiency [496, 497]. Remarkably, the cytoprotective role of HMS is not limited to protecting against ROS; however, also expands to facilitating the repair of DNA damage. In fact, in DNA damage, the ataxia telangiectasia, mutated (ATM) protein rapidly activates G6PD functions to hasten HMS for reducing ROS, enhancing nucleotide synthesis and permitting DNA repair with an efficient manner. Astonishingly, HMS also prompts the angiogenesis of tumors. Several earlier studies stated the tight association between angiogenesis through vascular endothelial growth factor (VEGF) and G6PD [498, 499]. Additionally, HMS stimulates tumor resistance to radiation and chemotherapy by numerous mechanisms. Firstly, HMS supplies cancerous cells with NAPDH that keeps them from ROS-induced cell death produced by radiation therapy and therapeutic agents [479]; secondly, HMS enables DNA damage repair by supplying material for nucleotide synthesis; thirdly, HMS decreases the intracellular concentrations of ROS by shifting cancer metabolism away from mitochondrial respiration, thus increasing tumor survival and endurance during radiation and chemotherapy treatments; lastly, NAPDH resulting from HMS, is an essential element for GSH generation that often works as a cleanser in detoxification reactions, allowing cancer cells to resist an assortment of chemotherapy treatments. In addition, increased G-6PD expression and HMS flux within cancer cells lead to increased levels of GSH and decreased drug accumulation in them [500].

In short, HMS is a vital metabolism supplying cancerous cells with R5P, NADPH and other important metabolites. NAPDH plays a critical role in counteracting biosynthetic reactions and ROS-induced oxidative stress. R5P is a key part of the production of nucleotides. Remarkably, the HMS influence on carcinogenesis is in excess of more than oxidative resistance. In fact, up-regulation of HMS enhances cancerous cell immortality, propagation, spreading, invasion, angiogenic changes, and chemotherapeutic and radiation resistance. For that reason, elevation and activation of HMS enzymes, like G6PD or TKTL, are often noticed in malignance, aggression, proliferation, invasion, and therapeutic resistance of cancerous tissues [479]. The fresh, exhilarating findings of HMS unlock novel treatment windows but correspondingly need additional studies to polish rational approaches for effective and precise aiming to this vigorous metabolism within cancerous cells.

Lipid Metabolism

The increased rate of lipid metabolism is another significant feature of cancer metabolism, being documented as the noticeable hallmark in cellular transformation. Lipids are a miscellaneous set of molecules, including triglycerides, fats, cholesterols, cholesteryl esters, and phospholipids (Fig. **4.6d**) [501, 502]. Lipids are essential building blocks of new cells and organelles; they form the main component of plasma membranes (phospholipid bilayer), certain fat-soluble vitamins, and hormones (steroid hormones, like cholesterol). Therefore, lipids implement numerous roles within the body, from supplying energy to muscles to making hormones [503]. Synthesis of lipids is a multiple-step process including a number of enzymes like acetyl-CoA carboxylase (ACC), ATP citrate lyase (ACLY), fatty acid synthase (FASN), and stearoyl-CoA desaturase (SCD). The procedure of lipid synthesis starts with the ACC enzyme that converts acetyl-CoA to malonyl-CoA. A sequence of condensation reactions by FASN produces saturated fatty acids (Fas). SCD catalyzes the production of de-saturated Fas.

In rapidly proliferating cancer cells, there is a frequent up-regulation of *de novo* FA synthesis to fulfill their requests for lipids [501, 504, 505]. ACLY, is an enzyme involved in the *de novo* FAs synthesis, converting citrate derived within mitochondria to oxaloacetate and cytosolic acetyl-CoA. Hence, ACLY associates *de novo* lipid synthesis pathway to the Krebs cycle and gluconeogenesis [506]. A variety of study research has confirmed that overexpression levels of ACLY are linked to lymph node metastasis and advanced stages of cancer in tissue samples from patients with gastric adenocarcinoma [507]. However, microRNA-22 (miR-22) targets ACLY, and overwhelms cancer invasion and proliferation within the lung, bone, prostate, and cervical cancerous cells [508]. Additional investigation exhibits that ACLY is essential for low-molecular-weight (LMW) isoform of cyclin E mediated transformation, invasion, and migration, of cancerous breast cells *in vitro* along with tumor development *in vivo* [509]. FASN, catalyzing the last step in the synthesis of FA is frequently expressed at high levels in human oncogenesis [510, 511]. Its rise is detected in prostate, breast, and other types of cancer [512-514]. FASN inhibition suppresses the migration and invasion of hepatocellular carcinoma (HCC) cells [510]. ACC is the regulatory enzyme in FA synthesis. ACC activates the carboxylation of acetyl-CoA to form malonyl-CoA. In patients with squamous cell cancer (SCC) of the neck and head, there is a relationship between phosphorylated AMP-activated protein kinase and expression of ACC, and the therapeutic consequence is that extraordinary phosphorylated-ACC expression is related to poorer general *survivability* within patients [515]. Likewise, the up-regulation of ACC1expression has been observed in patients with HCC, and its up-regulation is also considerably linked to disease recurrence and worse general immortalization within HCC patients [516]. In addition, ACC is essential for tumorigenesis because ACC inhibition ends cancer growth and prompts prostate cancer apoptosis [517].

In addition, the synthesis of cholesterol or the mevalonic acid pathway is an essential feature of lipogenesis as cholesterol is a key metabolite of the membrane fluidity, membrane governing, and lipid rafts construction. Cholesterol biosynthesis deregulation is associated with cell transformation [518]. Remarkably, statin suppression of HMGCR, a vital enzyme of cholesterol synthesis, significantly improves the chemotherapies efficiency in patients with HCC [519], acute myeloid leukemia [520], and other types of cancer over epigenetic programming modification [521].

The expression of enzymes implicated in fatty acid and cholesterol biosynthesis is controlled by the major transcription factor, sterol regulatory element-binding protein (SREBPs). SREBPs are 125 kDa proteins that need an endoplasmic reticulum protein cleavage for activation [504]. Whereas SREBP1 regulates fatty acid, triacylglycerol and phospholipid generation, SREBP2 controls cholesterol synthesis [522]. In fact, SREBPs are regulated by oncogenes and tumor suppressors. For instance, AMP-activated protein kinase (AMPK) suppresses the activation of SREBP and inhibits ACC [523], thus keeping the synthesis of lipids in check. Mutants of p53 coordinate with SREBP to transactivate enzymes of cholesterol synthesis [524]. On the other hand, loss of retinoblastoma protein (pRb) upregulates SREBP1 and SREBP2, thus activating Ras signaling [525]. Of note, SREBPs1 and 2 are frequently overexpressed in cancerous cells [512] and perform a vital role in their survival [526].

Extreme lipogenesis participates in carcinogenesis. Obesity has been well recognized to increase cancer risk [504]. Indeed, insulin resistance is induced by a high level of lipid concentrations within muscle and liver cells, by deteriorating insulin signaling and decreasing glucose absorption. Moreover, high-level secretion of insulin and insulin-like growth factors by Insulin resistance forcing is very supportive for cancer cell proliferation and survival [527, 528]. As well as, obesity enhances inflammatory responses that participate in insulin resistance and carcinogenesis [529]. Carcinogenic trends might be reversed by dietary restriction; however, in certain cases, such as in overactivity of PI3K/Akt signaling is overactivated, the influence of dietary restriction to suppress tumors decreases [530]. Decreasing the levels of circulating insulin-like growth factors and insulin as a result of nutrient restriction is a possible explanation of the impact of dietary restriction on tumor suppression. However, the deficiency of insulin signaling may be compensated by the activation of PI3K/Akt signaling [531].

Amino Acid Metabolism

Amino acids are considered one of the most important nutrients for biosynthesis, as they are involved in most cellular metabolism. Amino acids are an ultimate requirement for tumor cell proliferation, as a result of their feature as the most essential nutrients. Moreover, a minor change in the metabolic reactions may have an influence on the synthesis of amino acids. Amino acid, glutamine, is another main fuel for carcinoma, even though it is a nonessential amino acid [532, 533]. In tumor cells, it is a major mitochondrial amino acid needed to maintain the integrity and potential of the mitochondrial membrane and to create NADPH [443].

Besides glycolysis, several tumors depend on glutamine catabolism 'glutaminolysis' to fuel their cellular metabolic pathways and bioenergetics. Glutamine catabolism is a sequence of metabolic reactions that catabolize glutamine by the action of glutaminase, which catalyzes the conversion of glutamine to glutamic acid and NH_3. Glutamic acid is then transformed to α-KG and enters the krebs cycle [534]. Glutaminolysis products are essential to fuel the TCA cycle of tumor cells. TCA cycle intermediates can be utilized for the biosynthesis of amino acids, lipids, cholesterol, and other important nutrients [532]. Furthermore, NADH and $FADH_2$ generated from the krebs cycle supply electrons for RC for ATP generation. Consequently, like to glycolytic pathway, glutamine catabolism provides cancerous cells with ATP as well as critical precursors for accelerated proliferation and continuous biosynthetic pathways [443].

The upregulation of glutaminolysis in tumor cells is intermediated by c-Myc [532, 535]. Several studies prove that c-Myc stimulates the uptake of glutamine and its catabolism. Indeed, two essential glutamine transporters on the cellular plasma membrane, *ASCT2* and *SN2,* are transactivated by c-Myc [536]. In addition, c-Myc inhibits miR-23a/b to upregulate the expression of glutaminase [537], which is a vital enzyme of glutamine catabolism. Hence, c-Myc is an essential glutaminolysis stimulator within the cancerous transformation. Remarkably, c-Myc makes cancerous cells dependent on glutaminolysis, which unlocks a novel anticancer curative window to selectively inhibit and eradicate these cells [538, 539]. Assured cancer cells are described as 'glutamine addiction', the capacity of cancerous cells to show a great degree of glutamine uptake. Catabolic glutamine is raised in definite cancer types [540]. Evidence shows the role of glutamate and glutamate receptors in neuroblastoma, human rhabdomyosarcoma/ medulloblastoma, thyroid cancer, astrocytoma, lung carcinoma, plasma, and myeloma, lung carcinoma, Glioblastoma, colorectal cancer, breast carcinoma, and T-cell leukemia [541].

Serine, another significant non-essential amino acid, which contributes to nucleotide biosynthesis, has been publicized to be up-regulated in breast carcinoma [542, 543]. Research works in melanoma melanocytes have confirmed that considerable portions of serine are transformed into glycine [544]. Glycine, one of the modest and other non-essential amino acids, has also been involved in tumor [545]. It is an important component of proteins that construct tissues as well as organs. Glycine is the greatest plentiful type of amino acid within the body as well as one of the main essential regulators of the inflammatory response [546, 547]. Metabolism of glycine has also been verified to be upregulated in adenocarcinoma, squamous cell carcinoma, and large cell carcinoma [543]. Several studies have elucidated that glycine promotes cancer cell proliferation, and tumor cells glycine deficiency indicated a significant decline in cell growth [548]. Glycine, serine, and vitamin B9 (folate) are constitutively bioactive in numerous tumor cells [543, 549].

Mitochondria and its Central Role in Carcinogenesis

Metabolism in mitochondria has appeared as the main target for anti-cancer drugs [426]. Mitochondria are significant biosynthetic and bioenergetics organelles; they produce ATP and most of the intermediates that are needed in the biosynthesis of different macromolecules. Additionally, mitochondria participate and contribute to ROS generation, apoptosis regulation, calcium homeostasis, and cell signaling pathways [424, 425]. Mitochondria with numerous degrees of aberrations have been recognized within cancer cells. This observation makes mitochondria properly targeted by the therapeutic intervention [427, 428]. As well as, it has been noticed that different types of cancer involve alterations in nuclear and mitochondria, such as single nucleotide polymorphisms (SNPs), and deletions/insertions [550]. Moreover, as mitochondria constantly generate ROS species, their DNA is always exposed to oxidative impairment and stress by ROS. Earlier studies have explored the influence of alterations of mitochondrial DNA in proliferating and invading tumor cells [551]. Within growing mutations, the capacity of mitochondrial respiration has been shown to decline gradually [552]. As well as, faults in the mitochondrial RC may either inhibit or promote apoptosis [553]. Osellame *et al.* demonstrated that apoptosis initiation and ROS production are thoroughly interconnected with mitochondria [554]. As well as, it has been recognized that loss of permeability in the mitochondrial outer membrane is a special characteristic of intrinsic apoptosis [554]. Through the past 10 years, the influence of polyamines in the stimulation of apoptotic pathways has been the center of clinical examinations [555]. Additionally, ROS may be mediated in anti- and pro-apoptotic effects [556]. Recently, Novel associates between mitochondria and polyamines have been displayed in a brief manner through a review article by

Grancara *et al.* [557]. Growing attention has been considered to understanding multifaceted mitochondrial biology, which participates in tumorigenesis. Mitochondria act as a fundamental hub for cell metabolism, cell survival, as well as cell death processes. Taking into account the role of mitochondria in multiple facets *via* carcinogenesis, targeting mitochondria might exist as a nominal approach to anti-cancer therapy.

Metabolic Alteration by p53

p53, an important tumor suppressor and transcription factor, counters stress circumstances by arresting the cell cycle, prompting DNA repair, or causing cell death. Its actions on energy metabolic and biosynthetic pathways are also important, including stimulation of SCO_2 (synthesis of cytochrome c oxidase 2) that is required for mitochondrial respiration, and TIGAR (TP53-induced glycolysis and apoptosis regulator) that stops glycolysis and directs glucose to the pentose phosphate pathway [558]. A lately illustrated metabolic role for p53 in cancerous cells has suggested an interesting possibility for treatment against p53-null tumors. Maddocks *et al.* showed that HCT116 tumors in mice, and mainly those lacking p53, established hindered growth on the exclusion of the non-essential amino acid serine from the diet. As a result of less serine in p53-null cells than normal cells under serine-starving conditions, the team demonstrated that p53 must play a role in assisting cells to acclimatize to low-serine situations [559]. Consequently, p53, to some extent, supports cell proliferation in the counter of serine starving conditions by restoring GSH levels rather than preserving nucleotide biosynthesis.

On the other hand, p53-null cells do not ever make this crucial move. Consuming oxygen remains high, G1 arrest is not efficient, and these cells preserve pumping serine into the nucleotide biosynthesis pathway instead of generating more GSH. Growing ROS levels are not counteracted by GSH; consequently, these cells fail to proliferate. The propositions for treatment of p53-null tumors are thrilling and credibly far-reaching, since p53 loss is a hallmark of numerous various types of cancers. The authors' alert that other genetic mutations could totally counter sensitivity to serine reduction, however, further work will requisite to be carried out to confirm if targeting serine is an effective method to fight these cancerous transformations.

Metabolic Alteration by Kras

Mutation of K-ras oncogene is involved in 17-25% of carcinogenesis, and recent studies have exposed numerous roles for this oncogene in the regulation of metabolic pathways within cancer cells. In pancreatic adenocarcinoma (PDAC) cells mainly, K-ras manages several important metabolic effects that upgrade the progress of these cellular alterations, counting effects on glucose uptake and flux, and change of catabolic pathway of glutamine. Both of the studies detailed below afford solid leads for scientists seeking to find out approaches to control PDAC, a predominantly lethal disease in serious need of novel therapeutic choices [560].

Regarding the role of K-ras in glucose metabolic and biosynthetic pathways, Ying *et al.* presented that in an inducible, tissue-specific model of Kras exemplification in PDAC carcinogenesis, K-ras had all the earmarks of being involved in driving the expression of genes in various biosynthesis pathways, incorporating genes included in steroid and pyrimidine biosynthetic pathway [560]. K-ras similarly stimulate flux of glycolysis at the gene expression and protein level, as measured by glucose uptake, expression of glycolytic rate-limiting enzymes, locality of intermediates of glycolysis, and lactate generation. Moreover, K-ras unregulated Gfpt1, the first enzyme within the hexosamine biosynthesis pathway (HBP), completely affect glycosylation.

As a result of Kras activity, Glucose, more abundant, was regulated into the non-oxidative arm of the HMS. Flux into the non-oxidative HMS extended R-5ph generation for combination into DNA and RNA synthesis while leaving the oxidative arm of the HMS pathway, which is involved in redox balance through NADPH generation, untouched. Obstructing this pathway reduced Kras-dependent carcinogenesis, presenting that Kras's role in ribose synthesis is elementary for maintaining PDAC carcinogenesis. Furthermore, knockdown experiments displayed the involved signaling pathways, representing that both MAPK and Myc are implicated in Kras's effects on the HBP and HMS [560].

In addition, K-ras is significantly included in regulating glutamine metabolism in PDAC cells. Son *et al.* established that carcinogenic K-ras controls the expression of key genes to switch to a glutamine-utilizing transaminase pathway, which cellular PDAC requires; however, not healthy cells for growth and preservation of redox balance [561]. Glutamine is required for PDAC growth; conversely, even though GLUD1-Glutamate dehydrogenase 1 is the traditional metabolism pathway used by various other cancer cells, the team's results point out that PDAC cells require both alpha-KG and NEAA to rescue growth upon glutamine deprivation, suggesting that PDAC cells utilized transaminases for glutamine metabolic pathway instead. Absolutely, knocking down the aspartate transaminase (GOT1) inhibited PDAC development and had munificent values for oxaloacetate, aspartate levels, and reduced glutathione.

Concluding Remarks

In most types of cancer cells, metabolic reprogramming is documented as one of the hallmarks of cancerogenesis. Increased glucose consumption, lactate production, HMS, metabolism of lipids, and synthesis of amino acids are frequently detected in metabolomics in nearly all cancerous cells. This sort of metabolomics of cancer cells is suggested to sustain their prompt cell development [562]. Glycolysis with great level rates produces lactic acid (the Warburg effect or aerobic glycolysis) to discriminate tumor 'proliferating' cells from healthy 'nonproliferating' cells [436]. Glucose is a significant energy source for tumor cells, and a precursor for supplying several intermediates-mediated metabolisms that are utilized in the biosynthesis of nucleotides, lipids, and amino-acids. Glutamine functions as an additional significant source of cancer fuel [533]. Glutamine moves to the mitochondria in order to refill the intermediates of the Krebs cycle [540] by creating α-KG, succinic acid, fumaric acid, and eventually malic acid. Greatly growing cancerous cells own a great request for the fast production of macromolecules [501, 504]. In addition, cancer cells divert carbon from the glycolytic pathway into the HMS [480] for macromolecule synthesis, like nucleic acids. As well as, acetyl-coA and citrate are important intermediates for lipogenesis [508, 509]. Since there is an interconnection between these metabolic pathways, comprehension machinery pathways causing this metabolic reprogramming in cancerous cells are of the highest significance. The current topic article, cancer cell differentiation, proliferation, and metastasis, results from the contribution of core misregulated metabolic pathways. In addition, the vital mitochondrial roles in coordinating the dysregulation of metabolism were outlined. The nearby association among these metabolic routes and the mitochondrial role and oxidation-reduction control within cancerous cells is a hopeful delineation for targeting the development of cancers. Consequently, aiming these essential mitochondrial metabolic pathways and/or their enzymes could display a novel and valid cancer treatment strategy.

CONCLUSION

The disturbances in the regulatory interactions of adjacent normal tissues of the host surrounding tumor environment, chronic inflammation and genomic instability are essential factors that influence the tumor initiation in the target tissue, tumor development, invasion and metastasis.

CONSENT FOR PUBLICATION

Not applicable.

CONFLICT OF INTEREST

The author declares no conflict of interest, financial or otherwise.

ACKNOWLEDGEMENTS

We thank King Abdullah International Medical Research Center (KAIMRC), Um Al Qura University and King Saud University for their technical support.

REFERENCES

[1] Clarke MF, Dick JE, Dirks PB, *et al.* Cancer stem cells-perspectives on current status and future directions: AACR Workshop on cancer stem cells. Cancer Res 2006; 66(19): 9339-44. [http://dx.doi.org/10.1158/0008-5472.CAN-06-3126] [PMID: 16990346]

[2] De Francesco EM, Sotgia F, Lisanti MP. Cancer stem cells (CSCs): metabolic strategies for their identification and eradication. Biochem J 2018; 475(9): 1611-34. [http://dx.doi.org/10.1042/BCJ20170164] [PMID: 29743249]

[3] Evans SMBR, Gatenby R, Hendrix MJ, Hill R, Lee WM. Biology of cancer.Interventional Oncology: Principles and Practice. Cambridge: Cambridge University Press 2008; pp. 3-22. [http://dx.doi.org/10.1017/CBO9780511722226.002]

[4] Papaccio F, Paino F, Regad T, Papaccio G, Desiderio V, Tirino V. Concise Review: Cancer Cells, Cancer Stem Cells, and Mesenchymal Stem Cells: Influence in Cancer Development. Stem Cells Transl Med 2017; 6(12): 2115-25. [http://dx.doi.org/10.1002/sctm.17-0138] [PMID: 29072369]

[5] Jain SRK, Agrawal AK, Vaidya A. Basic pathology and etiology of tumor Nanotechnology applications for cancer chemotherapy. Elsevier 2020; pp. 1-29.

[6] Roger JB. King MWR Cancer Biology. UK: Pearson Prentice Hall 2006.

[7] Reya T, Morrison SJ, Clarke MF, Weissman IL. Stem cells, cancer, and cancer stem cells. Nature 2001; 414(6859): 105-11. [http://dx.doi.org/10.1038/35102167] [PMID: 11689955]

[8] Kamalabadi-Farahani M, Kia V. High percentage of cancer stem cells in metastatic locations; a comment on a claim "variation in cancer risk among tissues can be explained by the number of stem cell divisions". Med Hypotheses 2020; 144: 110170. [http://dx.doi.org/10.1016/j.mehy.2020.110170] [PMID: 32795837]

[9] Xue WZ, Wang BB, Zhao XL, *et al.* Rhodamine hydrazone as a lysosome-targetable pH biomarker for the selective differentiation of cancer cells from normal cells. Inorg Chem Commun 2020; 122: 108260. [http://dx.doi.org/10.1016/j.inoche.2020.108260]

[10] Chan-Penebre E, Kuplast KG, Majer CR, *et al.* A selective inhibitor of PRMT5 with in vivo and in vitro potency in MCL models. Nat Chem Biol 2015; 11(6): 432-7. [http://dx.doi.org/10.1038/nchembio.1810] [PMID: 25915199]

[11] He L, Hu Z, Sun Y, *et al.* PRMT1 is critical to FEN1 expression and drug resistance in lung cancer cells. DNA Repair (Amst) 2020; 95: 102953. [http://dx.doi.org/10.1016/j.dnarep.2020.102953] [PMID: 32861926]

[12] Schatton T, Frank NY, Frank MH. Identification and targeting of cancer stem cells. BioEssays 2009; 31(10): 1038-49. [http://dx.doi.org/10.1002/bies.200900058] [PMID: 19708024]

[13] Borah A, Raveendran S, Rochani A, Maekawa T, Kumar DS. Targeting self-renewal pathways in

cancer stem cells: clinical implications for cancer therapy. Oncogenesis 2015; 4: e117. [http://dx.doi.org/10.1038/oncsis.2015.35] [PMID: 26619402]

[14] Carson-Walter EB, Watkins DN, Nanda A, Vogelstein B, Kinzler KW, St Croix B. Cell surface tumor endothelial markers are conserved in mice and humans. Cancer Res 2001; 61(18): 6649-55. [PMID: 11559528]

[15] Mekler LB. Hybridization of transformed cells with lymphocytes as 1 of the probable causes of the progression leading to the development of metastatic malignant cells. Vestn Akad Med Nauk SSSR 1971; 26(8): 80-9. [PMID: 4944404]

[16] Al-Hajj M, Becker MW, Wicha M, Weissman I, Clarke MF. Therapeutic implications of cancer stem cells. Curr Opin Genet Dev 2004; 14(1): 43-7. [http://dx.doi.org/10.1016/j.gde.2003.11.007] [PMID: 15108804]

[17] Bergsmedh A, Szeles A, Henriksson M, *et al.* Horizontal transfer of oncogenes by uptake of apoptotic bodies. Proc Natl Acad Sci USA 2001; 98(11): 6407-11. [http://dx.doi.org/10.1073/pnas.101129998] [PMID: 11353826]

[18] Afify S, Seno M. Conversion of Stem Cells to Cancer Stem Cells: Undercurrent of Cancer Initiation. Cancers (Basel) 2019; 11(3): E345. [http://dx.doi.org/10.3390/cancers11030345] [PMID: 30862050]

[19] Cao D, Cao D. The origin of cancer stem cells. Front Biosci (Schol Ed) 2012; S4(3): 819-30. [http://dx.doi.org/10.2741/s302] [PMID: 22202093]

[20] Majeti R, Chao MP, Alizadeh AA, *et al.* CD47 is an adverse prognostic factor and therapeutic antibody target on human acute myeloid leukemia stem cells. Cell 2009; 138(2): 286-99. [http://dx.doi.org/10.1016/j.cell.2009.05.045] [PMID: 19632179]

[21] Stephen BW, Jens-Peter V, Andrew JG, *et al.* The CD47-signal regulatory protein alpha (SIRPa) interaction is a therapeutic target for human solid tumors. Proceedings of the National Academy of Sciences - Proc Natl Acad Sci 2012; 109(17): 6662-7. [http://dx.doi.org/10.1073/pnas.1121623109]

[22] McCracken MN, George BM, Kao KS, Marjon KD, Raveh T, Weissman IL. Normal and Neoplastic Stem Cells. Cold Spring Harb Symp Quant Biol 2016; 81: 1-9. [http://dx.doi.org/10.1101/sqb.2016.81.030965] [PMID: 28416577]

[23] Escribano J, Chen MB, Moeendarbary E, *et al.* Balance of mechanical forces drives endothelial gap formation and may facilitate cancer and immune-cell extravasation. PLOS Comput Biol 2019; 15(5): e1006395. [http://dx.doi.org/10.1371/journal.pcbi.1006395] [PMID: 31048903]

[24] Dudley AC. Tumor endothelial cells. Cold Spring Harb Perspect Med 2012; 2(3): a006536. [http://dx.doi.org/10.1101/cshperspect.a006536] [PMID: 22393533]

[25] Hynes RO. The extracellular matrix: not just pretty fibrils. Science 2009; 326(5957): 1216-9. [http://dx.doi.org/10.1126/science.1176009] [PMID: 19965464]

[26] Wagner MJ, Ravi V, Menter DG, Sood AK. Endothelial cell malignancies: new insights from the laboratory and clinic. NPJ Precis Oncol 2017; 1(1): 11. [http://dx.doi.org/10.1038/s41698-017-0013-2] [PMID: 29872699]

[27] Ravi V, Patel S. Vascular Sarcomas. Curr Oncol Rep 2013; 15(4): 347-55. [http://dx.doi.org/10.1007/s11912-013-0328-2] [PMID: 23852636]

[28] Guo T, Zhang L, Chang NE, Singer S, Maki RG, Antonescu CR. Consistent MYC and FLT4 gene amplification in radiation-induced angiosarcoma but not in other radiation-associated atypical vascular lesions. Genes Chromosomes Cancer 2011; 50(1): 25-33. [http://dx.doi.org/10.1002/gcc.20827] [PMID: 20949568]

[29] Ohga N, Ishikawa S, Maishi N, *et al.* Heterogeneity of tumor endothelial cells: comparison between tumor endothelial cells isolated from high- and low-metastatic tumors. Am J Pathol 2012; 180(3): 1294-307.
[http://dx.doi.org/10.1016/j.ajpath.2011.11.035] [PMID: 22245217]

[30] Hida K, Maishi N, Torii C, Hida Y. Tumor angiogenesis—characteristics of tumor endothelial cells. Int J Clin Oncol 2016; 21(2): 206-12.
[http://dx.doi.org/10.1007/s10147-016-0957-1] [PMID: 26879652]

[31] Hida K, Maishi N, Annan D, Hida Y. Contribution of Tumor Endothelial Cells in Cancer Progression. Int J Mol Sci 2018; 19(5): E1272.
[http://dx.doi.org/10.3390/ijms19051272] [PMID: 29695087]

[32] Bjarnadóttir TK, Fredriksson R, Höglund PJ, Gloriam DE, Lagerström MC, Schiöth HB. The human and mouse repertoire of the adhesion family of G-protein-coupled receptors. Genomics 2004; 84(1): 23-33.
[http://dx.doi.org/10.1016/j.ygeno.2003.12.004] [PMID: 15203201]

[33] Vargas M, Karamsetty R, Leppla SH, Chaudry GJ. Broad expression analysis of human ANTXR1/TEM8 transcripts reveals differential expression and novel splizce variants. PLoS One 2012; 7(8): e43174.
[http://dx.doi.org/10.1371/journal.pone.0043174] [PMID: 22912819]

[34] Hong YK, Lee YC, Cheng TL, *et al.* Tumor Endothelial Marker 1 (TEM1/Endosialin/CD248) Enhances Wound Healing by Interacting with Platelet-Derived Growth Factor Receptors. J Invest Dermatol 2019; 139(10): 2204-2214.e7.
[http://dx.doi.org/10.1016/j.jid.2019.03.1149] [PMID: 30986375]

[35] Kalluri R. Basement membranes: structure, assembly and role in tumour angiogenesis. Nat Rev Cancer 2003; 3(6): 422-33.
[http://dx.doi.org/10.1038/nrc1094] [PMID: 12778132]

[36] Nishida N, Yano H, Nishida T, Kamura T, Kojiro M. Angiogenesis in cancer. Vasc Health Risk Manag 2006; 2(3): 213-9.
[http://dx.doi.org/10.2147/vhrm.2006.2.3.213] [PMID: 17326328]

[37] Gerhardt H, Golding M, Fruttiger M, *et al.* VEGF guides angiogenic sprouting utilizing endothelial tip cell filopodia. J Cell Biol 2003; 161(6): 1163-77.
[http://dx.doi.org/10.1083/jcb.200302047] [PMID: 12810700]

[38] Hellström M, Phng LK, Hofmann JJ, *et al.* Dll4 signalling through Notch1 regulates formation of tip cells during angiogenesis. Nature 2007; 445(7129): 776-80.
[http://dx.doi.org/10.1038/nature05571] [PMID: 17259973]

[39] Shibuya M, Claesson-Welsh L. Signal transduction by VEGF receptors in regulation of angiogenesis and lymphangiogenesis. Exp Cell Res 2006; 312(5): 549-60.
[http://dx.doi.org/10.1016/j.yexcr.2005.11.012] [PMID: 16336962]

[40] Antonescu CR, Yoshida A, Guo T, *et al.* KDR activating mutations in human angiosarcomas are sensitive to specific kinase inhibitors. Cancer Res 2009; 69(18): 7175-9.
[http://dx.doi.org/10.1158/0008-5472.CAN-09-2068] [PMID: 19723655]

[41] Jin SW, Patterson C. The opening act: vasculogenesis and the origins of circulation. Arterioscler Thromb Vasc Biol 2009; 29(5): 623-9.
[http://dx.doi.org/10.1161/ATVBAHA.107.161539] [PMID: 19008532]

[42] Burri PH, Hlushchuk R, Djonov V. Intussusceptive angiogenesis: Its emergence, its characteristics, and its significance. Dev Dyn 2004; 231(3): 474-88.
[http://dx.doi.org/10.1002/dvdy.20184] [PMID: 15376313]

[43] Armulik A, Abramsson A, Betsholtz C. Endothelial/pericyte interactions. Circ Res 2005; 97(6): 512-23.

[http://dx.doi.org/10.1161/01.RES.0000182903.16652.d7] [PMID: 16166562]

[44] Hall AP. Review of the pericyte during angiogenesis and its role in cancer and diabetic retinopathy. Toxicol Pathol 2006; 34(6): 763-75.
[http://dx.doi.org/10.1080/01926230600936290] [PMID: 17162534]

[45] Gaengel K, Genové G, Armulik A, Betsholtz C. Endothelial-mural cell signaling in vascular development and angiogenesis. Arterioscler Thromb Vasc Biol 2009; 29(5): 630-8.
[http://dx.doi.org/10.1161/ATVBAHA.107.161521] [PMID: 19164813]

[46] Armulik A, Genové G, Betsholtz C. Pericytes: developmental, physiological, and pathological perspectives, problems, and promises. Dev Cell 2011; 21(2): 193-215.
[http://dx.doi.org/10.1016/j.devcel.2011.07.001] [PMID: 21839917]

[47] Hwa C, Aird WC. The history of the capillary wall: doctors, discoveries, and debates. Am J Physiol Heart Circ Physiol 2007; 293(5): H2667-79.
[http://dx.doi.org/10.1152/ajpheart.00704.2007] [PMID: 17693543]

[48] Krueger M, Bechmann I. CNS pericytes: Concepts, misconceptions, and a way out. Glia 2010; 58(1): 1-10.
[http://dx.doi.org/10.1002/glia.20898] [PMID: 19533601]

[49] Grant RI, Hartmann DA, Underly RG, Berthiaume AA, Bhat NR, Shih AY. Organizational hierarchy and structural diversity of microvascular pericytes in adult mouse cortex. J Cereb Blood Flow Metab 2019; 39(3): 411-25.
[http://dx.doi.org/10.1177/0271678X17732229] [PMID: 28933255]

[50] Attwell D, Mishra A, Hall CN, O'Farrell FM, Dalkara T. What is a pericyte? J Cereb Blood Flow Metab 2016; 36(2): 451-5.
[http://dx.doi.org/10.1177/0271678X15610340] [PMID: 26661200]

[51] Stallcup WB. The NG2 proteoglycan: past insights and future prospects. J Neurocytol 2002; 31(6/7): 423-35.
[http://dx.doi.org/10.1023/A:1025731428581] [PMID: 14501214]

[52] Lindahl P, Johansson BR, Levéen P, Betsholtz C. Pericyte loss and microaneurysm formation in PDGF-B-deficient mice. Science 1997; 277(5323): 242-5.
[http://dx.doi.org/10.1126/science.277.5323.242] [PMID: 9211853]

[53] Bernard-Patrzynski F, Lécuyer MA, Puscas I, *et al.* Isolation of endothelial cells, pericytes and astrocytes from mouse brain. PLoS One 2019; 14(12): e0226302.
[http://dx.doi.org/10.1371/journal.pone.0226302] [PMID: 31851695]

[54] Bergers G, Song S. The role of pericytes in blood-vessel formation and maintenance. Neuro-oncol 2005; 7(4): 452-64.
[http://dx.doi.org/10.1215/S1152851705000232] [PMID: 16212810]

[55] Kunisaki Y, Bruns I, Scheiermann C, *et al.* Arteriolar niches maintain haematopoietic stem cell quiescence. Nature 2013; 502(7473): 637-43.
[http://dx.doi.org/10.1038/nature12612] [PMID: 24107994]

[56] Kidd S, Spaeth E, Watson K, *et al.* Origins of the tumor microenvironment: quantitative assessment of adipose-derived and bone marrow-derived stroma. PLoS One 2012; 7(2): e30563.
[http://dx.doi.org/10.1371/journal.pone.0030563] [PMID: 22363446]

[57] Wang HH, Cui YL, Zaorsky NG, *et al.* Mesenchymal stem cells generate pericytes to promote tumor recurrence via vasculogenesis after stereotactic body radiation therapy. Cancer Lett 2016; 375(2): 349-59.
[http://dx.doi.org/10.1016/j.canlet.2016.02.033] [PMID: 26996301]

[58] Bussard KM, Mutkus L, Stumpf K, Gomez-Manzano C, Marini FC. Tumor-associated stromal cells as key contributors to the tumor microenvironment. Breast Cancer Res 2016; 18(1): 84.
[http://dx.doi.org/10.1186/s13058-016-0740-2] [PMID: 27515302]

[59] Cheng L, Huang Z, Zhou W, *et al.* Glioblastoma stem cells generate vascular pericytes to support vessel function and tumor growth. Cell 2013; 153(1): 139-52. [http://dx.doi.org/10.1016/j.cell.2013.02.021] [PMID: 23540695]

[60] Song S, Ewald AJ, Stallcup W, Werb Z, Bergers G. PDGFRβ+ perivascular progenitor cells in tumours regulate pericyte differentiation and vascular survival. Nat Cell Biol 2005; 7(9): 870-9. [http://dx.doi.org/10.1038/ncb1288] [PMID: 16113679]

[61] Morikawa S, Baluk P, Kaidoh T, Haskell A, Jain RK, McDonald DM. Abnormalities in pericytes on blood vessels and endothelial sprouts in tumors. Am J Pathol 2002; 160(3): 985-1000. [http://dx.doi.org/10.1016/S0002-9440(10)64920-6] [PMID: 11891196]

[62] Eberhard A, Kahlert S, Goede V, Hemmerlein B, Plate KH, Augustin HG. Heterogeneity of angiogenesis and blood vessel maturation in human tumors: implications for antiangiogenic tumor therapies. Cancer Res 2000; 60(5): 1388-93. [PMID: 10728704]

[63] Abramsson A, Berlin Ö, Papayan H, Paulin D, Shani M, Betsholtz C. Analysis of mural cell recruitment to tumor vessels. Circulation 2002; 105(1): 112-7. [http://dx.doi.org/10.1161/hc0102.101437] [PMID: 11772885]

[64] Hosaka K, Yang Y, Seki T, *et al.* Pericyte–fibroblast transition promotes tumor growth and metastasis. Proc Natl Acad Sci USA 2016; 113(38): E5618-27. [http://dx.doi.org/10.1073/pnas.1608384113] [PMID: 27608497]

[65] Balkwill F, Mantovani A. Inflammation and cancer: back to Virchow? Lancet 2001; 357(9255): 539-45. [http://dx.doi.org/10.1016/S0140-6736(00)04046-0] [PMID: 11229684]

[66] Karin M. Nuclear factor-κB in cancer development and progression. Nature 2006; 441(7092): 431-6. [http://dx.doi.org/10.1038/nature04870] [PMID: 16724054]

[67] Mantovani A, Allavena P, Sica A, Balkwill F. Cancer-related inflammation. Nature 2008; 454(7203): 436-44. [http://dx.doi.org/10.1038/nature07205] [PMID: 18650914]

[68] de Visser KE, Eichten A, Coussens LM. Paradoxical roles of the immune system during cancer development. Nat Rev Cancer 2006; 6(1): 24-37. [http://dx.doi.org/10.1038/nrc1782] [PMID: 16397525]

[69] Alpert L, Yassan L, Poon R, *et al.* Targeted mutational analysis of inflammatory bowel disease–associated colorectal cancers. Hum Pathol 2019; 89: 44-50. [http://dx.doi.org/10.1016/j.humpath.2019.04.013] [PMID: 31054900]

[70] Lopes de Oliveira GA, Alarcón de la Lastra C, Rosillo MÁ, *et al.* Preventive effect of bergenin against the development of TNBS-induced acute colitis in rats is associated with inflammatory mediators inhibition and NLRP3/ASC inflammasome signaling pathways. Chem Biol Interact 2019; 297: 25-33. [http://dx.doi.org/10.1016/j.cbi.2018.10.020] [PMID: 30365937]

[71] Condeelis J, Pollard JW. Macrophages: obligate partners for tumor cell migration, invasion, and metastasis. Cell 2006; 124(2): 263-6. [http://dx.doi.org/10.1016/j.cell.2006.01.007] [PMID: 16439202]

[72] Komohara Y, Jinushi M, Takeya M. Clinical significance of macrophage heterogeneity in human malignant tumors. Cancer Sci 2014; 105(1): 1-8. [http://dx.doi.org/10.1111/cas.12314] [PMID: 24168081]

[73] Ruffell B, Coussens LM. Macrophages and therapeutic resistance in cancer. Cancer Cell 2015; 27(4): 462-72. [http://dx.doi.org/10.1016/j.ccell.2015.02.015] [PMID: 25858805]

[74] Giraldo NA, Sanchez-Salas R, Peske JD, *et al.* The clinical role of the TME in solid cancer. Br J

Cancer 2019; 120(1): 45-53.
[http://dx.doi.org/10.1038/s41416-018-0327-z] [PMID: 30413828]

[75] Hanahan D, Coussens LM. Accessories to the crime: functions of cells recruited to the tumor microenvironment. Cancer Cell 2012; 21(3): 309-22.
[http://dx.doi.org/10.1016/j.ccr.2012.02.022] [PMID: 22439926]

[76] Solinas G, Germano G, Mantovani A, Allavena P. Tumor-associated macrophages (TAM) as major players of the cancer-related inflammation. J Leukoc Biol 2009; 86(5): 1065-73.
[http://dx.doi.org/10.1189/jlb.0609385] [PMID: 19741157]

[77] Weber CE, Kuo PC. The tumor microenvironment. Surg Oncol 2012; 21(3): 172-7.
[http://dx.doi.org/10.1016/j.suronc.2011.09.001] [PMID: 21963199]

[78] Murdoch C, Muthana M, Coffelt SB, Lewis CE. The role of myeloid cells in the promotion of tumour angiogenesis. Nat Rev Cancer 2008; 8(8): 618-31.
[http://dx.doi.org/10.1038/nrc2444] [PMID: 18633355]

[79] Zhang W, Wang L, Zhou D, Cui Q, Zhao D, Wu Y. Expression of tumor-associated macrophages and vascular endothelial growth factor correlates with poor prognosis of peripheral T-cell lymphoma, not otherwise specified. Leuk Lymphoma 2011; 52(1): 46-52.
[http://dx.doi.org/10.3109/10428194.2010.529204] [PMID: 21077742]

[80] Mathias RA, Gopal SK, Simpson RJ. Contribution of cells undergoing epithelial–mesenchymal transition to the tumour microenvironment. J Proteomics 2013; 78: 545-57.
[http://dx.doi.org/10.1016/j.jprot.2012.10.016] [PMID: 23099347]

[81] Cano RLELH. Introduction to T and B lymphocytes.Autoimmunity: From Bench to Bedside. Bogota, Colombia: El Rosario University Press 2013.

[82] Alberts BJA, Lewis J, *et al.* Lymphocytes and the Cellular Basis of Adaptive Immunity. 4th ed. Molecular Biology of the Cell. New York: Garland Science; 2002.

[83] Gutcher I, Becher B. APC-derived cytokines and T cell polarization in autoimmune inflammation. J Clin Invest 2007; 117(5): 1119-27.
[http://dx.doi.org/10.1172/JCI31720] [PMID: 17476341]

[84] Sakaguchi S, Sakaguchi N, Asano M, Itoh M, Toda M. Immunologic self-tolerance maintained by activated T cells expressing IL-2 receptor alpha-chains (CD25). Breakdown of a single mechanism of self-tolerance causes various autoimmune diseases. Journal of immunology 1995; 155(3): 1151-64.

[85] Fantini MC, Favale A, Onali S, Facciotti F. Tumor Infiltrating Regulatory T Cells in Sporadic and Colitis-Associated Colorectal Cancer: The Red Little Riding Hood and the Wolf. Int J Mol Sci 2020; 21(18): 6744.
[http://dx.doi.org/10.3390/ijms21186744] [PMID: 32937953]

[86] Whiteside TL. FOXP3+ Treg as a therapeutic target for promoting anti-tumor immunity. Expert Opin Ther Targets 2018; 22(4): 353-63.
[http://dx.doi.org/10.1080/14728222.2018.1451514] [PMID: 29532697]

[87] Chaudhary B, Elkord E, Regulatory T. Regulatory T Cells in the Tumor Microenvironment and Cancer Progression: Role and Therapeutic Targeting. Vaccines (Basel) 2016; 4(3): 28.
[http://dx.doi.org/10.3390/vaccines4030028] [PMID: 27509527]

[88] Jameson SC, Masopust D. Understanding Subset Diversity in T Cell Memory. Immunity 2018; 48(2): 214-26.
[http://dx.doi.org/10.1016/j.immuni.2018.02.010] [PMID: 29466754]

[89] Mueller SN, Mackay LK. Tissue-resident memory T cells: local specialists in immune defence. Nat Rev Immunol 2016; 16(2): 79-89.
[http://dx.doi.org/10.1038/nri.2015.3] [PMID: 26688350]

[90] Park SL, Gebhardt T, Mackay LK. Tissue-Resident Memory T Cells in Cancer Immunosurveillance.

Trends Immunol 2019; 40(8): 735-47.
[http://dx.doi.org/10.1016/j.it.2019.06.002] [PMID: 31255505]

[91] Kumar BV, Connors TJ, Farber DL, Human T. Human T Cell Development, Localization, and Function throughout Life. Immunity 2018; 48(2): 202-13.
[http://dx.doi.org/10.1016/j.immuni.2018.01.007] [PMID: 29466753]

[92] Kaech SM, Wherry EJ. Heterogeneity and cell-fate decisions in effector and memory CD8+ T cell differentiation during viral infection. Immunity 2007; 27(3): 393-405.
[http://dx.doi.org/10.1016/j.immuni.2007.08.007] [PMID: 17892848]

[93] Sallusto F, Lanzavecchia A, Araki K, Ahmed R. From vaccines to memory and back. Immunity 2010; 33(4): 451-63.
[http://dx.doi.org/10.1016/j.immuni.2010.10.008] [PMID: 21029957]

[94] Ho AW, Kupper TS. T cells and the skin: from protective immunity to inflammatory skin disorders. Nat Rev Immunol 2019; 19(8): 490-502.
[http://dx.doi.org/10.1038/s41577-019-0162-3] [PMID: 30992525]

[95] Macallan D, Borghans J, Asquith B, Human T. Human T Cell Memory: A Dynamic View. Vaccines (Basel) 2017; 5(1).
[http://dx.doi.org/10.3390/vaccines5010005] [PMID: 28165397]

[96] Akdis M, Palomares O, van de Veen W, van Splunter M, Akdis CA. TH17 and TH22 cells: a confusion of antimicrobial response with tissue inflammation versus protection. J Allergy Clin Immunol 2012; 129(6): 1438-49.
[http://dx.doi.org/10.1016/j.jaci.2012.05.003]

[97] Zhu J. T Helper Cell Differentiation, Heterogeneity, and Plasticity. Cold Spring Harb Perspect Biol 2018; 10(10): a030338.
[http://dx.doi.org/10.1101/cshperspect.a030338] [PMID: 28847903]

[98] Hsieh CS, Macatonia SE, Tripp CS, Wolf SF, O'Garra A, Murphy KM. Development of TH1 CD4+ T cells through IL-12 produced by Listeria-induced macrophages. Science 1993; 260(5107): 547-9.
[http://dx.doi.org/10.1126/science.8097338] [PMID: 8097338]

[99] Manetti R, Parronchi P, Giudizi MG, *et al.* Natural killer cell stimulatory factor (interleukin 12 [IL-12]) induces T helper type 1 (Th1)-specific immune responses and inhibits the development of IL-4-producing Th cells. J Exp Med 1993; 177(4): 1199-204.
[http://dx.doi.org/10.1084/jem.177.4.1199] [PMID: 8096238]

[100] Dardalhon V, Awasthi A, Kwon H, *et al.* IL-4 inhibits TGF-β-induced Foxp3+ T cells and, together with TGF-β, generates IL-9+ IL-10+ Foxp3− effector T cells. Nat Immunol 2008; 9(12): 1347-55.
[http://dx.doi.org/10.1038/ni.1677] [PMID: 18997793]

[101] Saraiva M, Christensen JR, Veldhoen M, Murphy TL, Murphy KM, O'Garra A. Interleukin-10 production by Th1 cells requires interleukin-12-induced STAT4 transcription factor and ERK MAP kinase activation by high antigen dose. Immunity 2009; 31(2): 209-19.
[http://dx.doi.org/10.1016/j.immuni.2009.05.012] [PMID: 19646904]

[102] Goswami R, Kaplan MH. Gcn5 is required for PU.1-dependent IL-9 induction in Th9 cells. J Immunol 2012; 189(6): 3026-33.
[http://dx.doi.org/10.4049/jimmunol.1201496] [PMID: 22904310]

[103] Goswami R, Jabeen R, Yagi R, *et al.* STAT6-dependent regulation of Th9 development. J Immunol 2012; 188(3): 968-75.
[http://dx.doi.org/10.4049/jimmunol.1102840] [PMID: 22180613]

[104] Zhu X, Zhu J. CD4 T Helper Cell Subsets and Related Human Immunological Disorders. Int J Mol Sci 2020; 21(21): 8011.
[http://dx.doi.org/10.3390/ijms21218011] [PMID: 33126494]

[105] Tesmer LA, Lundy SK, Sarkar S, Fox DA. Th17 cells in human disease. Immunol Rev 2008; 223(1):

87-113.
[http://dx.doi.org/10.1111/j.1600-065X.2008.00628.x] [PMID: 18613831]

[106] Burkett PR, Lee Y, Peters A, Kuchroo VK. Th17 and Th22 Cells. Encyclopedia of Immunobiology. Oxford: Academic Press 2016; pp. 307-18.
[http://dx.doi.org/10.1016/B978-0-12-374279-7.08004-8]

[107] Coffelt SB, Lewis CE, Naldini L, Brown JM, Ferrara N, De Palma M. Elusive identities and overlapping phenotypes of proangiogenic myeloid cells in tumors. Am J Pathol 2010; 176(4): 1564-76.
[http://dx.doi.org/10.2353/ajpath.2010.090786] [PMID: 20167863]

[108] Qian BZ, Pollard JW. Macrophage diversity enhances tumor progression and metastasis. Cell 2010; 141(1): 39-51.
[http://dx.doi.org/10.1016/j.cell.2010.03.014] [PMID: 20371344]

[109] Valenti R, Huber V, Iero M, Filipazzi P, Parmiani G, Rivoltini L. Tumor-released microvesicles as vehicles of immunosuppression. Cancer Res 2007; 67(7): 2912-5.
[http://dx.doi.org/10.1158/0008-5472.CAN-07-0520] [PMID: 17409393]

[110] Baranyi U, Winter B, Gugerell A, *et al.* Primary Human Fibroblasts in Culture Switch to a Myofibroblast-Like Phenotype Independently of TGF Beta. Cells 2019; 8(7): E721.
[http://dx.doi.org/10.3390/cells8070721] [PMID: 31337073]

[111] Marsh T, Pietras K, McAllister SS. Fibroblasts as architects of cancer pathogenesis. Biochim Biophys Acta Mol Basis Dis 2013; 1832(7): 1070-8.
[http://dx.doi.org/10.1016/j.bbadis.2012.10.013] [PMID: 23123598]

[112] Gabbiani G, Ryan GB, Majno G. Presence of modified fibroblasts in granulation tissue and their possible role in wound contraction. Experientia 1971; 27(5): 549-50.
[http://dx.doi.org/10.1007/BF02147594] [PMID: 5132594]

[113] Majno G, Gabbiani G, Hirschel BJ, Ryan GB, Statkov PR. Contraction of granulation tissue in vitro: similarity to smooth muscle. Science 1971; 173(3996): 548-50.
[http://dx.doi.org/10.1126/science.173.3996.548] [PMID: 4327529]

[114] Hinz B, Celetta G, Tomasek JJ, Gabbiani G, Chaponnier C. Alpha-smooth muscle actin expression upregulates fibroblast contractile activity. Mol Biol Cell 2001; 12(9): 2730-41.
[http://dx.doi.org/10.1091/mbc.12.9.2730] [PMID: 11553712]

[115] Tomasek JJ, Gabbiani G, Hinz B, Chaponnier C, Brown RA. Myofibroblasts and mechano-regulation of connective tissue remodelling. Nat Rev Mol Cell Biol 2002; 3(5): 349-63.
[http://dx.doi.org/10.1038/nrm809] [PMID: 11988769]

[116] Li B, Wang JHC. Fibroblasts and myofibroblasts in wound healing: Force generation and measurement. J Tissue Viability 2011; 20(4): 108-20.
[http://dx.doi.org/10.1016/j.jtv.2009.11.004] [PMID: 19995679]

[117] Sandberg TP, Stuart MPME, Oosting J, Tollenaar RAEM, Sier CFM, Mesker WE. Increased expression of cancer-associated fibroblast markers at the invasive front and its association with tumor-stroma ratio in colorectal cancer. BMC Cancer 2019; 19(1): 284.
[http://dx.doi.org/10.1186/s12885-019-5462-2] [PMID: 30922247]

[118] Kalluri R. The biology and function of fibroblasts in cancer. Nat Rev Cancer 2016; 16(9): 582-98.
[http://dx.doi.org/10.1038/nrc.2016.73] [PMID: 27550820]

[119] Lecomte J, Masset A, Blacher S, *et al.* Bone marrow-derived myofibroblasts are the providers of pro-invasive matrix metalloproteinase 13 in primary tumor. Neoplasia 2012; 14(10): 943-51.
[http://dx.doi.org/10.1593/neo.121092] [PMID: 23097628]

[120] Tremblay G. Stromal aspects of breast carcinoma. Exp Mol Pathol 1979; 31(1): 248-60.
[http://dx.doi.org/10.1016/0014-4800(79)90026-1] [PMID: 222605]

[121] Ishii G, Ochiai A, Neri S. Phenotypic and functional heterogeneity of cancer-associated fibroblast within the tumor microenvironment. Adv Drug Deliv Rev 2016; 99(Pt B): 186-96. [http://dx.doi.org/10.1016/j.addr.2015.07.007]

[122] LeBleu VS, Kalluri R. A peek into cancer-associated fibroblasts: origins, functions and translational impact. Dis Model Mech 2018; 11(4): dmm029447. [http://dx.doi.org/10.1242/dmm.029447] [PMID: 29686035]

[123] Balzar M, Winter MJ, de Boer CJ, Litvinov SV. The biology of the 17–1A antigen (Ep-CAM). J Mol Med (Berl) 1999; 77(10): 699-712. [http://dx.doi.org/10.1007/s001099900038] [PMID: 10606205]

[124] Huang L, Yang Y, Yang F, *et al.* Functions of EpCAM in physiological processes and diseases (Review). Int J Mol Med 2018; 42(4): 1771-85. [http://dx.doi.org/10.3892/ijmm.2018.3764] [PMID: 30015855]

[125] Xing F, Saidou J, Watabe K. Cancer associated fibroblasts (CAFs) in tumor microenvironment. Front Biosci 2010; 15(1): 166-79. [http://dx.doi.org/10.2741/3613] [PMID: 20036813]

[126] Sukowati CHC, Anfuso B, Crocé LS, Tiribelli C. The role of multipotent cancer associated fibroblasts in hepatocarcinogenesis. BMC Cancer 2015; 15(1): 188. [http://dx.doi.org/10.1186/s12885-015-1196-y] [PMID: 25879842]

[127] Nurmik M, Ullmann P, Rodriguez F, Haan S, Letellier E. In search of definitions: Cancer-associated fibroblasts and their markers. Int J Cancer 2020; 146(4): 895-905. [http://dx.doi.org/10.1002/ijc.32193] [PMID: 30734283]

[128] Orimo A, Weinberg RA. Heterogeneity of stromal fibroblasts in tumor. Cancer Biol Ther 2007; 6(4): 618-9. [http://dx.doi.org/10.4161/cbt.6.4.4255] [PMID: 18027438]

[129] Bu L, Baba H, Yoshida N, *et al.* Biological heterogeneity and versatility of cancer-associated fibroblasts in the tumor microenvironment. Oncogene 2019; 38(25): 4887-901. [http://dx.doi.org/10.1038/s41388-019-0765-y] [PMID: 30816343]

[130] Santi A, Kugeratski FG, Zanivan S. Cancer Associated Fibroblasts: The Architects of Stroma Remodeling. Proteomics 2018; 18(5-6): 1700167. [http://dx.doi.org/10.1002/pmic.201700167] [PMID: 29280568]

[131] Reagan MR, Kaplan DL. Concise review: Mesenchymal stem cell tumor-homing: detection methods in disease model systems. Stem Cells 2011; 29(6): 920-7. [http://dx.doi.org/10.1002/stem.645] [PMID: 21557390]

[132] Quante M, Tu SP, Tomita H, *et al.* Bone marrow-derived myofibroblasts contribute to the mesenchymal stem cell niche and promote tumor growth. Cancer Cell 2011; 19(2): 257-72. [http://dx.doi.org/10.1016/j.ccr.2011.01.020] [PMID: 21316604]

[133] Fiori ME, Di Franco S, Villanova L, Bianca P, Stassi G, De Maria R. Cancer-associated fibroblasts as abettors of tumor progression at the crossroads of EMT and therapy resistance. Mol Cancer 2019; 18(1): 70. [http://dx.doi.org/10.1186/s12943-019-0994-2] [PMID: 30927908]

[134] Kuzet SE, Gaggioli C. Fibroblast activation in cancer: when seed fertilizes soil. Cell Tissue Res 2016; 365(3): 607-19. [http://dx.doi.org/10.1007/s00441-016-2467-x] [PMID: 27474009]

[135] Calvo F, Ege N, Grande-Garcia A, *et al.* Mechanotransduction and YAP-dependent matrix remodelling is required for the generation and maintenance of cancer-associated fibroblasts. Nat Cell Biol 2013; 15(6): 637-46. [http://dx.doi.org/10.1038/ncb2756] [PMID: 23708000]

[136] Paget S. The distribution of secondary growths in cancer of the breast. 1889. Cancer Metastasis Rev 1989; 8(2): 98-101.
[PMID: 2673568]

[137] Balkwill FR, Capasso M, Hagemann T. The tumor microenvironment at a glance. The Company of Biologists Ltd 2012.
[http://dx.doi.org/10.1242/jcs.116392]

[138] Gascard P, Tlsty TD. Carcinoma-associated fibroblasts: orchestrating the composition of malignancy. Genes Dev 2016; 30(9): 1002-19.
[http://dx.doi.org/10.1101/gad.279737.116] [PMID: 27151975]

[139] Mishra PJ, Mishra PJ, Humeniuk R, *et al.* Carcinoma-associated fibroblast-like differentiation of human mesenchymal stem cells. Cancer Res 2008; 68(11): 4331-9.
[http://dx.doi.org/10.1158/0008-5472.CAN-08-0943] [PMID: 18519693]

[140] Radisky DC, Kenny PA, Bissell MJ. Fibrosis and cancer: Do myofibroblasts come also from epithelial cells via EMT? J Cell Biochem 2007; 101(4): 830-9.
[http://dx.doi.org/10.1002/jcb.21186] [PMID: 17211838]

[141] Desmoulière A, Guyot C, Gabbiani G. The stroma reaction myofibroblast: a key player in the control of tumor cell behavior. Int J Dev Biol 2004; 48(5-6): 509-17.
[http://dx.doi.org/10.1387/ijdb.041802ad] [PMID: 15349825]

[142] Orimo A, Weinberg RA. Stromal fibroblasts in cancer: a novel tumor-promoting cell type. Cell Cycle 2006; 5(15): 1597-601.
[http://dx.doi.org/10.4161/cc.5.15.3112] [PMID: 16880743]

[143] Haslene-Hox H, Oveland E, Berg KC, *et al.* A new method for isolation of interstitial fluid from human solid tumors applied to proteomic analysis of ovarian carcinoma tissue. PLoS One 2011; 6(4): e19217.
[http://dx.doi.org/10.1371/journal.pone.0019217] [PMID: 21541282]

[144] Takabe K, Spiegel S. Export of sphingosine-1-phosphate and cancer progression. J Lipid Res 2014; 55(9): 1839-46.
[http://dx.doi.org/10.1194/jlr.R046656] [PMID: 24474820]

[145] Wiig H, Swartz MA. Interstitial fluid and lymph formation and transport: physiological regulation and roles in inflammation and cancer. Physiol Rev 2012; 92(3): 1005-60.
[http://dx.doi.org/10.1152/physrev.00037.2011] [PMID: 22811424]

[146] Jahanban-Esfahlan R, Seidi K, Banimohamad-Shotorbani B, Jahanban-Esfahlan A, Yousefi B. Combination of nanotechnology with vascular targeting agents for effective cancer therapy. J Cell Physiol 2018; 233(4): 2982-92.
[http://dx.doi.org/10.1002/jcp.26051] [PMID: 28608554]

[147] Jahanban-Esfahlan R, Seidi K, Zarghami N. Tumor vascular infarction: prospects and challenges. Int J Hematol 2017; 105(3): 244-56.
[http://dx.doi.org/10.1007/s12185-016-2171-3] [PMID: 28044258]

[148] Spill F, Reynolds DS, Kamm RD, Zaman MH. Impact of the physical microenvironment on tumor progression and metastasis. Curr Opin Biotechnol 2016; 40: 41-8.
[http://dx.doi.org/10.1016/j.copbio.2016.02.007] [PMID: 26938687]

[149] Del Prete A, Schioppa T, Tiberio L, Stabile H, Sozzani S. Leukocyte trafficking in tumor microenvironment. Curr Opin Pharmacol 2017; 35: 40-7.
[http://dx.doi.org/10.1016/j.coph.2017.05.004] [PMID: 28577499]

[150] Frisch J, Angenendt A, Hoth M, Prates Roma L, Lis A. STIM-Orai Channels and Reactive Oxygen Species in the Tumor Microenvironment. Cancers (Basel) 2019; 11(4): 457.
[http://dx.doi.org/10.3390/cancers11040457] [PMID: 30935064]

[151] Dominiak A, Chełstowska B, Olejarz W, Nowicka G. Communication in the cancer microenvironment as a target for therapeutic interventions. Cancers (Basel) 2020; 12(5): 1232. [http://dx.doi.org/10.3390/cancers12051232]

[152] Jahanban-Esfahlan R, Seidi K, Monhemi H, *et al.* RGD delivery of truncated coagulase to tumor vasculature affords local thrombotic activity to induce infarction of tumors in mice. Sci Rep 2017; 7(1): 8126. [http://dx.doi.org/10.1038/s41598-017-05326-9] [PMID: 28811469]

[153] Orr JW. The changes antecedent to tumour formation during the treatment of mouse skin with carcinogenic hydrocarbons. J Pathol Bacteriol 1938; 46(3): 495-515. [http://dx.doi.org/10.1002/path.1700460310]

[154] Tarin D. Tissue interactions in carcinogenesis. Academic Press 1972.

[155] Folkman J. Angiogenesis. Annu Rev Med. 2006;57:1-18. [http://dx.doi.org/10.1146/annurev.med.57.121304.131306] [PMID: 16409133]

[156] Tarin D. Sequential electron microscopical study of experimental mouse skin carcinogenesis. Int J Cancer 1967; 2(3): 195-211. [http://dx.doi.org/10.1002/ijc.2910020302] [PMID: 6041987]

[157] Tarin D. Fine structure of murine mammary tumours: the relationship between epithelium and connective tissue in neoplasms induced by various agents. Br J Cancer 1969; 23(2): 417-25. [http://dx.doi.org/10.1038/bjc.1969.54] [PMID: 5788050]

[158] Tarin D. Cell and tissue interactions in carcinogenesis and metastasis and their clinical significance. Semin Cancer Biol 2011; 21(2): 72-82. [http://dx.doi.org/10.1016/j.semcancer.2010.12.006] [PMID: 21147229]

[159] Tarin D. Inappropriate gene expression in human cancer and its far-reaching biological and clinical significance. Cancer Metastasis Rev 2012; 31(1-2): 21-39. [http://dx.doi.org/10.1007/s10555-011-9326-8] [PMID: 22138779]

[160] Billingham RE, Orr JW, Woodhouse DL. Transplantation of skin components during chemical carcinogenesis with 20-methylcholanthrene. Br J Cancer 1951; 5(4): 417-32. [http://dx.doi.org/10.1038/bjc.1951.48] [PMID: 14904839]

[161] Paino F, La Noce M, Di Nucci D, *et al.* Human adipose stem cell differentiation is highly affected by cancer cells both *in vitro* and *in vivo*: implication for autologous fat grafting. Cell Death Dis 2018; 8(1): e2568. [http://dx.doi.org/10.1038/cddis.2016.308]

[162] Guan J, Chen J. Mesenchymal stem cells in the tumor microenvironment. Biomed Rep 2013; 1(4): 517-21. [http://dx.doi.org/10.3892/br.2013.103] [PMID: 24648978]

[163] Relation T, Dominici M, Horwitz EM. Concise review: an (im) penetrable shield: how the tumor microenvironment protects cancer stem cells. Stem Cells 2017; 35(5): 1123-30. [http://dx.doi.org/10.1002/stem.2596] [PMID: 28207184]

[164] Lackie J. Cytokines. Oxford University Press; 2010.

[165] Cytokine. In: Wilkins WKHLW, Ed. Stedman's Medical Dictionary. 28th ed. Philadelphia, PA, USA2006.

[166] Kowal J, Tkach M, Théry C. Biogenesis and secretion of exosomes. Curr Opin Cell Biol 2014; 29: 116-25. [http://dx.doi.org/10.1016/j.ceb.2014.05.004] [PMID: 24959705]

[167] Li I, Nabet BY. Exosomes in the tumor microenvironment as mediators of cancer therapy resistance. Mol Cancer 2019; 18(1): 32. [http://dx.doi.org/10.1186/s12943-019-0975-5] [PMID: 30823926]

[168] Saigusa D, Okudaira M, Wang J, *et al.* Simultaneous quantification of sphingolipids in small quantities of liver by LC-MS/MS. Mass Spectrometry 2014; 3(3): S0046.

[169] Kasuga K, Suga T, Mano N. Bioanalytical insights into mediator lipidomics. J Pharm Biomed Anal 2015; 113: 151-62.
[http://dx.doi.org/10.1016/j.jpba.2015.02.011] [PMID: 25769667]

[170] Nagahashi M, Hait NC, Maceyka M, *et al.* Sphingosine-1-phosphate in chronic intestinal inflammation and cancer. Adv Biol Regul 2014; 54: 112-20.
[http://dx.doi.org/10.1016/j.jbior.2013.10.001] [PMID: 24210073]

[171] Fernández-Messina L, Ashiru O, Boutet P, *et al.* Differential mechanisms of shedding of the glycosylphosphatidylinositol (GPI)-anchored NKG2D ligands. J Biol Chem 2010; 285(12): 8543-51.
[http://dx.doi.org/10.1074/jbc.M109.045906] [PMID: 20080967]

[172] Raneros AB, Minguela A, Rodriguez RM, *et al.* Increasing TIMP3 expression by hypomethylating agents diminishes soluble MICA, MICB and ULBP2 shedding in acute myeloid leukemia, facilitating NK cell-mediated immune recognition. Oncotarget 2017; 8(19): 31959-76.
[http://dx.doi.org/10.18632/oncotarget.16657] [PMID: 28404876]

[173] Rabinovich GA, Gabrilovich D, Sotomayor EM. Immunosuppressive strategies that are mediated by tumor cells. Annu Rev Immunol 2007; 25(1): 267-96.
[http://dx.doi.org/10.1146/annurev.immunol.25.022106.141609] [PMID: 17134371]

[174] Nausch N, Cerwenka A. NKG2D ligands in tumor immunity. Oncogene 2008; 27(45): 5944-58.
[http://dx.doi.org/10.1038/onc.2008.272] [PMID: 18836475]

[175] Cox MB, Johnson JL. Evidence for Hsp90 Co-chaperones in Regulating Hsp90 Function and Promoting Client Protein Folding.Chaperones: Methods and Protocols. New York, NY: Springer New York 2018; pp. 397-422.
[http://dx.doi.org/10.1007/978-1-4939-7477-1_28]

[176] Gonzalez M, De Brasi C, Ferri C, Bengió R, Bianchini M, Larripa I. *CAMKIIγ, HSP70* and *HSP90* transcripts are differentially expressed in chronic myeloid leukemia cells from patients with resistant mutated disease. Leuk Lymphoma 2014; 55(9): 2101-8.
[http://dx.doi.org/10.3109/10428194.2013.861070] [PMID: 24206096]

[177] Biaoxue R, Xiling J, Shuanying Y, *et al.* Upregulation of Hsp90-beta and annexin A1 correlates with poor survival and lymphatic metastasis in lung cancer patients. J Exp Clin Cancer Res 2012; 31(1): 70.
[http://dx.doi.org/10.1186/1756-9966-31-70] [PMID: 22929401]

[178] Becker B, Multhoff G, Farkas B, *et al.* Induction of Hsp90 protein expression in malignant melanomas and melanoma metastases. Exp Dermatol 2004; 13(1): 27-32.
[http://dx.doi.org/10.1111/j.0906-6705.2004.00114.x] [PMID: 15009113]

[179] Yano M, Naito Z, Yokoyama M, *et al.* Expression of hsp90 and cyclin D1 in human breast cancer. Cancer Lett 1999; 137(1): 45-51.
[http://dx.doi.org/10.1016/S0304-3835(98)00338-3] [PMID: 10376793]

[180] Zhang S, Guo S, Li Z, Li D, Zhan Q. High expression of HSP90 is associated with poor prognosis in patients with colorectal cancer. PeerJ 2019; 7: e7946.
[http://dx.doi.org/10.7717/peerj.7946]

[181] Taha EA, Ono K, Eguchi T. Roles of Extracellular HSPs as Biomarkers in Immune Surveillance and Immune Evasion. Int J Mol Sci 2019; 20(18): 4588.
[http://dx.doi.org/10.3390/ijms20184588] [PMID: 31533245]

[182] Chauvin JM, Zarour HM. TIGIT in cancer immunotherapy. J Immunother Cancer 2020; 8(2): e000957.
[http://dx.doi.org/10.1136/jitc-2020-000957] [PMID: 32900861]

[183] Nagumo Y, Iguchi-Manaka A, Yamashita-Kanemaru Y, *et al.* Increased CD112 expression in

methylcholanthrene-induced tumors in CD155-deficient mice. PloS one 2014; 9(11): e112415. [http://dx.doi.org/10.1371/journal.pone.0112415]

[184] Masson D, Jarry A, Baury B, *et al.* Overexpression of the *CD155* gene in human colorectal carcinoma. Gut 2001; 49(2): 236-40. [http://dx.doi.org/10.1136/gut.49.2.236] [PMID: 11454801]

[185] Carlsten M, Björkström NK, Norell H, *et al.* DNAX accessory molecule-1 mediated recognition of freshly isolated ovarian carcinoma by resting natural killer cells. Cancer Res 2007; 67(3): 1317-25. [http://dx.doi.org/10.1158/0008-5472.CAN-06-2264] [PMID: 17283169]

[186] Lopez M, Aoubala M, Jordier F, Isnardon D, Gomez S, Dubreuil P. The human poliovirus receptor related 2 protein is a new hematopoietic/endothelial homophilic adhesion molecule. Blood 1998; 92(12): 4602-11. [http://dx.doi.org/10.1182/blood.V92.12.4602] [PMID: 9845526]

[187] Iguchi-Manaka A, Okumura G, Ichioka E, *et al.* High expression of soluble CD155 in estrogen receptor-negative breast cancer. Breast Cancer 2020; 27(1): 92-9. [http://dx.doi.org/10.1007/s12282-019-00999-8] [PMID: 31372841]

[188] Henke E, Nandigama R, Ergün S. Extracellular matrix in the tumor microenvironment and its impact on cancer therapy. Front Mol Biosci 2020; 6: 160. [http://dx.doi.org/10.3389/fmolb.2019.00160] [PMID: 32118030]

[189] Conti JA, Kendall TJ, Bateman A, *et al.* The desmoplastic reaction surrounding hepatic colorectal adenocarcinoma metastases aids tumor growth and survival via alphav integrin ligation. Clin Cancer Res 2008; 14(20): 6405-13. [http://dx.doi.org/10.1158/1078-0432.CCR-08-0816] [PMID: 18927279]

[190] Schober M, Jesenofsky R, Faissner R, *et al.* Desmoplasia and chemoresistance in pancreatic cancer. Cancers (Basel) 2014; 6(4): 2137-54. [http://dx.doi.org/10.3390/cancers6042137] [PMID: 25337831]

[191] Tarin D. Clinical and biological implications of the tumor microenvironment. Cancer Microenviron 2012; 5(2): 95-112. [http://dx.doi.org/10.1007/s12307-012-0099-6] [PMID: 22782446]

[192] Roschke AV, Kirsch IR. Targeting karyotypic complexity and chromosomal instability of cancer cells. Curr Drug Targets 2010; 11(10): 1341-50. [http://dx.doi.org/10.2174/1389450111007011341] [PMID: 20840077]

[193] Al-Sohaily S, Biankin A, Leong R, Kohonen-Corish M, Warusavitarne J. Molecular pathways in colorectal cancer. J Gastroenterol Hepatol 2012; 27(9): 1423-31. [http://dx.doi.org/10.1111/j.1440-1746.2012.07200.x] [PMID: 22694276]

[194] Yao Y, Dai W. Genomic instability and cancer. J Carcinog Mutagen 2014; 5. [PMID: 25541596]

[195] Dipple A. DNA adducts of chemical carcinogens. Carcinogenesis 1995; 16(3): 437-41. [http://dx.doi.org/10.1093/carcin/16.3.437] [PMID: 7697795]

[196] Negrini S, Gorgoulis VG, Halazonetis TD. Genomic instability — an evolving hallmark of cancer. Nat Rev Mol Cell Biol 2010; 11(3): 220-8. [http://dx.doi.org/10.1038/nrm2858] [PMID: 20177397]

[197] Abbas T, Keaton MA, Dutta A. Genomic instability in cancer. Cold Spring Harb Perspect Biol 2013; 5(3): a012914. [http://dx.doi.org/10.1101/cshperspect.a012914] [PMID: 23335075]

[198] Shen Z. Genomic instability and cancer: an introduction. J Mol Cell Biol 2011; 3(1): 1-3. [http://dx.doi.org/10.1093/jmcb/mjq057] [PMID: 21278445]

[199] Wenzel ES, Singh AT. Cell-cycle checkpoints and aneuploidy on the path to cancer. in vivo 2018;

32(1): 1-5.

[200] Schafer KA. The cell cycle: a review. Vet Pathol 1998; 35(6): 461-78. [http://dx.doi.org/10.1177/030098589803500601] [PMID: 9823588]

[201] Baserga R. A study of nucleic acid synthesis in ascites tumor cells by two-emulsion autoradiography. J Cell Biol 1962; 12(3): 633-7. [http://dx.doi.org/10.1083/jcb.12.3.633] [PMID: 13865584]

[202] Swaffer MP, Jones AW, Flynn HR, Snijders AP, Nurse P. CDK substrate phosphorylation and ordering the cell cycle. Cell 2016; 167(7): 1750-61. [http://dx.doi.org/10.1016/j.cell.2016.11.034]

[203] Fisher RP. The CDK network: linking cycles of cell division and gene expression. Genes Cancer 2012; 3(11-12): 731-8. [http://dx.doi.org/10.1177/1947601912473308] [PMID: 23634260]

[204] Hindley C, Philpott A. The cell cycle and pluripotency. Biochem J 2013; 451(2): 135-43. [http://dx.doi.org/10.1042/BJ20121627] [PMID: 23535166]

[205] Hwang HC, Clurman BE. Cyclin E in normal and neoplastic cell cycles. Oncogene 2005; 24(17): 2776-86. [http://dx.doi.org/10.1038/sj.onc.1208613] [PMID: 15838514]

[206] Xuereb J, Blundell R. The Role of Cell Cycle Regulation in Cancer. Res J Biologic Sci 2008; 3 (2): 251-7.

[207] Sherr CJ, Roberts JM. Living with or without cyclins and cyclin-dependent kinases. Genes Dev 2004; 18(22): 2699-711. [http://dx.doi.org/10.1101/gad.1256504] [PMID: 15545627]

[208] Cappell SD, Chung M, Jaimovich A, Spencer SL, Meyer T. Irreversible APCCdh1 inactivation underlies the point of no return for cell-cycle entry. Cell 2016; 166(1): 167-80. [http://dx.doi.org/10.1016/j.cell.2016.05.077] [PMID: 27368103]

[209] Cappell SD, Mark KG, Garbett D, Pack LR, Rape M, Meyer T. EMI1 switches from being a substrate to an inhibitor of APC/C^{CDH1} to start the cell cycle. Nature 2018; 558(7709): 313-7. [http://dx.doi.org/10.1038/s41586-018-0199-7] [PMID: 29875408]

[210] Satyanarayana A, Kaldis P. Mammalian cell-cycle regulation: several Cdks, numerous cyclins and diverse compensatory mechanisms. Oncogene 2009; 28(33): 2925-39. [http://dx.doi.org/10.1038/onc.2009.170] [PMID: 19561645]

[211] Chang DC, Xu N, Luo KQ. Degradation of cyclin B is required for the onset of anaphase in Mammalian cells. J Biol Chem 2003; 278(39): 37865-73. [http://dx.doi.org/10.1074/jbc.M306376200] [PMID: 12865421]

[212] Al-Tassan N, Chmiel NH, Maynard J, *et al.* Inherited variants of MYH associated with somatic G:C→T:A mutations in colorectal tumors. Nat Genet 2002; 30(2): 227-32. [http://dx.doi.org/10.1038/ng828] [PMID: 11818965]

[213] Dworaczek H, Xiao W. Xeroderma pigmentosum: a glimpse into nucleotide excision repair, genetic instability, and cancer. Critical Reviews™ in Oncogenesis 2007; 13(2) [http://dx.doi.org/10.1615/CritRevOncog.v13.i2.20]

[214] Lee HC, Yin PH, Lin JC, *et al.* Mitochondrial genome instability and mtDNA depletion in human cancers. Ann N Y Acad Sci 2005; 1042(1): 109-22. [http://dx.doi.org/10.1196/annals.1338.011] [PMID: 15965052]

[215] Loeb LA. A mutator phenotype in cancer. Cancer Res 2001; 61(8): 3230-9. [PMID: 11309271]

[216] Pikor L, Thu K, Vucic E, Lam W. The detection and implication of genome instability in cancer. Cancer Metastasis Rev 2013; 32(3-4): 341-52.

[http://dx.doi.org/10.1007/s10555-013-9429-5] [PMID: 23633034]

[217] Yamamoto H, Imai K. Microsatellite instability: an update. Arch Toxicol 2015; 89(6): 899-921. [http://dx.doi.org/10.1007/s00204-015-1474-0] [PMID: 25701956]

[218] Li K, Luo H, Huang L, Luo H, Zhu X. Microsatellite instability: a review of what the oncologist should know. Cancer Cell Int 2020; 20(1): 16. [http://dx.doi.org/10.1186/s12935-019-1091-8] [PMID: 31956294]

[219] Lower SS, McGurk MP, Clark AG, Barbash DA. Satellite DNA evolution: old ideas, new approaches. Curr Opin Genet Dev 2018; 49: 70-8. [http://dx.doi.org/10.1016/j.gde.2018.03.003] [PMID: 29579574]

[220] Garrido-Ramos M. Satellite DNA: an evolving topic. Genes (Basel) 2017; 8(9): 230. [http://dx.doi.org/10.3390/genes8090230] [PMID: 28926993]

[221] Halling KC, Harper J, Moskaluk CA, *et al.* Origin of microsatellite instability in gastric cancer. Am J Pathol 1999; 155(1): 205-11. [http://dx.doi.org/10.1016/S0002-9440(10)65114-0] [PMID: 10393852]

[222] Kim WS, Park C, Hong SK, Park BK, Kim HS, Park K. Microsatellite instability(MSI) in non-small cell lung cancer(NSCLC) is highly associated with transforming growth factor-beta type II receptor(TGF-beta RII) frameshift mutation. Anticancer Res 2000; 20(3A): 1499-502. [PMID: 10928062]

[223] Zaanan A, Meunier K, Sangar F, Fléjou JF, Praz F. Microsatellite instability in colorectal cancer: from molecular oncogenic mechanisms to clinical implications. Cell Oncol (Dordr) 2011; 34(3): 155-76. [http://dx.doi.org/10.1007/s13402-011-0024-x] [PMID: 21484480]

[224] Bronner CE, Baker SM, Morrison PT, *et al.* Mutation in the DNA mismatch repair gene homologue hMLH1 is associated with hereditary non-polyposis colon cancer. Nature 1994; 368(6468): 258-61. [http://dx.doi.org/10.1038/368258a0] [PMID: 8145827]

[225] Papadopoulos N, Nicolaides NC, Wei YF, *et al.* Mutation of a mutL homolog in hereditary colon cancer. Science 1994; 263(5153): 1625-9. [http://dx.doi.org/10.1126/science.8128251] [PMID: 8128251]

[226] Issa JP. CpG island methylator phenotype in cancer. Nat Rev Cancer 2004; 4(12): 988-93. [http://dx.doi.org/10.1038/nrc1507] [PMID: 15573120]

[227] Goel A, Nagasaka T, Arnold CN, *et al.* The CpG island methylator phenotype and chromosomal instability are inversely correlated in sporadic colorectal cancer. Gastroenterology 2007; 132(1): 127-38. [http://dx.doi.org/10.1053/j.gastro.2006.09.018] [PMID: 17087942]

[228] Ward R, Meagher A, Tomlinson I, *et al.* Microsatellite instability and the clinicopathological features of sporadic colorectal cancer. Gut 2001; 48(6): 821-9. [http://dx.doi.org/10.1136/gut.48.6.821] [PMID: 11358903]

[229] Ogino S, Nosho K, Kirkner GJ, *et al.* CpG island methylator phenotype, microsatellite instability, BRAF mutation and clinical outcome in colon cancer. Gut 2009; 58(1): 90-6. [http://dx.doi.org/10.1136/gut.2008.155473] [PMID: 18832519]

[230] Vilar E, Gruber SB. Microsatellite instability in colorectal cancer—the stable evidence. Nat Rev Clin Oncol 2010; 7(3): 153-62. [http://dx.doi.org/10.1038/nrclinonc.2009.237] [PMID: 20142816]

[231] Shen C, Wang X, Tian L, Che G. Microsatellite alteration in multiple primary lung cancer. J Thorac Dis 2014; 6(10): 1499-505. [PMID: 25364529]

[232] Chang L, Chang M, Chang HM, Chang F. Microsatellite instability: a predictive biomarker for cancer immunotherapy. Appl Immunohistochem Mol Morphol 2018; 26(2): e15-21.

[http://dx.doi.org/10.1097/PAI.0000000000000575] [PMID: 28877075]

[233] Warth A, Körner S, Penzel R, *et al.* Microsatellite instability in pulmonary adenocarcinomas: a comprehensive study of 480 cases. Virchows Arch 2016; 468(3): 313-9. [http://dx.doi.org/10.1007/s00428-015-1892-7] [PMID: 26637197]

[234] Soca-Chafre G, Montiel-Dávalos A, Rosa-Velázquez IADL, Caro-Sánchez CHS, Peña-Nieves A, Arrieta O. Multiple molecular targets associated with genomic instability in lung cancer. International journal of genomics 2019; 2019 [http://dx.doi.org/10.1155/2019/9584504]

[235] Takamochi K, Takahashi F, Suehara Y, *et al.* DNA mismatch repair deficiency in surgically resected lung adenocarcinoma: Microsatellite instability analysis using the Promega panel. Lung Cancer 2017; 110: 26-31. [http://dx.doi.org/10.1016/j.lungcan.2017.05.016] [PMID: 28676214]

[236] Gagos S, Irminger-Finger I. Chromosome instability in neoplasia: chaotic roots to continuous growth. Int J Biochem Cell Biol 2005; 37(5): 1014-33. [http://dx.doi.org/10.1016/j.biocel.2005.01.003] [PMID: 15743675]

[237] Rao CV, Yamada HY, Yao Y, Dai W. Enhanced genomic instabilities caused by deregulated microtubule dynamics and chromosome segregation: a perspective from genetic studies in mice. Carcinogenesis 2009; 30(9): 1469-74. [http://dx.doi.org/10.1093/carcin/bgp081] [PMID: 19372138]

[238] Bakhoum SF, Silkworth WT, Nardi IK, Nicholson JM, Compton DA, Cimini D. The mitotic origin of chromosomal instability. Curr Biol 2014; 24(4): R148-9. [http://dx.doi.org/10.1016/j.cub.2014.01.019] [PMID: 24556433]

[239] Geigl JB, Obenauf AC, Schwarzbraun T, Speicher MR. Defining 'chromosomal instability'. Trends Genet 2008; 24(2): 64-9. [http://dx.doi.org/10.1016/j.tig.2007.11.006] [PMID: 18192061]

[240] McGranahan N, Burrell RA, Endesfelder D, Novelli MR, Swanton C. Cancer chromosomal instability: therapeutic and diagnostic challenges. EMBO Rep 2012; 13(6): 528-38. [http://dx.doi.org/10.1038/embor.2012.61] [PMID: 22595889]

[241] Walther A, Houlston R, Tomlinson I. Association between chromosomal instability and prognosis in colorectal cancer: a meta-analysis. Gut 2008; 57(7): 941-50. [http://dx.doi.org/10.1136/gut.2007.135004] [PMID: 18364437]

[242] Lee AJX, Endesfelder D, Rowan AJ, *et al.* Chromosomal instability confers intrinsic multidrug resistance. Cancer Res 2011; 71(5): 1858-70. [http://dx.doi.org/10.1158/0008-5472.CAN-10-3604] [PMID: 21363922]

[243] Solomon DA, Kim T, Diaz-Martinez LA, *et al.* Mutational inactivation of STAG2 causes aneuploidy in human cancer. Science 2011; 333(6045): 1039-43. [http://dx.doi.org/10.1126/science.1203619] [PMID: 21852505]

[244] Levitt NC, Hickson ID. Caretaker tumour suppressor genes that defend genome integrity. Trends Mol Med 2002; 8(4): 179-86. [http://dx.doi.org/10.1016/S1471-4914(02)02298-0] [PMID: 11927276]

[245] O'Sullivan RJ, Karlseder J. Telomeres: protecting chromosomes against genome instability. Nat Rev Mol Cell Biol 2010; 11(3): 171-81. [http://dx.doi.org/10.1038/nrm2848] [PMID: 20125188]

[246] Hanks S, Coleman K, Reid S, *et al.* Constitutional aneuploidy and cancer predisposition caused by biallelic mutations in BUB1B. Nat Genet 2004; 36(11): 1159-61. [http://dx.doi.org/10.1038/ng1449] [PMID: 15475955]

[247] Hackett JA, Greider CW. Balancing instability: dual roles for telomerase and telomere dysfunction in tumorigenesis. Oncogene 2002; 21(4): 619-26.

[http://dx.doi.org/10.1038/sj.onc.1205061] [PMID: 11850787]

[248] Vitre BD, Cleveland DW. Centrosomes, chromosome instability (CIN) and aneuploidy. Curr Opin Cell Biol 2012; 24(6): 809-15.
[http://dx.doi.org/10.1016/j.ceb.2012.10.006] [PMID: 23127609]

[249] Ertych N, Stolz A, Stenzinger A, *et al.* Increased microtubule assembly rates influence chromosomal instability in colorectal cancer cells. Nat Cell Biol 2014; 16(8): 779-91.
[http://dx.doi.org/10.1038/ncb2994] [PMID: 24976383]

[250] Burrell RA, McClelland SE, Endesfelder D, *et al.* Replication stress links structural and numerical cancer chromosomal instability. Nature 2013; 494(7438): 492-6.
[http://dx.doi.org/10.1038/nature11935] [PMID: 23446422]

[251] Pampalona J, Soler D, Genescà A, Tusell L. Whole chromosome loss is promoted by telomere dysfunction in primary cells. Genes Chromosomes Cancer 2010; 49(4): NA.
[http://dx.doi.org/10.1002/gcc.20749] [PMID: 20088004]

[252] Crasta K, Ganem NJ, Dagher R, *et al.* DNA breaks and chromosome pulverization from errors in mitosis. Nature 2012; 482(7383): 53-8.
[http://dx.doi.org/10.1038/nature10802] [PMID: 22258507]

[253] Baylin SB, Ohm JE. Epigenetic gene silencing in cancer–a mechanism for early oncogenic pathway addiction? Nat Rev Cancer 2006; 6(2): 107-16.
[http://dx.doi.org/10.1038/nrc1799]

[254] Malkin D. Li-Fraumeni Syndrome. Genes Cancer 2011; 2(4): 475-84.
[http://dx.doi.org/10.1177/1947601911413466] [PMID: 21779515]

[255] Zhang XP, Liu F, Wang W. Two-phase dynamics of p53 in the DNA damage response. Proc Natl Acad Sci USA 2011; 108(22): 8990-5.
[http://dx.doi.org/10.1073/pnas.1100600108] [PMID: 21576488]

[256] Bhatti S, Kozlov S, Farooqi AA, Naqi A, Lavin M, Khanna KK. ATM protein kinase: the linchpin of cellular defenses to stress. Cell Mol Life Sci 2011; 68(18): 2977-3006.
[http://dx.doi.org/10.1007/s00018-011-0683-9] [PMID: 21533982]

[257] Smith J, Tho LM, Xu N, Gillespie DA. The ATM-Chk2 and ATR-Chk1 pathways in DNA damage signaling and cancer. Adv Cancer Res 2010; 108: 73-112.
[http://dx.doi.org/10.1016/B978-0-12-380888-2.00003-0] [PMID: 21034966]

[258] Lowe SW, Sherr CJ. Tumor suppression by Ink4a–Arf: progress and puzzles. Curr Opin Genet Dev 2003; 13(1): 77-83.
[http://dx.doi.org/10.1016/S0959-437X(02)00013-8] [PMID: 12573439]

[259] Palmero I, Pantoja C, Serrano M. p19ARF links the tumour suppressor p53 to Ras. Nature 1998; 395(6698): 125-6.
[http://dx.doi.org/10.1038/25870] [PMID: 9744268]

[260] Zindy F, Eischen CM, Randle DH, *et al.* Myc signaling via the ARF tumor suppressor regulates p53-dependent apoptosis and immortalization. Genes Dev 1998; 12(15): 2424-33.
[http://dx.doi.org/10.1101/gad.12.15.2424] [PMID: 9694806]

[261] Weiss E, Winey M. The Saccharomyces cerevisiae spindle pole body duplication gene MPS1 is part of a mitotic checkpoint. J Cell Biol 1996; 132(1): 111-23.
[http://dx.doi.org/10.1083/jcb.132.1.111] [PMID: 8567717]

[262] Cahill DP, Lengauer C, Yu J, *et al.* Mutations of mitotic checkpoint genes in human cancers. Nature 1998; 392(6673): 300-3.
[http://dx.doi.org/10.1038/32688] [PMID: 9521327]

[263] Olesen SH, Thykjaer T, Ørntoft TF. Mitotic checkpoint genes hBUB1, hBUB1B, hBUB3 and TTK in human bladder cancer, screening for mutations and loss of heterozygosity. Carcinogenesis 2001;

22(5): 813-5.
[http://dx.doi.org/10.1093/carcin/22.5.813] [PMID: 11323402]

[264] Resnick TD, Satinover DL, MacIsaac F, *et al.* INCENP and Aurora B promote meiotic sister chromatid cohesion through localization of the Shugoshin MEI-S332 in Drosophila. Dev Cell 2006; 11(1): 57-68.
[http://dx.doi.org/10.1016/j.devcel.2006.04.021] [PMID: 16824953]

[265] Takaki T, Trenz K, Costanzo V, Petronczki M. Polo-like kinase 1 reaches beyond mitosis—cytokinesis, DNA damage response, and development. Curr Opin Cell Biol 2008; 20(6): 650-60.
[http://dx.doi.org/10.1016/j.ceb.2008.10.005] [PMID: 19000759]

[266] Mistry HB, MacCallum DE, Jackson RC, Chaplain MA, Davidson FA. A pharmacodynamic model of Aurora kinase inhibitors in the spindle assembly checkpoint. Front Biosci 2010; 15(1): 249-58.
[http://dx.doi.org/10.2741/3619] [PMID: 20036819]

[267] Liu ST, Zhang H. The mitotic checkpoint complex (MCC): looking back and forth after 15 years. AIMS Mol Sci 2016; 3(4): 597-634.
[http://dx.doi.org/10.3934/molsci.2016.4.597] [PMID: 28920074]

[268] Londoño-Vallejo JA, Wellinger RJ. Telomeres and telomerase dance to the rhythm of the cell cycle. Trends Biochem Sci 2012; 37(9): 391-9.
[http://dx.doi.org/10.1016/j.tibs.2012.05.004] [PMID: 22727244]

[269] Reddel RR, Bryan TM. Alternative lengthening of telomeres: dangerous road less travelled. Lancet 2003; 361(9372): 1840-1.
[http://dx.doi.org/10.1016/S0140-6736(03)13538-6] [PMID: 12788566]

[270] Fouladi B, Sabatier L, Miller D, Pottier G, Murnane JP. The relationship between spontaneous telomere loss and chromosome instability in a human tumor cell line. Neoplasia 2000; 2(6): 540-54.
[http://dx.doi.org/10.1038/sj.neo.7900107] [PMID: 11228547]

[271] Sabatier L, Ricoul M, Pottier G, Murnane JP. The loss of a single telomere can result in instability of multiple chromosomes in a human tumor cell line. Mol Cancer Res 2005; 3(3): 139-50.
[http://dx.doi.org/10.1158/1541-7786.MCR-04-0194] [PMID: 15798094]

[272] Maser RS, DePinho RA. Connecting chromosomes, crisis, and cancer. Science 2002; 297(5581): 565-9.
[http://dx.doi.org/10.1126/science.297.5581.565] [PMID: 12142527]

[273] Rampazzo E, Bertorelle R, Serra L, *et al.* Relationship between telomere shortening, genetic instability, and site of tumour origin in colorectal cancers. Br J Cancer 2010; 102(8): 1300-5.
[http://dx.doi.org/10.1038/sj.bjc.6605644] [PMID: 20386541]

[274] Rudolph KL, Chang S, Lee HW, *et al.* Longevity, stress response, and cancer in aging telomerase-deficient mice. Cell 1999; 96(5): 701-12.
[http://dx.doi.org/10.1016/S0092-8674(00)80580-2] [PMID: 10089885]

[275] Hahn WC, Counter CM, Lundberg AS, Beijersbergen RL, Brooks MW, Weinberg RA. Creation of human tumour cells with defined genetic elements. Nature 1999; 400(6743): 464-8.
[http://dx.doi.org/10.1038/22780] [PMID: 10440377]

[276] Ferguson LR, Chen H, Collins AR, *et al.* Genomic instability in human cancer: Molecular insights and opportunities for therapeutic attack and prevention through diet and nutrition Seminars in cancer biology. Elsevier 2015; pp. S5-S24.

[277] Mitchell JR, Hoeijmakers JHJ, Niedernhofer LJ. Divide and conquer: nucleotide excision repair battles cancer and ageing. Curr Opin Cell Biol 2003; 15(2): 232-40.
[http://dx.doi.org/10.1016/S0955-0674(03)00018-8] [PMID: 12648680]

[278] Nouspikel TP, Hyka-Nouspikel N, Hanawalt PC. Transcription domain-associated repair in human cells. Mol Cell Biol 2006; 26(23): 8722-30.

[http://dx.doi.org/10.1128/MCB.01263-06] [PMID: 17015469]

[279] Sancar A, Lindsey-Boltz LA, Ünsal-Kaçmaz K, Linn S. Molecular mechanisms of mammalian DNA repair and the DNA damage checkpoints. Annu Rev Biochem 2004; 73(1): 39-85. [http://dx.doi.org/10.1146/annurev.biochem.73.011303.073723] [PMID: 15189136]

[280] Houtgraaf JH, Versmissen J, van der Giessen WJ. A concise review of DNA damage checkpoints and repair in mammalian cells. Cardiovasc Revasc Med 2006; 7(3): 165-72. [http://dx.doi.org/10.1016/j.carrev.2006.02.002] [PMID: 16945824]

[281] Aguilera A, Gómez-González B. Genome instability: a mechanistic view of its causes and consequences. Nat Rev Genet 2008; 9(3): 204-17. [http://dx.doi.org/10.1038/nrg2268] [PMID: 18227811]

[282] Lindahl T. An N-glycosidase from *Escherichia coli* that releases free uracil from DNA containing deaminated cytosine residues. Proc Natl Acad Sci USA 1974; 71(9): 3649-53. [http://dx.doi.org/10.1073/pnas.71.9.3649] [PMID: 4610583]

[283] de Boer J, Hoeijmakers JHJ. Nucleotide excision repair and human syndromes. Carcinogenesis 2000; 21(3): 453-60. [http://dx.doi.org/10.1093/carcin/21.3.453] [PMID: 10688865]

[284] Nilsen H, Krokan HE. Base excision repair in a network of defence and tolerance. Carcinogenesis 2001; 22(7): 987-98. [http://dx.doi.org/10.1093/carcin/22.7.987] [PMID: 11408341]

[285] Maynard S, Schurman SH, Harboe C, de Souza-Pinto NC, Bohr VA. Base excision repair of oxidative DNA damage and association with cancer and aging. Carcinogenesis 2008; 30(1): 2-10. [http://dx.doi.org/10.1093/carcin/bgn250] [PMID: 18978338]

[286] Rouleau M, Patel A, Hendzel MJ, Kaufmann SH, Poirier GG. PARP inhibition: PARP1 and beyond. Nat Rev Cancer 2010; 10(4): 293-301. [http://dx.doi.org/10.1038/nrc2812] [PMID: 20200537]

[287] Larsen E, Gran C, Sæther BE, Seeberg E, Klungland A. Proliferation failure and gamma radiation sensitivity of Fen1 null mutant mice at the blastocyst stage. Mol Cell Biol 2003; 23(15): 5346-53. [http://dx.doi.org/10.1128/MCB.23.15.5346-5353.2003] [PMID: 12861020]

[288] Farrington SM, Tenesa A, Barnetson R, *et al.* Germline susceptibility to colorectal cancer due to base-excision repair gene defects. Am J Hum Genet 2005; 77(1): 112-9. [http://dx.doi.org/10.1086/431213] [PMID: 15931596]

[289] Barnetson RA, Devlin L, Miller J, *et al.* Germline mutation prevalence in the base excision repair gene, *MYH*, in patients with endometrial cancer. Clin Genet 2007; 72(6): 551-5. [http://dx.doi.org/10.1111/j.1399-0004.2007.00900.x] [PMID: 17956577]

[290] Mahjabeen I, Masood N, Baig RM, *et al.* Novel mutations of OGG1 base excision repair pathway gene in laryngeal cancer patients. Fam Cancer 2012; 11(4): 587-93. [http://dx.doi.org/10.1007/s10689-012-9554-2] [PMID: 22829015]

[291] Shinmura K, Tao H, Goto M, *et al.* Inactivating mutations of the human base excision repair gene NEIL1 in gastric cancer. Carcinogenesis 2004; 25(12): 2311-7. [http://dx.doi.org/10.1093/carcin/bgh267] [PMID: 15319300]

[292] Kunkel TA. Evolving views of DNA replication (in) fidelity Cold Spring Harbor symposia on quantitative biology. Cold Spring Harbor Laboratory Press 2009; pp. 91-101.

[293] Albertson TM, Ogawa M, Bugni JM, *et al.* DNA polymerase ε and δ proofreading suppress discrete mutator and cancer phenotypes in mice. Proc Natl Acad Sci USA 2009; 106(40): 17101-4. [http://dx.doi.org/10.1073/pnas.0907147106] [PMID: 19805137]

[294] Sengupta S, Chakrabarti S, Roy A, Panda CK, Roychoudhury S. Inactivation of human mutL homolog 1 and mutS homolog 2 genes in head and neck squamous cell carcinoma tumors and leukoplakia

samples by promoter hypermethylation and its relation with microsatellite instability phenotype. Cancer 2007; 109(4): 703-12.
[http://dx.doi.org/10.1002/cncr.22430] [PMID: 17219447]

[295] Modrich P. Mechanisms in eukaryotic mismatch repair. J Biol Chem 2006; 281(41): 30305-9.
[http://dx.doi.org/10.1074/jbc.R600022200] [PMID: 16905530]

[296] Kunkel TA, Erie DA. Eukaryotic mismatch repair in relation to DNA replication. Annu Rev Genet 2015; 49(1): 291-313.
[http://dx.doi.org/10.1146/annurev-genet-112414-054722] [PMID: 26436461]

[297] Ciccia A, Elledge SJ. The DNA damage response: making it safe to play with knives. Mol Cell 2010; 40(2): 179-204.
[http://dx.doi.org/10.1016/j.molcel.2010.09.019] [PMID: 20965415]

[298] Moynahan ME, Jasin M. Mitotic homologous recombination maintains genomic stability and suppresses tumorigenesis. Nat Rev Mol Cell Biol 2010; 11(3): 196-207.
[http://dx.doi.org/10.1038/nrm2851] [PMID: 20177395]

[299] Willers H, Pfäffle HN, Zou L. Targeting homologous recombination repair in cancer DNA Repair in Cancer Therapy. Elsevier 2012; pp. 119-60.
[http://dx.doi.org/10.1016/B978-0-12-384999-1.10007-1]

[300] Helleday T, Lo J, Vangent D, Engelward B. DNA double-strand break repair: From mechanistic understanding to cancer treatment. DNA Repair (Amst) 2007; 6(7): 923-35.
[http://dx.doi.org/10.1016/j.dnarep.2007.02.006] [PMID: 17363343]

[301] Yun H, Kim K. Ku complex suppresses recombination in the absence of MRX activity during budding yeast meiosis. BMB Rep 2019; 52(10): 607-12.
[http://dx.doi.org/10.5483/BMBRep.2019.52.10.245] [PMID: 30940321]

[302] Davis AJ, Chen DJ. DNA double strand break repair via non-homologous end-joining. Transl Cancer Res 2013; 2(3): 130-43.
[PMID: 24000320]

[303] Li X, Heyer WD. Homologous recombination in DNA repair and DNA damage tolerance. Cell Res 2008; 18(1): 99-113.
[http://dx.doi.org/10.1038/cr.2008.1] [PMID: 18166982]

[304] Hong S, Joo JH, Yun H, Kleckner N, Kim KP. Recruitment of Rec8, Pds5 and Rad61/Wapl to meiotic homolog pairing, recombination, axis formation and S-phase. Nucleic Acids Res 2019; 47(22): gkz903.
[http://dx.doi.org/10.1093/nar/gkz903] [PMID: 31617566]

[305] Hall JM, Lee MK, Newman B, *et al.* Linkage of early-onset familial breast cancer to chromosome 17q21. Science 1990; 250(4988): 1684-9.
[http://dx.doi.org/10.1126/science.2270482] [PMID: 2270482]

[306] Ford D, Easton DF, Bishop DT, Narod SA, Goldgar DE. Risks of cancer in BRCA1-mutation carriers. Lancet 1994; 343(8899): 692-5.
[http://dx.doi.org/10.1016/S0140-6736(94)91578-4] [PMID: 7907678]

[307] Wooster R, Neuhausen SL, Mangion J, *et al.* Localization of a breast cancer susceptibility gene, BRCA2, to chromosome 13q12-13. Science 1994; 265(5181): 2088-90.
[http://dx.doi.org/10.1126/science.8091231] [PMID: 8091231]

[308] Chen S, Parmigiani G. Meta-Analysis of *BRCA1* and *BRCA2* Penetrance. J Clin Oncol 2007; 25(11): 1329-33.
[http://dx.doi.org/10.1200/JCO.2006.09.1066] [PMID: 17416853]

[309] Friedenson B. BRCA1 and BRCA2 pathways and the risk of cancers other than breast or ovarian. MedGenMed 2005; 7(2): 60.
[PMID: 16369438]

[310] Kee Y, D'Andrea AD. Expanded roles of the Fanconi anemia pathway in preserving genomic stability. Genes Dev 2010; 24(16): 1680-94.
[http://dx.doi.org/10.1101/gad.1955310] [PMID: 20713514]

[311] Tischkowitz M, Xia B. PALB2/FANCN: recombining cancer and Fanconi anemia. Cancer Res 2010; 70(19): 7353-9.
[http://dx.doi.org/10.1158/0008-5472.CAN-10-1012] [PMID: 20858716]

[312] Chirnomas D, Taniguchi T, de la Vega M, *et al.* Chemosensitization to cisplatin by inhibitors of the Fanconi anemia/BRCA pathway. Mol Cancer Ther 2006; 5(4): 952-61.
[http://dx.doi.org/10.1158/1535-7163.MCT-05-0493] [PMID: 16648566]

[313] Stracker TH, Roig I, Knobel PA, Marjanović M. The ATM signaling network in development and disease. Front Genet 2013; 4: 37.
[http://dx.doi.org/10.3389/fgene.2013.00037] [PMID: 23532176]

[314] Yichao H and Gabriele B. Tumors vs. Chronic Wounds: An Immune Cell's Perspective. Front Immunol 2019. doi: 10.3389/fimmu.2019.02178

[315] Peiris-Pagès M, Harper SJ, Bates DO, Ramani P. Balance of pro-*versus* anti-angiogenic splice isoforms of vascular endothelial growth factor as a regulator of neuroblastoma growth. J Pathol 2010; 222(2): 138-47.

[316] Mantovani A, Allavena P, Sica A, Balkwill F. Cancer-related inflammation. Nature. 2008; 454(7203): 436-44.

[317] Chen L, Deng H, Cui H, *et al.* Inflammatory responses and inflammation-associated diseases in organs. Oncotarget 2018; 9(6): 7204-18.
[http://dx.doi.org/10.18632/oncotarget.23208] [PMID: 29467962]

[318] Serhan CN. Pro-resolving lipid mediators are leads for resolution physiology. Nature 2014; 510(7503): 92-101.
[http://dx.doi.org/10.1038/nature13479] [PMID: 24899309]

[319] Buckley CD, Gilroy DW, Serhan CN. Proresolving lipid mediators and mechanisms in the resolution of acute inflammation. Immunity 2014; 40(3): 315-27.
[http://dx.doi.org/10.1016/j.immuni.2014.02.009] [PMID: 24656045]

[320] Zhang Q, Zhu B, Li Y. Resolution of cancer-promoting inflammation: a new approach for anticancer therapy. Front Immunol 2017; 8: 71.
[http://dx.doi.org/10.3389/fimmu.2017.00071] [PMID: 28210259]

[321] Heppner FL, Ransohoff RM, Becher B. Immune attack: the role of inflammation in Alzheimer disease. Nat Rev Neurosci 2015; 16(6): 358-72.
[http://dx.doi.org/10.1038/nrn3880] [PMID: 25991443]

[322] Aggarwal BB. Nuclear factor-κB. Cancer Cell 2004; 6(3): 203-8.
[http://dx.doi.org/10.1016/j.ccr.2004.09.003] [PMID: 15380510]

[323] Sorriento D, Iaccarino G. Inflammation and Cardiovascular Diseases: The Most Recent Findings. Int J Mol Sci 2019; 20(16): 3879.
[http://dx.doi.org/10.3390/ijms20163879] [PMID: 31395800]

[324] Rutter M, Saunders B, Wilkinson K, *et al.* Severity of inflammation is a risk factor for colorectal neoplasia in ulcerative colitis. Gastroenterology 2004; 126(2): 451-9.
[http://dx.doi.org/10.1053/j.gastro.2003.11.010] [PMID: 14762782]

[325] Guerra C, Schuhmacher AJ, Cañamero M, *et al.* Chronic pancreatitis is essential for induction of pancreatic ductal adenocarcinoma by K-Ras oncogenes in adult mice. Cancer Cell 2007; 11(3): 291-302.
[http://dx.doi.org/10.1016/j.ccr.2007.01.012] [PMID: 17349585]

[326] Greene ER, Huang S, Serhan CN, Panigrahy D. Regulation of inflammation in cancer by eicosanoids.

Prostaglandins Other Lipid Mediat 2011; 96(1-4): 27-36.
[http://dx.doi.org/10.1016/j.prostaglandins.2011.08.004] [PMID: 21864702]

[327] Guerra C, Collado M, Navas C, *et al.* Pancreatitis-induced inflammation contributes to pancreatic cancer by inhibiting oncogene-induced senescence. Cancer Cell 2011; 19(6): 728-39.
[http://dx.doi.org/10.1016/j.ccr.2011.05.011] [PMID: 21665147]

[328] Colotta F, Allavena P, Sica A, Garlanda C, Mantovani A. Cancer-related inflammation, the seventh hallmark of cancer: links to genetic instability. Carcinogenesis 2009; 30(7): 1073-81.
[http://dx.doi.org/10.1093/carcin/bgp127] [PMID: 19468060]

[329] Ferlay J, Soerjomataram I, Dikshit R, *et al.* Cancer incidence and mortality worldwide: Sources, methods and major patterns in GLOBOCAN 2012. Int J Cancer 2015; 136(5): E359-86.
[http://dx.doi.org/10.1002/ijc.29210] [PMID: 25220842]

[330] Siegel RL, Miller KD, Jemal A. Cancer statistics, 2016. CA Cancer J Clin 2016; 66(1): 7-30.
[http://dx.doi.org/10.3322/caac.21332] [PMID: 26742998]

[331] Hosseini H, Obradović MMS, Hoffmann M, *et al.* Early dissemination seeds metastasis in breast cancer. Nature 2016; 540(7634): 552-8.
[http://dx.doi.org/10.1038/nature20785] [PMID: 27974799]

[332] Gonzalez H, Hagerling C, Werb Z. Roles of the immune system in cancer: from tumor initiation to metastatic progression. Genes Dev 2018; 32(19-20): 1267-84.
[http://dx.doi.org/10.1101/gad.314617.118] [PMID: 30275043]

[333] Chambers AF, Werb Z. Invasion and metastasis—recent advances and future challenges. Springer 2015.
[http://dx.doi.org/10.1007/s00109-015-1269-z]

[334] Gonzalez H, Robles I, Werb Z. Innate and acquired immune surveillance in the postdissemination phase of metastasis. FEBS J 2018; 285(4): 654-64.
[http://dx.doi.org/10.1111/febs.14325] [PMID: 29131550]

[335] Hanahan D, Weinberg RA. Hallmarks of cancer: the next generation. Cell 2011; 144(5): 646-74.
[http://dx.doi.org/10.1016/j.cell.2011.02.013] [PMID: 21376230]

[336] Lu H, Ouyang W, Huang C. Inflammation, a key event in cancer development. Mol Cancer Res 2006; 4(4): 221-33.
[http://dx.doi.org/10.1158/1541-7786.MCR-05-0261] [PMID: 16603636]

[337] Coussens LM, Werb Z. Inflammation and cancer. Nature 2002; 420(6917): 860-7.
[http://dx.doi.org/10.1038/nature01322] [PMID: 12490959]

[338] Nathan C. Points of control in inflammation. Nature 2002; 420(6917): 846-52.
[http://dx.doi.org/10.1038/nature01320] [PMID: 12490957]

[339] Qu X, Tang Y, Hua S. Immunological approaches towards cancer and inflammation: a cross talk. Front Immunol 2018; 9: 563.
[http://dx.doi.org/10.3389/fimmu.2018.00563] [PMID: 29662489]

[340] Nickoloff BJ, Ben-Neriah Y, Pikarsky E. Inflammation and cancer: is the link as simple as we think? J Invest Dermatol 2005; 124(6): x-xiv.
[http://dx.doi.org/10.1111/j.0022-202X.2005.23724.x] [PMID: 15955081]

[341] Hussain SP, Amstad P, Raja K, *et al.* Increased p53 mutation load in noncancerous colon tissue from ulcerative colitis: A cancer-prone chronic inflammatory disease. Cancer Res 2000; 60(13): 3333-7.

[342] Beaugerie L, Svrcek M, Seksik P, *et al.* Risk of colorectal high-grade dysplasia and cancer in a prospective observational cohort of patients with inflammatory bowel disease. Gastroenterology 2013; 145(1): 166-75.
[http://dx.doi.org/10.1053/j.gastro.2013.03.044]

[343] Zeng M, Mao XH, Li JX, *et al.* Efficacy, safety, and immunogenicity of an oral recombinant

Helicobacter pylori vaccine in children in China: a randomised, double-blind, placebo-controlled, phase 3 trial. Lancet 2015; 386(10002): 1457-64.
[http://dx.doi.org/10.1016/S0140-6736(15)60310-5] [PMID: 26142048]

[344] Grivennikov SI, Greten FR, Karin M. Immunity, inflammation, and cancer. Cell 2010; 140(6): 883-99.
[http://dx.doi.org/10.1016/j.cell.2010.01.025] [PMID: 20303878]

[345] Schiffman M, Castle PE, Jeronimo J, Rodriguez AC, Wacholder S. Human papillomavirus and cervical cancer. Lancet 2007; 370(9590): 890-907.
[http://dx.doi.org/10.1016/S0140-6736(07)61416-0] [PMID: 17826171]

[346] Chua MLK, Wee JTS, Hui EP, Chan ATC. Nasopharyngeal carcinoma. Lancet 2016; 387(10022): 1012-24.
[http://dx.doi.org/10.1016/S0140-6736(15)00055-0] [PMID: 26321262]

[347] Wu S, Rhee KJ, Albesiano E, *et al.* A human colonic commensal promotes colon tumorigenesis via activation of T helper type 17 T cell responses. Nat Med 2009; 15(9): 1016-22.
[http://dx.doi.org/10.1038/nm.2015] [PMID: 19701202]

[348] Hoption Cann SA, van Netten JP, van Netten C. Dr William Coley and tumour regression: a place in history or in the future. Postgrad Med J 2003; 79(938): 672-80.
[PMID: 14707241]

[349] Rakoff-Nahoum S, Medzhitov R. Toll-like receptors and cancer. Nat Rev Cancer 2009; 9(1): 57-63.
[http://dx.doi.org/10.1038/nrc2541] [PMID: 19052556]

[350] Askeland EJ, Newton MR, O'Donnell MA, Luo Y. Bladder cancer immunotherapy: BCG and beyond. Adv Urol 2012; 2012: 181987.
[http://dx.doi.org/10.1155/2012/181987]

[351] Shalapour S, Karin M. Immunity, inflammation, and cancer: an eternal fight between good and evil. J Clin Invest 2015; 125(9): 3347-55.
[http://dx.doi.org/10.1172/JCI80007] [PMID: 26325032]

[352] Frisch M, Biggar RJ, Engels EA, Goedert JJ. Association of cancer with AIDS-related immunosuppression in adults. JAMA 2001; 285(13): 1736-45.
[http://dx.doi.org/10.1001/jama.285.13.1736] [PMID: 11277828]

[353] Thun MJ, Henley SJ, Patrono C. Nonsteroidal anti-inflammatory drugs as anticancer agents: mechanistic, pharmacologic, and clinical issues. J Natl Cancer Inst 2002; 94(4): 252-66.
[http://dx.doi.org/10.1093/jnci/94.4.252] [PMID: 11854387]

[354] Waldner MJ, Neurath MF. Colitis-associated cancer: the role of T cells in tumor development Seminars in immunopathology. Springer 2009; pp. 249-56.

[355] Jess T, Simonsen J, Jørgensen KT, Pedersen BV, Nielsen NM, Frisch M. Decreasing risk of colorectal cancer in patients with inflammatory bowel disease over 30 years. Gastroenterology 2012; 143(2): 375-81.
[http://dx.doi.org/10.1053/j.gastro.2012.04.016]

[356] Punturieri A, Szabo E, Croxton TL, Shapiro SD, Dubinett SM. Lung cancer and chronic obstructive pulmonary disease: needs and opportunities for integrated research. J Natl Cancer Inst 2009; 101(8): 554-9.
[http://dx.doi.org/10.1093/jnci/djp023] [PMID: 19351920]

[357] Dostert C, Pétrilli V, Van Bruggen R, Steele C, Mossman BT, Tschopp J. Innate immune activation through Nalp3 inflammasome sensing of asbestos and silica. Science 2008; 320(5876): 674-7.
[http://dx.doi.org/10.1126/science.1156995] [PMID: 18403674]

[358] Tuncman G, Hirosumi J, Solinas G, Chang L, Karin M, Hotamisligil GS. Functional *in vivo* interactions between JNK1 and JNK2 isoforms in obesity and insulin resistance. Proc Natl Acad Sci USA 2006; 103(28): 10741-6.
[http://dx.doi.org/10.1073/pnas.0603509103] [PMID: 16818881]

[359] Sjöström L, Narbro K, Sjöström CD, *et al.* Effects of bariatric surgery on mortality in Swedish obese subjects. N Engl J Med 2007; 357(8): 741-52. [http://dx.doi.org/10.1056/NEJMoa066254] [PMID: 17715408]

[360] Park EJ, Lee JH, Yu GY, *et al.* Dietary and genetic obesity promote liver inflammation and tumorigenesis by enhancing IL-6 and TNF expression. Cell 2010; 140(2): 197-208. [http://dx.doi.org/10.1016/j.cell.2009.12.052] [PMID: 20141834]

[361] Rodier F, Coppé JP, Patil CK, *et al.* Persistent DNA damage signalling triggers senescence-associated inflammatory cytokine secretion. Nat Cell Biol 2009; 11(8): 973-9. [http://dx.doi.org/10.1038/ncb1909] [PMID: 19597488]

[362] Freund A, Orjalo AV, Desprez PY, Campisi J. Inflammatory networks during cellular senescence: causes and consequences. Trends Mol Med 2010; 16(5): 238-46. [http://dx.doi.org/10.1016/j.molmed.2010.03.003] [PMID: 20444648]

[363] Del Prete A, Allavena P, Santoro G, Fumarulo R, Corsi MM, Mantovani A. Molecular pathways in cancer-related inflammation. Biochem Med (Zagreb) 2011; 21(3): 264-75. [http://dx.doi.org/10.11613/BM.2011.036] [PMID: 22420240]

[364] Soucek L, Lawlor ER, Soto D, Shchors K, Swigart LB, Evan GI. Mast cells are required for angiogenesis and macroscopic expansion of Myc-induced pancreatic islet tumors. Nat Med 2007; 13(10): 1211-8. [http://dx.doi.org/10.1038/nm1649] [PMID: 17906636]

[365] Theoharides TC. Mast cells and pancreatic cancer. N Engl J Med 2008; 358(17): 1860-1. [http://dx.doi.org/10.1056/NEJMcibr0801519] [PMID: 18434656]

[366] Vakkila J, Lotze MT. Inflammation and necrosis promote tumour growth. Nat Rev Immunol 2004; 4(8): 641-8. [http://dx.doi.org/10.1038/nri1415] [PMID: 15286730]

[367] Kim S, Takahashi H, Lin W-W, *et al.* Carcinoma-produced factors activate myeloid cells through TLR2 to stimulate metastasis. nature 2009; 457(7225): 102-6.

[368] Flier JS, Underhill LH, Dvorak HF. Tumors: wounds that do not heal. Similarities between tumor stroma generation and wound healing. N Engl J Med 1986; 315(26): 1650-9. [http://dx.doi.org/10.1056/NEJM198612253152606] [PMID: 3537791]

[369] Schäfer M, Werner S. Cancer as an overhealing wound: an old hypothesis revisited. Nat Rev Mol Cell Biol 2008; 9(8): 628-38. [http://dx.doi.org/10.1038/nrm2455] [PMID: 18628784]

[370] Zong WX, Thompson CB. Necrotic death as a cell fate. Genes Dev 2006; 20(1): 1-15. [http://dx.doi.org/10.1101/gad.1376506] [PMID: 16391229]

[371] Duprez L, Vanlangenakker N, Festjens N, Van Herreweghe F, Berghe TV, Vandenabeele P. Necrosis: Molecular Mechanisms and Physiological Roles Essentials of Apoptosis. Springer 2009; pp. 599-633. [http://dx.doi.org/10.1007/978-1-60327-381-7_27]

[372] Ammirante M, Luo JL, Grivennikov S, Nedospasov S, Karin M. B-cell-derived lymphotoxin promotes castration-resistant prostate cancer. Nature 2010; 464(7286): 302-5. [http://dx.doi.org/10.1038/nature08782] [PMID: 20220849]

[373] Zitvogel L, Apetoh L, Ghiringhelli F, Kroemer G. Immunological aspects of cancer chemotherapy. Nat Rev Immunol 2008; 8(1): 59-73. [http://dx.doi.org/10.1038/nri2216] [PMID: 18097448]

[374] DeNardo DG, PAndreu P, Coussens LM. Interactions between lymphocytes and myeloid cells regulate pro-versus anti-tumor immunity. Cancer Metastasis Rev 2010; 29(2): 309-16. [http://dx.doi.org/10.1007/s10555-010-9223-6]

[375] Copeland NG, Jenkins NA. Deciphering the genetic landscape of cancer – from genes to pathways.

Trends Genet 2009; 25(10): 455-62.
[http://dx.doi.org/10.1016/j.tig.2009.08.004] [PMID: 19818523]

[376] Wooster R, Bachman KE. Catalogue, cause, complexity and cure; the many uses of cancer genome sequence. Curr Opin Genet Dev 2010; 20(3): 336-41.
[http://dx.doi.org/10.1016/j.gde.2010.03.007] [PMID: 20382522]

[377] Siegel R, MA MS, Ahmedin Jemal DVM. Cancer Statistics. A Cancer Journal for Clinicians 2012; 62: 10-29.

[378] Wei EK, Wolin KY, Colditz GA. Time course of risk factors in cancer etiology and progression. J Clin Oncol 2010; 28(26): 4052-7.
[http://dx.doi.org/10.1200/JCO.2009.26.9324] [PMID: 20644083]

[379] Balkwill F, Charles KA, Mantovani A. Smoldering and polarized inflammation in the initiation and promotion of malignant disease. Cancer Cell 2005; 7(3): 211-7.
[http://dx.doi.org/10.1016/j.ccr.2005.02.013] [PMID: 15766659]

[380] DeNardo DG, Johansson M, Coussens LM. Immune cells as mediators of solid tumor metastasis. Cancer Metastasis Rev 2008; 27(1): 11-8.
[http://dx.doi.org/10.1007/s10555-007-9100-0] [PMID: 18066650]

[381] Tlsty TD, Coussens LM. Tumor stroma and regulation of cancer development. Annu Rev Pathol 2006; 1(1): 119-50.
[http://dx.doi.org/10.1146/annurev.pathol.1.110304.100224] [PMID: 18039110]

[382] Billottet C, Jouanneau J. Tumor-stroma interactions. Bull Cancer 2008; 95(1): 51-6.
[PMID: 18230570]

[383] Sharma P, Allison JP. The future of immune checkpoint therapy. Science 2015; 348(6230): 56-61.
[http://dx.doi.org/10.1126/science.aaa8172] [PMID: 25838373]

[384] Dunn GP, Old LJ, Schreiber RD. The three Es of cancer immunoediting. Annu Rev Immunol 2004; 22(1): 329-60.
[http://dx.doi.org/10.1146/annurev.immunol.22.012703.104803] [PMID: 15032581]

[385] Matsushita H, Vesely MD, Koboldt DC, *et al.* Cancer exome analysis reveals a T-cell-dependent mechanism of cancer immunoediting. Nature 2012; 482(7385): 400-4.
[http://dx.doi.org/10.1038/nature10755] [PMID: 22318521]

[386] Schreiber RD, Old LJ, Smyth MJ. Cancer immunoediting: integrating immunity's roles in cancer suppression and promotion. Science 2011; 331(6024): 1565-70.
[http://dx.doi.org/10.1126/science.1203486] [PMID: 21436444]

[387] Kim R. Cancer immunoediting: from immune surveillance to immune escape. Cancer Immunotherapy 2007; pp. 9-27.

[388] Mahoney KM, Rennert PD, Freeman GJ. Combination cancer immunotherapy and new immunomodulatory targets. Nat Rev Drug Discov 2015; 14(8): 561-84.
[http://dx.doi.org/10.1038/nrd4591] [PMID: 26228759]

[389] Moon EK, Langer CJ, Albelda SM. The era of checkpoint blockade in lung cancer: taking the brakes off the immune system. Ann Am Thorac Soc 2017; 14(8): 1248-60.
[http://dx.doi.org/10.1513/AnnalsATS.201702-152FR] [PMID: 28613923]

[390] Garrido F, Romero I, Aptsiauri N, Garcia-Lora AM. Generation of MHC class I diversity in primary tumors and selection of the malignant phenotype. Int J Cancer 2016; 138(2): 271-80.
[http://dx.doi.org/10.1002/ijc.29375] [PMID: 25471439]

[391] Mittal D, Gubin MM, Schreiber RD, Smyth MJ. New insights into cancer immunoediting and its three component phases—elimination, equilibrium and escape. Curr Opin Immunol 2014; 27: 16-25.
[http://dx.doi.org/10.1016/j.coi.2014.01.004] [PMID: 24531241]

[392] Beatty GL, Gladney WL. Immune escape mechanisms as a guide for cancer immunotherapy. Clin

Cancer Res 2015; 21(4): 687-92.
[http://dx.doi.org/10.1158/1078-0432.CCR-14-1860] [PMID: 25501578]

[393] Vinay DS, Ryan EP, Pawelec G, *et al.* Immune evasion in cancer: Mechanistic basis and therapeutic strategies Seminars in cancer biology. Elsevier 2015; pp. S185-98.

[394] Campoli M, Ferrone S. HLA antigen changes in malignant cells: epigenetic mechanisms and biologic significance. Oncogene 2008; 27(45): 5869-85.
[http://dx.doi.org/10.1038/onc.2008.273] [PMID: 18836468]

[395] Dong H, Strome SE, Salomao DR, *et al.* Tumor-associated B7-H1 promotes T-cell apoptosis: A potential mechanism of immune evasion. Nat Med 2002; 8(8): 793-800.
[http://dx.doi.org/10.1038/nm730] [PMID: 12091876]

[396] Hicklin DJ, Marincola FM, Ferrone S. HLA class I antigen downregulation in human cancers: T-cell immunotherapy revives an old story. Mol Med Today 1999; 5(4): 178-86.
[http://dx.doi.org/10.1016/S1357-4310(99)01451-3] [PMID: 10203751]

[397] Paul P, Rouas-Freiss N, Khalil-Daher I, *et al.* HLA-G expression in melanoma: A way for tumor cells to escape from immunosurveillance. Proc Natl Acad Sci USA 1998; 95(8): 4510-5.
[http://dx.doi.org/10.1073/pnas.95.8.4510] [PMID: 9539768]

[398] Wherry EJ, Kurachi M. Molecular and cellular insights into T cell exhaustion. Nat Rev Immunol 2015; 15(8): 486-99.
[http://dx.doi.org/10.1038/nri3862] [PMID: 26205583]

[399] Davoodzadeh Gholami M, kardar GA, Saeedi Y, Heydari S, Garssen J, Falak R. Exhaustion of T lymphocytes in the tumor microenvironment: Significance and effective mechanisms. Cell Immunol 2017; 322: 1-14.
[http://dx.doi.org/10.1016/j.cellimm.2017.10.002] [PMID: 29079339]

[400] Iwai Y, Hamanishi J, Chamoto K, Honjo T. Cancer immunotherapies targeting the PD-1 signaling pathway. J Biomed Sci 2017; 24(1): 26.
[http://dx.doi.org/10.1186/s12929-017-0329-9] [PMID: 28376884]

[401] Gasche JA, Hoffmann J, Boland CR, Goel A. Interleukin-6 promotes tumorigenesis by altering DNA methylation in oral cancer cells. Int J Cancer 2011; 129(5): 1053-63.
[http://dx.doi.org/10.1002/ijc.25764] [PMID: 21710491]

[402] Pálmai-Pallag T, Bachrati CZ. Inflammation-induced DNA damage and damage-induced inflammation: a vicious cycle. Microbes Infect 2014; 16(10): 822-32.
[http://dx.doi.org/10.1016/j.micinf.2014.10.001] [PMID: 25449753]

[403] Keeley EC, Mehrad B, Strieter RM. CXC chemokines in cancer angiogenesis and metastases. Adv Cancer Res 2010; 106: 91-111.
[http://dx.doi.org/10.1016/S0065-230X(10)06003-3] [PMID: 20399957]

[404] Vendramini-Costa DB, Carvalho JE. Molecular link mechanisms between inflammation and cancer. Curr Pharm Des 2012; 18(26): 3831-52.
[http://dx.doi.org/10.2174/138161212802083707] [PMID: 22632748]

[405] Toh B, Wang X, Keeble J, *et al.* Mesenchymal transition and dissemination of cancer cells is driven by myeloid-derived suppressor cells infiltrating the primary tumor. PLoS Biol 2011; 9(9): e1001162.
[http://dx.doi.org/10.1371/journal.pbio.1001162] [PMID: 21980263]

[406] Gabrilovich DI, Ostrand-Rosenberg S, Bronte V. Coordinated regulation of myeloid cells by tumours. Nat Rev Immunol 2012; 12(4): 253-68.
[http://dx.doi.org/10.1038/nri3175] [PMID: 22437938]

[407] Biswas SK, Allavena P, Mantovani A. Tumor-associated macrophages: functional diversity, clinical significance, and open questions Seminars in immunopathology. Springer 2013; pp. 585-600.

[408] Perwez Hussain S, Harris CC. Inflammation and cancer: An ancient link with novel potentials. Int J

Cancer 2007; 121(11): 2373-80.
[http://dx.doi.org/10.1002/ijc.23173] [PMID: 17893866]

[409] Serhan CN, de la Rosa X, Jouvene CC. Cutting edge: human vagus produces specialized proresolving mediators of inflammation with electrical stimulation reducing proinflammatory eicosanoids. J Immunol 2018; 201(11): 3161-5.
[http://dx.doi.org/10.4049/jimmunol.1800806] [PMID: 30355784]

[410] Azad N, Rojanasakul Y, Vallyathan V. Inflammation and lung cancer: roles of reactive oxygen/nitrogen species. J Toxicol Environ Health B Crit Rev 2008; 11(1): 1-15.
[http://dx.doi.org/10.1080/10937400701436460] [PMID: 18176884]

[411] Kraus S, Arber N. Inflammation and colorectal cancer. Curr Opin Pharmacol 2009; 9(4): 405-10.
[http://dx.doi.org/10.1016/j.coph.2009.06.006] [PMID: 19589728]

[412] Lin R, Zhang C, Zheng J, *et al.* Chronic inflammation-associated genomic instability paves the way for human esophageal carcinogenesis. Oncotarget 2016; 7(17): 24564-71.
[http://dx.doi.org/10.18632/oncotarget.8356] [PMID: 27028857]

[413] Chang CL, Marra G, Chauhan DP, *et al.* Oxidative stress inactivates the human DNA mismatch repair system. Am J Physiol Cell Physiol 2002; 283(1): C148-54.
[http://dx.doi.org/10.1152/ajpcell.00422.2001] [PMID: 12055083]

[414] Triantafillidis JK, Nasioulas G, Kosmidis PA. Colorectal cancer and inflammatory bowel disease: epidemiology, risk factors, mechanisms of carcinogenesis and prevention strategies. Anticancer Res 2009; 29(7): 2727-37.
[PMID: 19596953]

[415] Grimm M, Kim M, Rosenwald A, *et al.* Toll-like receptor (TLR) 7 and TLR8 expression on CD133+ cells in colorectal cancer points to a specific role for inflammation-induced TLRs in tumourigenesis and tumour progression. Eur J Cancer 2010; 46(15): 2849-57.
[http://dx.doi.org/10.1016/j.ejca.2010.07.017] [PMID: 20728343]

[416] Grivennikov SI, Karin M. Inflammation and oncogenesis: a vicious connection. Curr Opin Genet Dev 2010; 20(1): 65-71.
[http://dx.doi.org/10.1016/j.gde.2009.11.004] [PMID: 20036794]

[417] Guerra C, Barbacid M. Genetically engineered mouse models of pancreatic adenocarcinoma. Mol Oncol 2013; 7(2): 232-47.

[418] Liu S, Wu L-C, Pang J, *et al.* Sp1/NFκB/HDAC/miR-29b regulatory network in KIT-driven myeloid leukemia. Cancer Cell 2010; 17(4): 333-47.

[419] Shchors K, Shchors E, Rostker F, *et al.* The Myc-dependent angiogenic switch in tumors is mediated by interleukin 1β. Genes Dev 2006; 20(18): 2527-38.

[420] Solinas G, Germano G, Mantovani A. Tumor-associated macrophages (TAM) as major players of the cancer-related inflammation. J Leukoc Biol 2009; 86(5): 1065-73.

[421] Yu J, Vodyanik MA, Smuga-Otto K, *et al.* Induced pluripotent stem cell lines derived from human somatic cells. Science 2007; 318(5858): 1917-20.
[http://dx.doi.org/10.1126/science.1151526]

[422] Dang CV. Links between metabolism and cancer. Genes Dev 2012; 26(9): 877-90.
[http://dx.doi.org/10.1101/gad.189365.112] [PMID: 22549953]

[423] Ward PS, Thompson CB. Metabolic reprogramming: a cancer hallmark even warburg did not anticipate. Cancer Cell 2012; 21(3): 297-308.
[http://dx.doi.org/10.1016/j.ccr.2012.02.014] [PMID: 22439925]

[424] Detmer SA, Chan DC. Functions and dysfunctions of mitochondrial dynamics. Nat Rev Mol Cell Biol 2007; 8(11): 870-9.
[http://dx.doi.org/10.1038/nrm2275] [PMID: 17928812]

[425] McBride HM, Neuspiel M, Wasiak S. Mitochondria: more than just a powerhouse. Curr Biol 2006; 16(14): R551-60.
[http://dx.doi.org/10.1016/j.cub.2006.06.054] [PMID: 16860735]

[426] Weinberg SE, Chandel NS. Targeting mitochondria metabolism for cancer therapy. Nat Chem Biol 2015; 11(1): 9-15.
[http://dx.doi.org/10.1038/nchembio.1712] [PMID: 25517383]

[427] Wen S, Zhu D, Huang P. Targeting cancer cell mitochondria as a therapeutic approach. Future Med Chem 2013; 5(1): 53-67.
[http://dx.doi.org/10.4155/fmc.12.190] [PMID: 23256813]

[428] Wallace DC. Mitochondria and cancer. Nat Rev Cancer 2012; 12(10): 685-98.
[http://dx.doi.org/10.1038/nrc3365] [PMID: 23001348]

[429] Sreedhar A, Zhao Y. Dysregulated metabolic enzymes and metabolic reprogramming in cancer cells. Biomed Rep 2018; 8(1): 3-10.
[PMID: 29399334]

[430] Badrinath N, Yoo SY. Mitochondria in cancer: in the aspects of tumorigenesis and targeted therapy. Carcinogenesis 2018; 39(12): 1419-30.
[http://dx.doi.org/10.1093/carcin/bgy148] [PMID: 30357389]

[431] DeBerardinis R, Chandel N. Fundamentals of cancer metabolism. Sci Adv 2016; 2: e1600200.
[http://dx.doi.org/10.1126/sciadv.1600200]

[432] Warburg O. On the origin of cancer cells. Science 1956; 123(3191): 309-14.
[http://dx.doi.org/10.1126/science.123.3191.309] [PMID: 13298683]

[433] Visvader JE. Cells of origin in cancer. Nature 2011; 469(7330): 314-22.
[http://dx.doi.org/10.1038/nature09781] [PMID: 21248838]

[434] Jones RG, Thompson CBJG. Tumor suppressors and cell metabolism: A recipe for cancer growth. Genes Dev 2009; 23(5): 537-48.

[435] Semenza GL. Defining the role of hypoxia-inducible factor 1 in cancer biology and therapeutics. Oncogene 2010; 29(5): 625-34.
[http://dx.doi.org/10.1038/onc.2009.441]

[436] Vander Heiden MG, Cantley LC, Thompson CB. Understanding the Warburg effect: the metabolic requirements of cell proliferation. Science 2009; 324(5930): 1029-33.

[437] Lunt SY, Vander Heiden MG. Aerobic glycolysis: meeting the metabolic requirements of cell proliferation. Annu Rev Cell Dev Biol 2011; 27(1): 441-64.
[http://dx.doi.org/10.1146/annurev-cellbio-092910-154237] [PMID: 21985671]

[438] Deberardinis RJ. Is cancer a disease of abnormal cellular metabolism? New angles on an old idea. Genet Med 2008; 10(11): 767-77.
[http://dx.doi.org/10.1097/GIM.0b013e31818b0d9b] [PMID: 18941420]

[439] Seyfried TN, Shelton LM. Cancer as a metabolic disease. Nutr Metab (Lond) 2010; 7(1): 7.
[http://dx.doi.org/10.1186/1743-7075-7-7] [PMID: 20181022]

[440] Pelicano H, Martin DS, Xu R-H, Huang P. Glycolysis inhibition for anticancer treatment. Oncogene 2006; 25(34): 4633-46.
[http://dx.doi.org/10.1038/sj.onc.1209597] [PMID: 16892078]

[441] Chen Z, Lu W, Garcia-Prieto C, Huang P. The Warburg effect and its cancer therapeutic implications. J Bioenerg Biomembr 2007; 39(3): 267-74.
[http://dx.doi.org/10.1007/s10863-007-9086-x] [PMID: 17551814]

[442] DeBerardinis RJ, Sayed N, Ditsworth D, Thompson CB. Brick by brick: metabolism and tumor cell growth. Curr Opin Genet Dev 2008; 18(1): 54-61.

[http://dx.doi.org/10.1016/j.gde.2008.02.003] [PMID: 18387799]

[443] DeBerardinis RJ, Cheng T. Q's next: the diverse functions of glutamine in metabolism, cell biology and cancer. Oncogene 2010; 29(3): 313-24. [http://dx.doi.org/10.1038/onc.2009.358] [PMID: 19881548]

[444] Jones RG, Thompson CB. Tumor suppressors and cell metabolism: a recipe for cancer growth. Genes Dev 2009; 23(5): 537-48. [http://dx.doi.org/10.1101/gad.1756509] [PMID: 19270154]

[445] Kennedy KM, Dewhirst MW. Tumor metabolism of lactate: the influence and therapeutic potential for MCT and CD147 regulation. Future Oncol 2010; 6(1): 127-48. [http://dx.doi.org/10.2217/fon.09.145]

[446] Yeung SJ, Pan J, Lee MH. Roles of p53, MYC and HIF-1 in regulating glycolysis - the seventh hallmark of cancer. Cell Mol Life Sci 2008; 65(24): 3981-99. [http://dx.doi.org/10.1007/s00018-008-8224-x] [PMID: 18766298]

[447] Dang C. The interplay between MYC and HIF in the Warburg effect Oncogenes Meet Metabolism. Springer 2008; pp. 35-53. [http://dx.doi.org/10.1007/2789_2008_088]

[448] Dang CV, Le A, Gao P. MYC-induced cancer cell energy metabolism and therapeutic opportunities. Clin Cancer Res 2009; 15(21): 6479-83. [http://dx.doi.org/10.1158/1078-0432.CCR-09-0889] [PMID: 19861459]

[449] Lin J, Xia L, Liang J, *et al.* The roles of glucose metabolic reprogramming in chemo- and radio-resistance. J Exp Clin Cancer Res 2019; 38(1): 218. [http://dx.doi.org/10.1186/s13046-019-1214-z] [PMID: 31122265]

[450] Herrero P, Galíndez J, Ruiz N, Martínez-Campa C, Moreno F. Transcriptional regulation of the *Saccharomyces cerevisiae* HXK1,HXK2 andGLK1 genes. Yeast 1995; 11(2): 137-44. [http://dx.doi.org/10.1002/yea.320110205] [PMID: 7732723]

[451] Rempel A, Mathupala SP, Griffin CA, Hawkins AL, Pedersen PL. Glucose catabolism in cancer cells: amplification of the gene encoding type II hexokinase. Cancer Res 1996; 56(11): 2468-71. [PMID: 8653677]

[452] Zancan P, Sola-Penna M, Furtado CM, Da Silva D. Differential expression of phosphofructokinase-1 isoforms correlates with the glycolytic efficiency of breast cancer cells. Mol Genet Metab 2010; 100(4): 372-8. [http://dx.doi.org/10.1016/j.ymgme.2010.04.006] [PMID: 20483646]

[453] Clem BF, O'Neal J, Tapolsky G, *et al.* Targeting 6-phosphofructo-2-kinase (PFKFB3) as a therapeutic strategy against cancer. Mol Cancer Ther 2013; 12(8): 1461-70. [http://dx.doi.org/10.1158/1535-7163.MCT-13-0097] [PMID: 23674815]

[454] Moon JS, Jin WJ, Kwak JH, *et al.* Androgen stimulates glycolysis for *de novo* lipid synthesis by increasing the activities of hexokinase 2 and 6-phosphofructo-2-kinase/fructose-2,6-bisphosphatase 2 in prostate cancer cells. Biochem J 2011; 433(1): 225-33. [http://dx.doi.org/10.1042/BJ20101104] [PMID: 20958264]

[455] Li C, Xiao Z, Chen Z, *et al.* Proteome analysis of human lung squamous carcinoma. Proteomics 2006; 6(2): 547-58. [http://dx.doi.org/10.1002/pmic.200500256] [PMID: 16342241]

[456] Epner DE, Partin AW, Schalken JA, Isaacs JT, Coffey DS. Association of glyceraldehyde-3-phosphate dehydrogenase expression with cell motility and metastatic potential of rat prostatic adenocarcinoma. Cancer Res 1993; 53(9): 1995-7. [PMID: 8481901]

[457] Krasnov GS, Dmitriev AA, Snezhkina AV, Kudryavtseva AV. Deregulation of glycolysis in cancer: glyceraldehyde-3-phosphate dehydrogenase as a therapeutic target. Expert Opin Ther Targets 2013;

17(6): 681-93.
[http://dx.doi.org/10.1517/14728222.2013.775253] [PMID: 23445303]

[458] Azoitei N, Becher A, Steinestel K, *et al.* PKM2 promotes tumor angiogenesis by regulating HIF-1α through NF-κB activation. Mol Cancer 2016; 15(1): 3.
[http://dx.doi.org/10.1186/s12943-015-0490-2] [PMID: 26739387]

[459] Lu W, Cao Y, Zhang Y, *et al.* Up-regulation of PKM2 promote malignancy and related to adverse prognostic risk factor in human gallbladder cancer. Sci Rep 2016; 6(1): 26351.
[http://dx.doi.org/10.1038/srep26351] [PMID: 27283076]

[460] Le A, Cooper CR, Gouw AM, *et al.* Inhibition of lactate dehydrogenase A induces oxidative stress and inhibits tumor progression. Proc Natl Acad Sci USA 2010; 107(5): 2037-42.
[http://dx.doi.org/10.1073/pnas.0914433107] [PMID: 20133848]

[461] Taylor RW, Turnbull DM. Mitochondrial DNA mutations in human disease. Nat Rev Genet 2005; 6(5): 389-402.
[http://dx.doi.org/10.1038/nrg1606] [PMID: 15861210]

[462] Fliss MS, Usadel H, Caballero OL, *et al.* Facile detection of mitochondrial DNA mutations in tumors and bodily fluids. Science 2000; 287(5460): 2017-9.
[http://dx.doi.org/10.1126/science.287.5460.2017] [PMID: 10720328]

[463] Jakupciak JP, Maragh S, Markowitz ME, *et al.* Performance of mitochondrial DNA mutations detecting early stage cancer. BMC Cancer 2008; 8(1): 285.
[http://dx.doi.org/10.1186/1471-2407-8-285] [PMID: 18834532]

[464] Cardaci S, Ciriolo MR. TCA cycle defects and cancer: when metabolism tunes redox state. Int J Cell Biol 2012, Article ID 161837.
[http://dx.doi.org/10.1155/2012/161837]

[465] Todisco S, Convertini P, Iacobazzi V, Infantino V. TCA cycle rewiring as emerging metabolic signature of hepatocellular carcinoma. Cancers (Basel) 2019; 12(1): 68.
[http://dx.doi.org/10.3390/cancers12010068] [PMID: 31881713]

[466] Chen YB, Brannon AR, Toubaji A, *et al.* Hereditary leiomyomatosis and renal cell carcinoma syndrome-associated renal cancer: recognition of the syndrome by pathologic features and the utility of detecting aberrant succination by immunohistochemistry. Am J Surg Pathol 2014; 38(5): 627-37.
[http://dx.doi.org/10.1097/PAS.0000000000000163] [PMID: 24441663]

[467] Frezza C, Zheng L, Folger O, *et al.* Haem oxygenase is synthetically lethal with the tumour suppressor fumarate hydratase. Nature 2011; 477(7363): 225-8.
[http://dx.doi.org/10.1038/nature10363] [PMID: 21849978]

[468] Gaude E, Frezza C. Defects in mitochondrial metabolism and cancer. Cancer Metab 2014; 2(1): 10.
[http://dx.doi.org/10.1186/2049-3002-2-10] [PMID: 25057353]

[469] Neumann HP, Pawlu C, Pęczkowska M, *et al.* Distinct clinical features of paraganglioma syndromes associated with SDHB and SDHD gene mutations. JAMA 2004; 292(8): 943-51.
[http://dx.doi.org/10.1001/jama.292.8.943] [PMID: 15328326]

[470] Pollard PJ, Brière JJ, Alam NA, *et al.* Accumulation of Krebs cycle intermediates and over-expression of HIF1α in tumours which result from germline FH and SDH mutations. Hum Mol Genet 2005; 14(15): 2231-9.
[http://dx.doi.org/10.1093/hmg/ddi227] [PMID: 15987702]

[471] Habano W, Sugai T, Nakamura SI, *et al.* Reduced expression and loss of heterozygosity of the SDHD gene in colorectal and gastric cancer. Oncol Rep 2003; 10(5): 1375-80.
[http://dx.doi.org/10.3892/or.10.5.1375] [PMID: 12883710]

[472] Selak MA, Armour SM, MacKenzie ED, *et al.* Succinate links TCA cycle dysfunction to oncogenesis by inhibiting HIF-α prolyl hydroxylase. Cancer Cell 2005; 7(1): 77-85.
[http://dx.doi.org/10.1016/j.ccr.2004.11.022] [PMID: 15652751]

[473] Parsons DW, Jones S, Zhang X, *et al.* An integrated genomic analysis of human glioblastoma multiforme. Science 2008; 321(5897): 1807-2.

[474] Ducray F, Marie Y, Sanson M. IDH1 and IDH2 mutations in gliomas. N Engl J Med 2009; 360(21): 2248-9.
[http://dx.doi.org/10.1056/NEJMc090593] [PMID: 19469031]

[475] Yen KE, Bittinger MA, Su SM, Fantin VR. Cancer-associated IDH mutations: biomarker and therapeutic opportunities. Oncogene 2010; 29(49): 6409-17.
[http://dx.doi.org/10.1038/onc.2010.444] [PMID: 20972461]

[476] Dang L, White DW, Gross S, *et al.* Cancer-associated IDH1 mutations produce 2-hydroxyglutarate. Nature 2009; 462(7274): 739-44.
[http://dx.doi.org/10.1038/nature08617] [PMID: 19935646]

[477] Singh KK, Desouki MM, Franklin RB, Costello LC. Mitochondrial aconitase and citrate metabolism in malignant and nonmalignant human prostate tissues. Mol Cancer 2006; 5(1): 14.
[http://dx.doi.org/10.1186/1476-4598-5-14] [PMID: 16595004]

[478] Phan LM, Yeung S-CJ, Lee M-H. Cancer metabolic reprogramming: importance, main features, and potentials for precise targeted anti-cancer therapies. Cancer Biol Med 2014; 11(1): 1-19.
[PMID: 24738035]

[479] Riganti C, Gazzano E, Polimeni M, Aldieri E, Ghigo D. The pentose phosphate pathway: An antioxidant defense and a crossroad in tumor cell fate. Free Radic Biol Med 2012; 53(3): 421-36.
[http://dx.doi.org/10.1016/j.freeradbiomed.2012.05.006] [PMID: 22580150]

[480] Jiang P, Du W, Wu M. Regulation of the pentose phosphate pathway in cancer. Protein Cell 2014; 5(8): 592-602.
[http://dx.doi.org/10.1007/s13238-014-0082-8] [PMID: 25015087]

[481] Patra KC, Hay N. The pentose phosphate pathway and cancer. Trends Biochem Sci 2014; 39(8): 347-54.
[http://dx.doi.org/10.1016/j.tibs.2014.06.005] [PMID: 25037503]

[482] Jonas SK, Benedetto C, Flatman A, *et al.* Increased activity of 6-phosphogluconate dehydrogenase and glucose-6-phosphate dehydrogenase in purified cell suspensions and single cells from the uterine cervix in cervical intraepithelial neoplasia. Br J Cancer 1992; 66(1): 185-91.
[http://dx.doi.org/10.1038/bjc.1992.240] [PMID: 1637668]

[483] Yang H-C, Wu Y-H, Yen W-C, *et al.* The redox role of G6PD in cell growth, cell death, and cancer. Cells 2019; 8(9): 1055.
[http://dx.doi.org/10.3390/cells8091055] [PMID: 31500396]

[484] Lucarelli G, Galleggiante V, Rutigliano M, *et al.* Metabolomic profile of glycolysis and the pentose phosphate pathway identifies the central role of glucose-6-phosphate dehydrogenase in clear cell-renal cell carcinoma. Oncotarget 2015; 6(15): 13371-86.
[http://dx.doi.org/10.18632/oncotarget.3823] [PMID: 25945836]

[485] D'Alessandro A, Amelio I, Berkers CR, *et al.* Metabolic effect of TAp63α: enhanced glycolysis and pentose phosphate pathway, resulting in increased antioxidant defense. Oncotarget 2014; 5(17): 7722-33.
[http://dx.doi.org/10.18632/oncotarget.2300] [PMID: 25229745]

[486] Rotblat B, Agostini M, Niklison-Chirou MV, Amelio I, Willis AE, Melino G. Sustained protein synthesis and reduced eEF2K levels in TAp73^{-} mice brain: a possible compensatory mechanism. Cell Cycle 2018; 17(23): 2637-43.
[http://dx.doi.org/10.1080/15384101.2018.1553341] [PMID: 30507330]

[487] Sukhatme VP, Chan B. Glycolytic cancer cells lacking 6-phosphogluconate dehydrogenase metabolize glucose to induce senescence. FEBS Lett 2012; 586(16): 2389-95.
[http://dx.doi.org/10.1016/j.febslet.2012.05.052] [PMID: 22677172]

[488] Vizán P, Alcarraz-Vizán G, Díaz-Moralli S, Solovjeva ON, Frederiks WM, Cascante M. Modulation of pentose phosphate pathway during cell cycle progression in human colon adenocarcinoma cell line HT29. Int J Cancer 2009; 124(12): 2789-96.
[http://dx.doi.org/10.1002/ijc.24262] [PMID: 19253370]

[489] Hartmannsberger D, Mack B, Eggert C, *et al.* Transketolase-like protein 1 confers resistance to serum withdrawal in vitro. Cancer Lett 2011; 300(1): 20-9.
[http://dx.doi.org/10.1016/j.canlet.2010.08.017] [PMID: 20884117]

[490] Jiang P, Du W, Wang X, *et al.* p53 regulates biosynthesis through direct inactivation of glucose-6-phosphate dehydrogenase. Nat Cell Biol 2011; 13(3): 310-6.
[http://dx.doi.org/10.1038/ncb2172] [PMID: 21336310]

[491] Gao L, Mejías R, Echevarría M, López-Barneo J. Induction of the glucose-6-phosphate dehydrogenase gene expression by chronic hypoxia in PC12 cells. FEBS Lett 2004; 569(1-3): 256-60.
[http://dx.doi.org/10.1016/j.febslet.2004.06.004] [PMID: 15225644]

[492] Galtieri A, Tellone E, Ficarra S, *et al.* Resveratrol treatment induces redox stress in red blood cells: a possible role of caspase 3 in metabolism and anion transport. Biol Chem 2010; 391(9): 1057-65.
[http://dx.doi.org/10.1515/bc.2010.100] [PMID: 20536388]

[493] Nishimura M, Uyeda K. Purification and characterization of a novel xylulose 5-phosphate-activated protein phosphatase catalyzing dephosphorylation of fructose-6-phosphate,2-kinase:fructose-2,6-bisphosphatase. J Biol Chem 1995; 270(44): 26341-6.
[http://dx.doi.org/10.1074/jbc.270.44.26341] [PMID: 7592845]

[494] Tian WN, Braunstein LD, Apse K, *et al.* Importance of glucose-6-phosphate dehydrogenase activity in cell death. Am J Physiol Cell Physiol 1999; 276(5): C1121-31.
[http://dx.doi.org/10.1152/ajpcell.1999.276.5.C1121] [PMID: 10329961]

[495] Li D, Zhu Y, Tang Q, *et al.* A new G6PD knockdown tumor-cell line with reduced proliferation and increased susceptibility to oxidative stress. Cancer Biother Radiopharm 2009; 24(1): 81-90.
[http://dx.doi.org/10.1089/cbr.2008.0494] [PMID: 19243250]

[496] Fico A, Paglialunga F, Cigliano L, *et al.* Glucose-6-phosphate dehydrogenase plays a crucial role in protection from redox-stress-induced apoptosis. Cell Death Differ 2004; 11(8): 823-31.
[http://dx.doi.org/10.1038/sj.cdd.4401420] [PMID: 15044966]

[497] Pias EK, Yee Aw T. Apoptosis in mitotic competent undifferentiated cells is induced by cellular redox imbalance independent of reactive oxygen species production. FASEB J 2002; 16(8): 781-90.
[http://dx.doi.org/10.1096/fj.01-0784com] [PMID: 12039859]

[498] Leopold JA, Walker J, Scribner AW, *et al.* Glucose-6-phosphate dehydrogenase modulates vascular endothelial growth factor-mediated angiogenesis. J Biol Chem 2003; 278(34): 32100-6.
[http://dx.doi.org/10.1074/jbc.M301293200] [PMID: 12777375]

[499] Pan S, World CJ, Kovacs CJ, Berk BC. Glucose 6-phosphate dehydrogenase is regulated through c-Src-mediated tyrosine phosphorylation in endothelial cells. Arterioscler Thromb Vasc Biol 2009; 29(6): 895-901.
[http://dx.doi.org/10.1161/ATVBAHA.109.184812] [PMID: 19359662]

[500] Polimeni M, Voena C, Kopecka J, *et al.* Modulation of doxorubicin resistance by the glucose-6-phosphate dehydrogenase activity. Biochem J 2011; 439(1): 141-9.
[http://dx.doi.org/10.1042/BJ20102016] [PMID: 21679161]

[501] Baenke F, Peck B, Miess H, Schulze A. Hooked on fat: the role of lipid synthesis in cancer metabolism and tumour development. Dis Model Mech 2013; 6(6): 1353-63.
[http://dx.doi.org/10.1242/dmm.011338] [PMID: 24203995]

[502] Currie E, Schulze A, Zechner R, Walther TC, Farese RV Jr. Cellular fatty acid metabolism and cancer. Cell Metab 2013; 18(2): 153-61.
[http://dx.doi.org/10.1016/j.cmet.2013.05.017] [PMID: 23791484]

[503] Gurr MI, Harwood JL, Frayn KN. Lipid biochemistry. Springer 2002. [http://dx.doi.org/10.1002/9780470774366]

[504] Santos CR, Schulze A. Lipid metabolism in cancer. FEBS J 2012; 279(15): 2610-23. [http://dx.doi.org/10.1111/j.1742-4658.2012.08644.x] [PMID: 22621751]

[505] Kuhajda FP, Jenner K, Wood FD, *et al.* Fatty acid synthesis: a potential selective target for antineoplastic therapy. Proc Natl Acad Sci USA 1994; 91(14): 6379-83. [http://dx.doi.org/10.1073/pnas.91.14.6379] [PMID: 8022791]

[506] Bauer DE, Hatzivassiliou G, Zhao F, Andreadis C, Thompson CB. ATP citrate lyase is an important component of cell growth and transformation. Oncogene 2005; 24(41): 6314-22. [http://dx.doi.org/10.1038/sj.onc.1208773] [PMID: 16007201]

[507] Qian X, Hu J, Zhao J, Chen H. ATP citrate lyase expression is associated with advanced stage and prognosis in gastric adenocarcinoma. Int J Clin Exp Med 2015; 8(5): 7855-60. [PMID: 26221340]

[508] Xin M, Qiao Z, Li J, *et al.* miR-22 inhibits tumor growth and metastasis by targeting ATP citrate lyase: evidence in osteosarcoma, prostate cancer, cervical cancer and lung cancer. Oncotarget 2016; 7(28): 44252-65. [http://dx.doi.org/10.18632/oncotarget.10020] [PMID: 27317765]

[509] Lucenay KS, Doostan I, Karakas C, *et al.* Cyclin E associates with the lipogenic enzyme ATP-citrate lyase to enable malignant growth of breast cancer cells. Cancer Res 2016; 76(8): 2406-18. [http://dx.doi.org/10.1158/0008-5472.CAN-15-1646] [PMID: 26928812]

[510] Gong J, Shen S, Yang Y, *et al.* Inhibition of FASN suppresses migration, invasion and growth in hepatoma carcinoma cells by deregulating the HIF-1α/IGFBP1 pathway. Int J Oncol 2017; 50(3): 883-92. [http://dx.doi.org/10.3892/ijo.2017.3867] [PMID: 28197637]

[511] Ogino S, Kawasaki T, Ogawa A, Kirkner GJ, Loda M, Fuchs CS. Fatty acid synthase overexpression in colorectal cancer is associated with microsatellite instability, independent of CpG island methylator phenotype. Hum Pathol 2007; 38(6): 842-9. [http://dx.doi.org/10.1016/j.humpath.2006.11.018] [PMID: 17350669]

[512] Menendez JA, Lupu R. Fatty acid synthase and the lipogenic phenotype in cancer pathogenesis. Nat Rev Cancer 2007; 7(10): 763-77. [http://dx.doi.org/10.1038/nrc2222] [PMID: 17882277]

[513] Swinnen JV, Vanderhoydonc F, Elgamal AA, *et al.* Selective activation of the fatty acid synthesis pathway in human prostate cancer. Int J Cancer 2000; 88(2): 176-9. [http://dx.doi.org/10.1002/1097-0215(20001015)88:2<176::AID-IJC5>3.0.CO;2-3] [PMID: 11004665]

[514] Yoon S, Lee M-Y, Park S-W, Moon J-S, Koh Y-K, Ahn Y-H, *et al.* Upregulation of acetyl-CoA carboxylase α and fatty acid synthase by HER2 at translational level in breast cancer cells. J Biol Chem 2007; 282(36): 26122-31. [http://dx.doi.org/10.1074/jbc.M702854200]

[515] Su YW, Lin YH, Pai MH, *et al.* Association between phosphorylated AMP-activated protein kinase and acetyl-CoA carboxylase expression and outcome in patients with squamous cell carcinoma of the head and neck. PLoS One 2014; 9(4): e96183. [http://dx.doi.org/10.1371/journal.pone.0096183] [PMID: 24769813]

[516] Wang MD, Wu H, Fu GB, *et al.* Acetyl-coenzyme A carboxylase alpha promotion of glucose-mediated fatty acid synthesis enhances survival of hepatocellular carcinoma in mice and patients. Hepatology 2016; 63(4): 1272-86. [http://dx.doi.org/10.1002/hep.28415] [PMID: 26698170]

[517] Beckers A, Organe S, Timmermans L, *et al.* Chemical inhibition of acetyl-CoA carboxylase induces

growth arrest and cytotoxicity selectively in cancer cells. Cancer Res 2007; 67(17): 8180-7. [http://dx.doi.org/10.1158/0008-5472.CAN-07-0389] [PMID: 17804731]

[518] Clendening JW, Pandyra A, Boutros PC, *et al.* Dysregulation of the mevalonate pathway promotes transformation. Proc Natl Acad Sci USA 2010; 107(34): 15051-6. [http://dx.doi.org/10.1073/pnas.0910258107] [PMID: 20696928]

[519] Graf H, Jüngst C, Straub G, *et al.* Chemoembolization combined with pravastatin improves survival in patients with hepatocellular carcinoma. Digestion 2008; 78(1): 34-8. [http://dx.doi.org/10.1159/000156702] [PMID: 18797167]

[520] Kornblau SM, Banker DE, Stirewalt D, *et al.* Blockade of adaptive defensive changes in cholesterol uptake and synthesis in AML by the addition of pravastatin to idarubicin + high-dose Ara-C: a phase 1 study. Blood 2007; 109(7): 2999-3006. [http://dx.doi.org/10.1182/blood-2006-08-044446] [PMID: 17158228]

[521] Kodach LL, Jacobs RJ, Voorneveld PW, *et al.* Statins augment the chemosensitivity of colorectal cancer cells inducing epigenetic reprogramming and reducing colorectal cancer cell 'stemness' via the bone morphogenetic protein pathway. Gut 2011; 60(11): 1544-53. [http://dx.doi.org/10.1136/gut.2011.237495] [PMID: 21551187]

[522] Horton JD. Sterol regulatory element-binding proteins: transcriptional activators of lipid synthesis. Biochem Soc Trans 2002; 30(6): 1091-5. [http://dx.doi.org/10.1042/bst0301091] [PMID: 12440980]

[523] Hardie DG. AMP-activated/SNF1 protein kinases: conserved guardians of cellular energy. Nat Rev Mol Cell Biol 2007; 8(10): 774-85. [http://dx.doi.org/10.1038/nrm2249] [PMID: 17712357]

[524] Freed-Pastor WA, Mizuno H, Zhao X, *et al.* Mutant p53 disrupts mammary tissue architecture via the mevalonate pathway. Cell 2012; 148(1-2): 244-58. [http://dx.doi.org/10.1016/j.cell.2011.12.017] [PMID: 22265415]

[525] Shamma A, Takegami Y, Miki T, *et al.* Rb Regulates DNA damage response and cellular senescence through E2F-dependent suppression of N-ras isoprenylation. Cancer Cell 2009; 15(4): 255-69. [http://dx.doi.org/10.1016/j.ccr.2009.03.001] [PMID: 19345325]

[526] Guo D, Reinitz F, Youssef M, *et al.* An LXR agonist promotes glioblastoma cell death through inhibition of an EGFR/AKT/SREBP-1/LDLR-dependent pathway. Cancer Discov 2011; 1(5): 442-56. [http://dx.doi.org/10.1158/2159-8290.CD-11-0102] [PMID: 22059152]

[527] Samuel VT, Shulman GI. Mechanisms for insulin resistance: common threads and missing links. Cell 2012; 148(5): 852-71. [http://dx.doi.org/10.1016/j.cell.2012.02.017] [PMID: 22385956]

[528] Rosenzweig SA, Atreya HS. Defining the pathway to insulin-like growth factor system targeting in cancer. Biochem Pharmacol 2010; 80(8): 1115-24. [http://dx.doi.org/10.1016/j.bcp.2010.06.013] [PMID: 20599789]

[529] Shoelson SE, Lee J, Goldfine AB. Inflammation and insulin resistance. J Clin Invest 2006; 116(7): 1793-801. [http://dx.doi.org/10.1172/JCI29069] [PMID: 16823477]

[530] Kalaany NY, Sabatini DM. Tumours with PI3K activation are resistant to dietary restriction. Nature 2009; 458(7239): 725-31. [http://dx.doi.org/10.1038/nature07782] [PMID: 19279572]

[531] Sell Ch. Caloric restriction and insulin-like growth factors in aging and cancer. Horm Metab Res 2003; 35(11-12): 705-11. [PMID: 14710349]

[532] Dang CV. Glutaminolysis: Supplying carbon or nitrogen or both for cancer cells? Cell Cycle 2010; 9(19): 3884-6.

[http://dx.doi.org/10.4161/cc.9.19.13302] [PMID: 20948290]

[533] Wise DR, Thompson CB. Glutamine addiction: a new therapeutic target in cancer. Trends Biochem Sci 2010; 35(8): 427-33.
[http://dx.doi.org/10.1016/j.tibs.2010.05.003] [PMID: 20570523]

[534] DeBerardinis RJ, Lum JJ, Hatzivassiliou G, Thompson CB. The biology of cancer: metabolic reprogramming fuels cell growth and proliferation. Cell Metab 2008; 7(1): 11-20.
[http://dx.doi.org/10.1016/j.cmet.2007.10.002] [PMID: 18177721]

[535] Sandulache VC, Ow TJ, Pickering CR, *et al.* Glucose, not glutamine, is the dominant energy source required for proliferation and survival of head and neck squamous carcinoma cells. Cancer 2011; 117(13): 2926-38.
[http://dx.doi.org/10.1002/cncr.25868] [PMID: 21692052]

[536] Nicklin P, Bergman P, Zhang B, *et al.* Bidirectional transport of amino acids regulates mTOR and autophagy. Cell 2009; 136(3): 521-34.
[http://dx.doi.org/10.1016/j.cell.2008.11.044] [PMID: 19203585]

[537] Gangrade A, Calin GA. MicroRNAs and cancer hallmarks. Cancer Hallm 2013; 1(1): 50-7.
[http://dx.doi.org/10.1166/ch.2013.1005]

[538] Dang CV. Rethinking the Warburg effect with Myc micromanaging glutamine metabolism. Cancer Res 2010; 70(3): 859-62.
[http://dx.doi.org/10.1158/0008-5472.CAN-09-3556] [PMID: 20086171]

[539] Meng M, Chen S, Lao T, Liang D, Sang N. Nitrogen anabolism underlies the importance of glutaminolysis in proliferating cells. Cell Cycle 2010; 9(19): 3921-32.
[http://dx.doi.org/10.4161/cc.9.19.13139] [PMID: 20935507]

[540] Altman BJ, Stine ZE, Dang CV. From Krebs to clinic: glutamine metabolism to cancer therapy. Nat Rev Cancer 2016; 16(10): 619-34.
[http://dx.doi.org/10.1038/nrc.2016.71] [PMID: 27492215]

[541] Stepulak A, Luksch H, Gebhardt C, *et al.* Expression of glutamate receptor subunits in human cancers. Histochem Cell Biol 2009; 132(4): 435-45.
[http://dx.doi.org/10.1007/s00418-009-0613-1] [PMID: 19526364]

[542] Possemato R, Marks KM, Shaul YD, *et al.* Functional genomics reveal that the serine synthesis pathway is essential in breast cancer. Nature 2011; 476(7360): 346-50.
[http://dx.doi.org/10.1038/nature10350] [PMID: 21760589]

[543] Amelio I, Cutruzzolá F, Antonov A, Agostini M, Melino G. Serine and glycine metabolism in cancer. Trends Biochem Sci 2014; 39(4): 191-8.
[http://dx.doi.org/10.1016/j.tibs.2014.02.004] [PMID: 24657017]

[544] Locasale JW, Grassian AR, Melman T, *et al.* Phosphoglycerate dehydrogenase diverts glycolytic flux and contributes to oncogenesis. Nat Genet 2011; 43(9): 869-74.
[http://dx.doi.org/10.1038/ng.890] [PMID: 21804546]

[545] Jain M, Nilsson R, Sharma S, *et al.* Metabolite profiling identifies a key role for glycine in rapid cancer cell proliferation. Science 2012; 336(6084): 1040-4.
[http://dx.doi.org/10.1126/science.1218595] [PMID: 22628656]

[546] Cruz M, Maldonado-Bernal C, Mondragón-Gonzalez R, *et al.* Glycine treatment decreases proinflammatory cytokines and increases interferon-γ in patients with Type 2 diabetes. J Endocrinol Invest 2008; 31(8): 694-9.
[http://dx.doi.org/10.1007/BF03346417] [PMID: 18852529]

[547] Hasegawa S, Ichiyama T, Sonaka I, *et al.* Cysteine, histidine and glycine exhibit anti-inflammatory effects in human coronary arterial endothelial cells. Clin Exp Immunol 2012; 167(2): 269-74.
[http://dx.doi.org/10.1111/j.1365-2249.2011.04519.x] [PMID: 22236003]

[548] Locasale JW. Serine, glycine and one-carbon units: cancer metabolism in full circle. Nat Rev Cancer 2013; 13(8): 572-83.
[http://dx.doi.org/10.1038/nrc3557] [PMID: 23822983]

[549] Mattaini KR, Sullivan MR, Vander Heiden MG. The importance of serine metabolism in cancer. J Cell Biol 2016; 214(3): 249-57.
[http://dx.doi.org/10.1083/jcb.201604085] [PMID: 27458133]

[550] Tan D-J, Bai R-K, Wong L-JC. Comprehensive scanning of somatic mitochondrial DNA mutations in breast cancer. Cancer Res 2002; 62(4): 972-6.
[PMID: 11861366]

[551] Ishikawa K, Takenaga K, Akimoto M, *et al.* ROS-generating mitochondrial DNA mutations can regulate tumor cell metastasis. Science 2008; 320(5876): 661-4.
[http://dx.doi.org/10.1126/science.1156906] [PMID: 18388260]

[552] Swalwell H, Kirby DM, Blakely EL, *et al.* Respiratory chain complex I deficiency caused by mitochondrial DNA mutations. Eur J Hum Genet 2011; 19(7): 769-75.
[http://dx.doi.org/10.1038/ejhg.2011.18] [PMID: 21364701]

[553] Kwong JQ, Henning MS, Starkov AA, Manfredi G. The mitochondrial respiratory chain is a modulator of apoptosis. J Cell Biol 2007; 179(6): 1163-77.
[http://dx.doi.org/10.1083/jcb.200704059] [PMID: 18086914]

[554] Osellame LD, Blacker TS, Duchen MR. Cellular and molecular mechanisms of mitochondrial function. Best Pract Res Clin Endocrinol Metab 2012; 26(6): 711-23.
[http://dx.doi.org/10.1016/j.beem.2012.05.003] [PMID: 23168274]

[555] Agostinelli E, Tempera G, Molinari A, *et al.* The physiological role of biogenic amines redox reactions in mitochondria. New perspectives in cancer therapy. Amino Acids 2007; 33(2): 175-87.
[http://dx.doi.org/10.1007/s00726-007-0510-7] [PMID: 17390098]

[556] Shen YH, Wang XL, Wilcken DEL. Nitric oxide induces and inhibits apoptosis through different pathways. FEBS Lett 1998; 433(1-2): 125-31.
[http://dx.doi.org/10.1016/S0014-5793(98)00844-8] [PMID: 9738946]

[557] Grancara S, Ohkubo S, Artico M, *et al.* Milestones and recent discoveries on cell death mediated by mitochondria and their interactions with biologically active amines. Amino Acids 2016; 48(10): 2313-26.
[http://dx.doi.org/10.1007/s00726-016-2323-z] [PMID: 27619911]

[558] Bensaad K, Vousden KH. p53: new roles in metabolism. Trends Cell Biol 2007; 17(6): 286-91. [doi: 10.1016/j.tcb.2007.04.004].

[559] Maddocks OD, Berkers CR, Mason SM, *et al.* Serine starvation induces stress and p53-dependent metabolic remodelling in cancer cells. Nature 2013; 493(7433): 542-6.
[http://dx.doi.org/10.1038/nature11743]

[560] Ying H, Kimmelman AC, Lyssiotis CA, *et al.* Oncogenic Kras maintains pancreatic tumors through regulation of anabolic glucose metabolism. Cell 2012;149(3):656-70.
[http://dx.doi.org/10.1016/j.cell.2012.01.058]

[561] Son J, Lyssiotis CA, Ying H, *et al.* Glutamine supports pancreatic cancer growth through a KRAS-regulated metabolic pathway. Nature 2013; 496(7443): 101-5.
[http://dx.doi.org/10.1038/nature12040]

[562] Coller HA. Is cancer a metabolic disease? Am J Pathol 2014; 184(1): 4-17.
[http://dx.doi.org/10.1016/j.ajpath.2013.07.035] [PMID: 24139946]

CHAPTER 5

Growth Factors and Cancer

Aisha Al Anazi[1,*], Ravi Teja Chitturi Suryaprakash[2], Kate Shearston[2] and Omar Kujan[2]

[1] *Department of Paediatrics, Division of Endocrine and Diabetes, Prince Sultan Military Medical City, Riyadh, Saudi Arabia*

[2] *UWA Dental School, The University of Western Australia, Nedlands, 6009 WA, Australia*

Abstract: Cancer causes major patient morbidity and mortality and is a critical health concern worldwide. The recent GLOBOCAN 2019 factsheet recorded nearly 19.2 million new cancer cases, 9.9 million cancer deaths and 50.55 million people suffering from different kinds of cancer globally within 5 years after diagnosis. Growth factors (GF) are a group of proteins that can affect cellular processes, including differentiation, division, intravasation, extravasation and dissemination. The circulating tumor cells in the bloodstream can populate distant tissues and organs and believe to be the primary cause of metastasis. Extravasation is a crucial phase in the metastasis process, in which tumor cells leave the bloodstream and enter the host tissue. The progress of metastasis is triggered by the tendency of cancer cells to disseminate to target organs from the site of the primary tumor. Despite extensive basic scientific and clinical investigations, cancer is still a major clinical and public health problem. The development of cancer can be influenced by genetics, environmental factors, gene-environment interaction, lifestyle, age and a number of other factors. The harnessing and enhancement of the body's own cytotoxic cells to prevent basement membrane rupture and the intervening dissemination processes can provide useful insight into the development of cancer. The mutation in oncogenes and tumour suppressor genes, and chromosomal aberration is a cornerstones of the molecular basis of cancer. The basement Membrane (BM) acts as a cell invasion shield, thus identification of processes that underlie in breaching of BM can contribute to understanding the disease pathogenesis. TGF-β is known for its dual function; it requires inhibition in the advanced stage however, the growth inhibitory properties are displayed in the early stages of tumorigenesis. Therefore, inhibition of TGF-β signalling in the CD8+ T cell compartment may be necessary for tumor immunity to be restored. Quantitation of tumour cell dissemination is important and plays significant role in elucidating mechanisms of cancer and strategies for therapeutic intervention.

Keywords: Cancer, Growth Factors, Oncogenesis, Tyrosine Kinase Inhibitors.

[*] **Corresponding author Aisha Al Anazi:** Department of Paediatrics, Division of Endocrine and Diabetes, Prince Sultan Military Medical City, Riyadh, Saudi Arabia; Email: dr_aisha2005@hotmail.com

Faris Q.B. Alenzi (Ed.)

GROWTH FACTOR INDUCED BASEMENT MEMBRANE BREAKDOWN AND INVASION IN CANCER

Cancer, which causes major patient morbidity and mortality, is a critical health concern worldwide. Metastasis is a multistep process caused by tumor growth, angiogenesis, detachment of tumor cells, and invasion of the extracellular matrix that can lead to uncontrolled growth potential and metastasis into surrounding tissues [1]. Each of these steps is critical for the survival of tumor cells and the development of secondary lesions. Interactions between tumor cells and the host microenvironment influence tumor survival and development. Tumor invasion involves the disruption of the basement membrane and infiltration of the underlying stroma. Invasion necessitates significant changes in cell morphology and phenotype, especially in epithelial cells, which are the precursors of more than 90% of human cancers. It includes adhesion between cell-cell and cell-matrix could be responsible for the degradation of the matrix and cellular motility [2].

Tumor development is only permitted after the dissolution of the decorating secretory ducts of the basement membrane. Growth factors play a crucial role in the destruction of the basement membrane, the intrusion into adjacent tissues by cancer cells, the vascular or lymphatic networks (intravasation), as well as exit from the bloodstream (extravasation) and eventual invasion of distant organs [3]. In experimental data conducted on clinical specimens and ErbB-2/HER2-overexpression, spheroids resembling mammary ductal carcinoma *in situ* (DCIS) raised the likelihood that invasive growth was underpinned by TGF-β or 14-3-3-zeta adaptor overexpression [4, 5]. In *in vitro* models, TGF-β and other growth factors seem to have been involved in certain transformations. GFs have been shown to cause multiple adhesion molecular switches, such as a loss of epithelial E-cadherin and a gain of mesenchymal N-cadherin [6]. Tensin-3 is a connective protein that links the actin cytoskeleton and the extracellular matrix, which is replaced by tensin-4, resulting in the disruption of the bridge and facilitating cell migration [7]. In certain epithelial tumours, E-dual cadherin's growth arrest and adhesive functions are lost by mutational inactivation, transcriptional suppression, or extracellular cadherin domain proteolysis. A number of GFs, which include TGF-β, EGF, and Notch cleaved proteins, affect the expression of repressors of E-cadherin. Further, E-cadherin cleavage, ubiquitylation, and endocytosis may cause E-cadherin downregulation [8].

The degree and timing of invasion and metastasis may be affected by several factors, including genetic and epigenetic heterogeneity within the tumor, extrinsic factors and growth factors [9]. Growth factors and cytokines produced by the tumour microenvironment and tumour cells themselves, are the key extracellular triggers that control these migration programs and, thus, regulate strategies for adaptive invasion. They can work in an autocrine, paracrine or endocrine manner to orchestrate central cell functions, including proliferation, differentiation, apoptosis and cell migration [10]. Metastases are a major reason for the failure of modern cancer therapies and associated mortality and are caused by the detachment of malignant cells from the primary tumor site and colonisation of close and remote organ sites. Precise knowledge of the molecular mechanisms regulating each step of metastasis is required to understand the pathophysiology of cancer. Cancer metastasis is a multi-step process that comprises local invasion, neoangiogenesis, circulatory system survival, extravasation to the target organ, and so on. Tumor cells must remodel, or lose their basement barrier, in order to reach vessels and get access to distant organs [11]. Research so far has strongly suggested that the basement membrane acts as a cell invasion shield, therefore investigations into basement membrane invasion can provide useful insight into the development of cancer.

Growth Factor-Induced Basement Membrane Breakdown and Invasive Growth

Growth factors are small polypeptides that bind to kinase-activating transmembrane receptors to activate a certain set of intracellular signaling pathways. Examples include mitogen-activated protein kinase (MAPK), phosphatidylinositol 3-kinase (PI3K), phospholipase C-γ, and transcription factors, such as STATs or SMAD proteins [12, 13]. Growth factors encourage cell growth and proliferation, and are considered the main growth regulatory molecules for cells *in vitro* culture and likely *in vivo*. In culture conditions, non-transformed cells display an absolute necessity of growth factors for proliferation. And in most cases, more than one factor is needed. Growth factors are exhausted more quickly than other media components under standard culture conditions and hence rate limiting for proliferation. in neoplastic transformed cells, there is commonly a lack or reduced requirement for specific growth factors, which is the hall mark of cancer cells [12, 14]. The accumulation of genetic changes and genomic instability leads to tumorigenesis. Genomic instability describes a genome containing variation in a genetic sequence that may affect gene expression, and protein expression, known as mutation. It also includes epigenetic and chromosomal alteration [14]. Genomic instability is considered the cornerstone of the molecular classification of cancer. The most prevalent form of genomic instability is chromosomal instability, and the presence of a high degree of chromosome structural modifications has been reported in tumour cells [15]. A driver mutation is an alteration that gives cancer cells a selective advantage compared to other cells, leading to cell proliferation and tumor growth [16]. Previous studies suggested the role of GFs in the step-wise progression of cancers.

Insulin-like growth factor-1 (IGF-1) and epidermal growth factors (EGF) are polypeptide growth factors that play an important role in human physiology and have been linked to malignant transformation. IGF-I and EGF downstream signalling pathways play a direct role in the development of treatment-resistant disorder. Changes in the bioavailability of these GFs are a key contributor to disease progression [17]. Witsch *et al.* [12] have shown that somatic mutation that confers significant survival and growth benefits on activated cells. They have shown that EGF and IGF1 contribute to the clone-bearing mutation that is found frequently in intraluminal lesions, like *in situ* carcinoma or intraepithelial neoplasia surrounding the basal membrane, relating to the movement and invasion of cancer cells into adjacent tissues. This approach includes epithelial polarity loss, mesenchymal-like motility, and protease secretion. This crucial process of tumour growth is regulated by oncogenes and tumor suppressors, as well as a diverse range of GFs. Cancer cells enter lymphatic and blood vessels (extravasation) and leave (intravasation) to spread and metastasize to distant organs.

Macrophages, platelets, and endothelial cells all have supportive roles in extra- and intravasation. Chemotherapy and radiation are usually effective against micrometastases. However, the development of resistant clones is driven by the acquisition of new mutations and the capacity of cancer cells to generate GFs. In secondary tumors greater than 1mm, angiogenic processes are required to supply tumours with oxygen and nutrients. The GFs secreted by tumour and stromal cells, such as colony-stimulating factor, (CSF-1), EGF, growth factor for fibroblasts (FGF), heparin-binding EGF (HB-EGF), neuregulin (NRG), growth factor transformative (TGF), VEGF promote both the sprouting of existing arteries and the recruitment of bone marrow-derived endothelial progenitor cells. Relatively significant metastases occupy a distinct set of target organs in the final phase, but this may be preceded by a several-year latency period.

Intravasation

Intravasation is one of the earliest steps in the metastatic process, involving the transfer of tumor cells into adjacent endothelial or epithelial vessels [18, 19]. A single tumor cell goes through a series of events that leads to the creation of a secondary tumor. Intravasation, circulation, extravasation, and colonization are all part of the meta static cascade. Any intervention in these processes lowers the likelihood of metastasis [20]. The tumor cell's phenotype, the endothelium's local state, and the local microenvironment are indeed factors that influence the pace of intravasation [21].

Intravasation of post-EMT cells is critically promoted by paracrine contacts between cancer cells, macrophages, and endothelial cells. For example, mammary cancer cells release colony CSF1, which recruits tumor macrophages and boosts local production of GFs derived from macrophages [22].

Since macrophages are often located next to micro vessels, intravasation is intensified by this self-stimulatory loop. During tumour progression, the hypoxic and inflammatory circumstances that cause macrophages to secrete more TGF- In breast cancer cells, TGF-mediated angiopoietin-like 4 induction (ANGPTL4) induces tumor cells to remain in the lungs, whereas ANGPTL4 enhances tumor cells in the lungs [23]. Tumor cells bind to platelets while in circulation, particularly when stimulated by thrombin, thereby obtaining mitogenic stimuli (*e.g.,* PDGF and lysophosphatidic acid) and defence against natural killer cells [24]. Cancer-associated fibroblasts (CAFs) are another stromal type of pro-metastasis cytokines [25]. The importance of angiogenic, immunological, and hypoxic responses was found to be predictive in a gene expression signature based on laser stroma microdissection, which corresponded to clinical significance [26].

Role of Breaching of the Basement Membrane in Tumour Progression

Basement membranes are a specialized type of extracellular matrix (ECM) present in most of the tissue showing a wide variety of functions. The basement membrane serves a wide variety of functions for tissues, including tissue separation, barrier, and supply of an adhesive substrate for cells and signalling platform migration, polarization, differentiation, and tissue formation. They communicate with the actin cytoskeleton *via* integrins or other ECM receptors to mediate cell attachment and motility, as well as influence intracellular signaling cascades. They work as a reservoir for GFs and contribute their role in cell survival, migration, and proliferation. It includes transforming growth factor-β (TGF-β), fibroblast growth factor (FGF), vascular endothelial growth factor (VEGF), and heparin epidermal growth factor (HB-EGF) [27]. It plays a functional role in cell survival, migration, and proliferation, as well as protecting tissues from mechanical stress. During epithelial tumor formation, cancer cells, like normal epithelial cells, are kept inside the boundaries of the BM and therefore isolated from the surrounding stroma. Therefore, the BM protects from invasion and acts like a shield. There is an increase in stroma stiffness and an increase in the number of many types of cells, such as fibroblasts, macrophages, and pericytes. During tumor growth, natural developmental pathways are frequently hijacked. EMT, as well as decreased intercellular and cell-matrix adhesion, partially recapitulates embryonic processes [28, 29].

Despite the fact that tumor growth and normal morphogenetic processes have similar regulatory mechanisms, transcriptional dysregulation distinguishes tumor progression from developmental processes. Tumour development requires ECM modifications along with transcriptional and post-transcriptional acquisition by tumor cells of invading cellular machinery [30]. By this point, it is unknown whether the stability of the BM has changed or not. Finally, a mixture of events contributes to tumour invasions, such as the interaction between cancer and stromal cell, and contact through the BM. The BM is broken at this point hence, cancer cells invade and spread through the stroma of the tumor until they enter the blood or lymph vessels. Cancer cells will have to resolve two vascular BMs to disseminate and metastasize. To enter the blood vessel, first, they invade BM then, to exit the blood vessel followed by breaching the second BM, affecting other organs to form a secondary tumor [31]. Proteolytic degradation of BM, local displacement of BM by mechanical forces, and aberrant synthesis of BM are some of the mechanisms that have been proposed to explain this. BM degradation includes the development of invadopodia, a localized source of proteases causes matrix degradation. It includes matrix metalloproteinases (MMPs) such as serine protease seprase (FAP) and MT1-MMP (MMP14). *In-vitro* studies have shown the role of invadopodia in matrix degradation however, its role *in vivo* model needs further studies to draw any further conclusion. Dysregulation of proteases such as MMPs during tumour development promotes degradation and invasion of the BM [32]. MMPs are a class of proteolytic enzymes that can break many extracellular matrix constituents. MMPs have been shown to have a role in tumor invasion, neoangiogenesis, and metastasis in previous studies. Hence, it was considered an ideal pharmacological target for cancer therapy. Synthetic inhibitors of MMPs (MMPIs) were studied in multiple cancer types from the 1990s to early 2000. Unexpectedly, all the clinical trials of MMP inhibitors were largely ineffective, despite extremely encouraging preclinical results. The two main reasons were suggested for the failure of MMPIs in clinical trials. The first one, the MMPIs inhibitory effect in the initial trial resulting in blockage of MMPs and tumor progression. The other possible reason could be MMPs plays role in early tumor progression while MMPIs in late stage. Currently, more specific MMPIs are manufactured hence, clinical trial could be reconsidered. Since the basement membrane is an obstacle to the propagation of malignant cells, breaching and dysregulation of the basement membrane. Hence, these are hallmarks of many malignant tumors [33]. Tumour development requires ECM improvements along with transcriptional and post-transcriptional acquisition by tumour cells with invasive cellular machinery [30]. Invadopodia's structures are made up of membrane-associated F-actin that aid cell invasion by expressing proteolytic enzymes that breakdown ECM locally on the cell surface [34]. Invadopodia cell manifestation can be a part of natural morphogenetic processes such as axon guidance [35]. And can also be caused by a thick fibrilla in non-malignant cells. Invadopodia acquisition by tumor cells, however, represents a transcriptional and signalling transition. For local degradation, malignant cells also inject invadopodia into the BM as they develop adherence to the underlying stroma [36]. If they invade local protease activity, invasive cells may kill the basement membrane, consistent with a popular tumor histology feature: a decrease or total disappearance of the basement membrane [37]. Such as an invasive BM cell gives a poor prognosis [38].

The Transforming Growth Factor-β Induced Invasion

The transforming growth factor-β (TGF-β) is a member of cytokines' superfamily which also includes, activins, inhibins, nodal, growth and differentiation factors (GDFs), and bone morphogenetic proteins (BMPs) [39, 40]. In different cellular processes, each family member performs important roles consisting suppression of immune system, growth retardation, epithelial-mesenchymal transfer (EMT), cell migration, invasion, and remodelling of the extracellular matrix ECM [41, 42]. TGF-β also works as a tumour suppressor in the early stages of tumor development, while tumour cells can become immune to its antimitogenic effects in later phases and TGF-β can turn to a tumor promoter [42, 43]. TGF-β signaling enhances EMT in the later stages of cancer progression some of the markers such as mesenchymal markers like N-cadherin and vimentin have shown increased expression while decreased epithelial When adenocarcinoma cells are pre-treated with TGF-1 *in vitro* models, the metastatic potential is increased [44, 45]. TGF-treated carcinoma cells were found to be more invasive *in vitro* due to increased matrix metalloprotease expression, as well as increased tumor cell migration and invasion [46]. Several additional examples have shown over the past ten years that TGF-β1 has a disruptive ability and can accelerate both *in vitro* and *in vivo* malignant growth, invasion and metastasis [47]. TGF-β acts as both tumor suppressor and an effective tumour progression [48]. However, as the tumor grows, genetic and/or biochemical modifications allow TGF to promote tumor growth *via* its pleiotropic activities on both cancer cells and tumor forms of non-malignant stromal cells. The stimulation of TGF-β invasion and metastasis may have a greater therapeutic effect than its tumour-suppressive role, as most human tumors retain functionality.

TGF-β-Induced Epithelial to Mesenchymal Transformation

Reversible epithelial-to-mesenchymal transformation (EMT) is one feature of tumour cell biology which is believed to lead to metastasis. This is potentially a temporary differentiation event *in vivo* studies, inducing increased cell plasticity and encouraging cells to pass into circulation out of the primary tumor [49]. Fibroblastoid tumors of epithelial origin have been observed in both human and murine cancer tissue. There are some examples of tumor cells that may be able to undergo *in vitro* reversible EMT that may be beneficial for replication [50]. TGF has been shown to induce morphological changes in normal and transformed mammary epithelial cells in culture, which are characteristic of EMT [45]. This trans-differentiation is followed by a reorganization of the cytoskeleton actin, downregulation of adhesion expression and cytoskeleton E-cadherin, ZO-1, vinculin and keratin molecules and *de novo* expression of the vimentin mesenchymal marker [51, 52]. TGF-β was active in tumour resistance to treatment with tamoxifen. Later, dominant-negative TβRII has shown minor effect on the growth-suppressive activity of tamoxifen. In addition, transfected with a stable TβRII, TGF-β growth-resistant breast cancer cells restored TGF-β responsiveness without a difference in tamoxifen sensitivity, clearly demonstrating that tamoxifen works through a non-TGF-β-β reaction [53].

Elevated TGF-β expression was later shown to be held accountable for the failure of treatment with tamoxifen by virtue of immunosuppressive effects on NK cells. These findings highlight the importance of a complete understanding of cellular TGF activity before embarking on a new drug design aimed at subverting TGF-signaling pathways. In the late stage, cytostatic effects of TGF-β in cancer cells have been changed and TGF-β signalling function as a tumor promoter by stimulating the epithelial-to-mesenchymal transformation of cancer cells, by affecting angiogenesis, and by encouraging immune response avoidance [54].

Epigenetic Modification and Basement Membrane Invasion

In human cancers, transmembrane protein dysregulation of expression, epigenetic alterations and location of the proteins play a central role in metastasis. However, the exact mechanism and role of genetics and epigenetics in metastatic not yet completely known; it is suspected that the acquisition of the capacity to complete each phase causing metastasis is motivated by the accumulation of genetic mutations and epigenetic events that may contribute to the acquisition of metastatic characteristics by cells during the secondary tumour development period.

Epigenetics is the heritable and reversible changes in gene expression without any alteration in DNA sequence. Also, phenotypic changes occur, namely, without changes in genotype. The epigenetic changes are mainly due to DNA methylation, histone modification, nucleosome-remodelling, and non-coding RNAs. Depending on their functions, these changes may play a significant role in the initiation and maintenance of epigenetic repression or derepression of target genes [55, 56]. Epigenetic changes that cause tumor suppressor silencing or oncogene activation are supposed to play an important role in tumor development. Notably, during EMT and MET, several enzymes involving epigenetic modifications control the expression of the EMT marker E-cadherin, which is called a tumor suppressor [57, 58]. Recent studies have proposed the key function of histone-modifying enzymes in the epigenetic control of the expression of the EMT-TF gene [59, 60], confirming the pivotal role of epigenetic modification in the regulation of EMT-related factors, including EMT-TFs and EMT markers.

In conclusion, recent scientific advances in the field of different 'omics,' such as bioinformatics techniques, have made it possible to identify novel ECM genes and proteins at an unprecedented rate. The importance of many of these recently found genes to growth and disease, however, continues to be unravelled. Therefore, functional genomics and proteomics analyses of basement membrane proteins at the various stages of human development may be useful in the identification of disease biomarkers. Identification of processes that underlie the invasion of the basement membrane can provide useful insight into the development of cancer. Investigation for the source of specific ECM-degrading proteases and their role in the initiation of basement membrane breaching may signify the role of basement membrane breaching in cancer development.

To recognize various developmental and disease pathways, a deeper understanding of not only molecular signaling but also biomechanical processes would be required. Further research is needed to characterize the biophysical properties of the various basement membranes in relation to development and disease. Temporally and spatially regulated gene disruption would be important because, at the single-cell level, many developmental and disease pathways are precisely controlled. The ultimate aim of future studies will be to improve productive therapeutic techniques, such as helping to avoid breaches of the basement membrane in cancer. Additional potential treatment methods may help people suffering from disorders where the basement membrane plays a significant role in the development of pathogenesis and disease.

CURRENT UNDERSTANDING OF THE ROLE OF INTRAVASATION, EXTRAVASATION AND DISSEMINATION IN THE DEVELOPMENT OF CANCER

Intravasation

Intravasation is the invasion of cancer cells into a blood circulation or lymphatic channel through the basement membrane, followed by endothelial cell and cell junction disruption, which is critical for distant metastases. It can initiate the escape of cancerous cells from their primary sites. Micro vessel density and vasculature diameter are important vascular system parameters for intravasation; it has been proposed that the higher the intravasation rate, the larger the vessel diameter will be in particular cancers. Tumor microenvironment, proteases, signaling molecules, and environmental variables at the tumor and associated vasculature are some of the risk factors that lead to cancer cell intravasation [61, 62]. The presence of circulating tumor cells (CTCs) in the bloodstream is the direct result of intravasation (CTCs) and represents an intermediate stage of metastasis [63]. CTCs circulate as solitary cells or in clusters. Aceto *et al.* [64], reported that clusters affected the metastatic potential. It has a shorter half-life as compared to a single cell in the circulation (6–10 min for clusters *vs.* 25–30 min for single cells). The cells may develop metastatic tumors based on the number of CTCs. The metastatic breast cancer patients, the CTC value is >5 cells per 7.5 ml of blood which is above the threshold values [65].

Intravasations are also seen under normal physiological conditions. The entrance of the skin and mucous membranes of thymocytes or dendritic cells (DCs) into the bloodstream and lymph vessels may be considered a prototype of the intravasation of tumour cells during metastasis. The trans-endothelial movement of leukocytes from the site of inflammation represents a prototype of intravasation under the given pathological conditions [18]. Because most tumor cells have a diameter far greater than that of small capillaries, immediately after entering the circulatory system, they are likely to become stuck in the microvasculature [18]. Tumour cell clustering and the ability of certain tumour cells to form microaggregates with blood platelets will help encourage the rapid trapping of tumor cells [66]. It has been revealed that even clusters of CTC can cross capillary-sized vessels by rapid cell chain development and transient deformation of individual tumour cells.

The two-stage of intravasation must be distinguished. The first stage is marked by invasive tumor cell migration to the vessel wall, while the second stage is marked by infiltration through the vessel wall. Invasion into the pre-vascular zone occurs in response to chemotactic signals which are originating from the microenvironment. The first step in the intravasation of individual cells is through the mechanism of mesenchymal invasion, characterized by thick hard fibres in the extracellular matrix, which includes the movement of tumour cells through a loose extracellular matrix. Moreover, the high plasticity of the cells enables them to switch between mechanisms of motion several times [67, 68].

Tumor cells can more easily enter lymphatic vessels than blood vessels because lymphatic vcssels lack thick inter-endothelial junctions, and lymph circulation is slower than blood. In terms of both function and physiology, the lymphatic network is very different from the blood vasculature. Unlike most blood arteries, lymphatics begin as blind-ended capillaries that are freely permeable to fluids and feature pre-adapted discontinuous overlapping junctions for cell transit [69, 70]. Sleeman *et al.* [71], observed that tumour cells may enter the blood vessels directly from the lymph nodes. However, no association was found between the involvement of lymph nodes in lymphogenic metastasis and the emergence of hematogenous metastases. Hematogenous metastases have been indicated to occur in all primary tumours and lymph nodes [62].

Macrophage-Assisted Tumour Cell Intravasation

With the participation of tumour-associated macrophages, the movement of tumor cells into blood vessels continues. Metastasizing tumour cells are able to accelerate movement to blood vessels through type I collagen fibres due to chemotaxis, as seen by the 3D collagen fibre network model [72, 73]. The role of macrophages in intravasation has been supported by the fact their ablation from the tumour inhibits metastasis. Excessive CSF1 expression in tumour cells and EGF in macrophages have been found to be two indexed prognostic markers linked with unfavourable disease prognosis [73, 74]. Wyckoff *et al.* reported that pharmacological inhibition of EGFR signalling could block the intravasation of tumour cells, thereby corroborating the mechanism described above [75].

Intravasation of Tumour Cells Fusing with Macrophages

It is reasonable to expect that intravasation of hybrid CD45LCA+ tumour cells in metastatic breast cancer [76] and ascites in ovarian cancer could reverse trans-endothelial migration [77]. Since tumour cells may fuse with macrophages, it can be suggested that these hybrid cells acquire the properties like macrophage such as metalloproteinases and cytokines secretion, and the existence of typical ligands and receptors which may help in trans endothelial migration [76].

Intravasation Associated with Trogocytosis

There may be another process by which intravasation potential may be increased in tumour cells. Because neutrophils can take up ICAM1-containing endothelial cell membrane fragments *via* trogocytosis, it's possible that cancer cells can pick up ligands and receptors from nearby immune cells [78, 79]. It is important to explain how tumor cells are recruited to a vessel and consideration of mesenchymal and ameboid invasion processes in the penetration of the blood vessel. The presence of the hypothetical intravasation pathways proposed in this analysis should also be validated.

Extravasation

Extravasation is the critical step in the metastasis process in which tumor cells exit from the circulation to the host tissue. In this process, tumour cells invade from the interior of a vessel into the organ parenchyma. There are various mechanisms that can mediate and promote tumor cell extravasation [61]. If the cancer cell has reached a likely intravasation phase, it engages in long-term biochemical interactions with endothelial cells to strengthen adhesion and develop stronger connections, allowing it to extravasate through the endothelium and basement membrane [1, 80]. Tumor cell extravasation is thought to include adhesion to the endothelium, endothelial barrier modulation, and trans-endothelial migration to reach the concern tissues. Once arrested, often in narrow capillaries, tumor cells may migrate or proliferate inside blood vessels and then extravasate [81 - 83]. or transmigrate the endothelium as single cells [61, 81, 84, 85]. Paracellular migration, through which tumour cells migrate between two endothelial cells, tends to be the prevalent mode of extravasation, a mechanism involving cellular rearrangements and disturbance of inter-endothelial cell-cell junctions [85, 86]. In rare cases, tumor cells can migrate through the endothelium by invading individual cell bodies, a mechanism called transcellular migration, as shown by *in vitro* studies [87, 88].

Extravasation includes the interactions of ligand-receptor, chemokines, and circulating nontumor cells [66, 89]. Integrins play an important function in determining the location of extravasation and colonization [90]. The resemblance between cancer cell extravasation and trans endothelial leukocyte migration has been documented in several studies [91, 92]. In recent years, cancer cells have been demonstrated to cause endothelial cells to undergo programmed necrosis, allowing metastatic cells to spread. Endothelial necroptosis and metastatic extravasation were reduced when mice have given the receptor-interacting serine/threonine protein kinase (RIPK)-1 inhibitor necrostatin-1 or endothelial cell-specific RIPK3 deletion [93].

Tumor Cell Properties Promoting Extravasation

Tumour cells are able to facilitate their extravasation directly. Angiopoietin-like 4 (ANGPTL4) or its C-terminal fibrinogen-like domain (cANGPTL4), has been found to be secreted by breast cancer cells, to inhibit endothelial vascular tightness and adhesion junctions, and to enhance tumor cell extravasation and metastasis [23, 94].

Many ligands have been shown to regulate breast malignant cells extravasation, including epiregulin (EREG), heparin-binding EGF-like growth factor (HB-EGF), TGF, cyclooxygenase-2 (COX2), and MMP1 and MMP2. The basic processes remain uncertain, however. The extravasation and metastasis of melanoma cells are enhanced by osteonectin secretion (SPARC), which binds to VCAM-1 and facilitates actin remodelling and endothelial junction opening [95]. To connect with tumor cells and endothelial cells, extravasation requires the help of metastasis-promoting immune cells. Effective extravasation of tumor cells depends not only on tumour and endothelial cell connections, but also includes the intervention of other blood cells. It has been reported that eliminating or interfering with the function of specific cell types has a significant impact on tumor cell extravasation and subsequent metastatic growth [80]. The creation of NETs can encourage metastasis by various means such as its ability to trap circulating tumor cells has been demonstrated [96], a mechanism that can be regulated before or after extravasation by β1-integrin [97] and could promote adhesion to the endothelium. MMP-9, a matrix metalloproteinase released by neutrophils and detected on NETs, can promote extravasation by degrading the extract. The CC-chemokine ligand 2 (CCL2) and E-selectin release of CC-chemokine ligand 2 (CCL2) can also regulate extraversion and metastasis [98, 99]. Monocytes are drawn to metastatic locations and develop into metastasis-associated macrophages (MAMs), which promote tumor cell extravasation by releasing vascular endothelial growth factor (VEGF) [100]. *In vitro* research has revealed that tumor cells can promote endothelial leakiness and trans endothelial migration [101]. The multiple interaction modalities between tumor cells, endothelial cells, immune cells, and platelets most likely work together to modify the endothelium to facilitate tumor cell extravasation and metastasis in the early metastatic niche. The role of other blood constituents in particular phases of the extravasation mechanism is still being investigated [102].

Therapeutic Targets: Intravasation and Extravasation

It is suggested that an appropriate anti-metastatic motility target be used therapeutically in cancer patients to minimize disruption of migratory processes in the body, such as inflammation and wound healing [103]. The critical role of platelets in facilitating the survival of tumour cells in circulation, as well as the extravasation of tumor cells, indicates that anti-platelet drugs are promising to inhibit or limit metastasis, and this is confirmed by numerous pre-clinical trials [104]. Although one of the key mechanisms by which platelets increase metastasis is by protecting cancer cells from NK cell assaults. A combination of anti-platelet drugs and efforts to increase NK cell anti-tumor activity [105] could, on the other hand, have synergistic effects [105]. Several proteins that promote tumor cell survival or mediate tumor cell extravasation during the early phases of metastasis have been found in preclinical research over the last decade and could be used as preventative or therapeutic targets. Prostanoids are a large bioactive lipid family derived from cyclooxygenase-1 (COX-1) and COX-2 activity. Different clinical trials have demonstrated that low-dose aspirin reduces the likelihood of cancer metastasis, preferentially inhibiting platelet activity [106]. NSAIDs, including aspirin, have been reported to inhibit COX-1 and COX-2 leading to reduce metastasis [107, 108].

Extravasation of Leukocytes and Tumour Cells

Extravasation is a process of multiple stages that can be divided into various stages. The extravasation process begins with the rolling, low-affinity attachment of leukocytes and/or tumor cells, which is mediated by the selectin family of adhesion molecules. Rolling occurs when integrins and other adhesion molecules make a strong connection. In a process called diapedesis, leukocytes and tumour cells transmigrate *via* the vascular endothelium following adhesion. Leukocytes are capable of transmigrating through a paracellular or transcellular pathway guided by interactions of adhesion molecules [109]. In contrast to leukocytes, cancer cells are thought not to leave the endothelium intact after diapedesis. If one takes into account the size of tumor cells relative to leukocytes [109], this seems fair. N-cadherin [110] interactions are one of the few pathways conspired for diapedesis. This inadequacy in the knowledge of the means of tumor cell diapedesis should be subject to further study. This cascade is a biochemical pathway for leukocytes that they use to move to inflammatory sites. This mechanism allows tumor cells to disseminate throughout the body by allowing blood to circulate [109].

Dissemination

Metastasis development is triggered by the tendency of cancer cells to disseminate to target organs from the site of the primary tumour. Tumor cells are disseminated to areas in the body while in circulation. Ultimately, the spread of tumor cells to remote organs results in the majority of cancer-related deaths [18, 19]. Anatomical elements like blood and lymph flow in the circulatory system limit the process of diffusion. Metastasis is a multi-step procedure, which consists of the detachment of tumor cells from the primary tumor and then intravasation. Furthermore, extravasation allows the cells to circulate freely and reach neighboring lymph nodes or blood arteries [110]. Most tumours occur as a consequence of genetic modifications to cellular genes, which can be hereditary or arise spontaneously, for example, as a result of DNA damage caused by environmental carcinogens or mutations arising from replication errors [111]. All of the cells in a tumor come from a single cell, which repeatedly divides to produce a diverse population of cancer cells, only some of which contain genetic mutations that cause the cell to seed other tissues. In those cells that can break free and enter the bloodstream from the parent tumor, perhaps not more than 1 in 10,000 eventually ends up forming a new tumour at a distance [112]. The lungs are the first organ through which blood flows after it has passed through most of the other organs, hence, they are the most prevalent location of metastasis [61]. The adhesion and extravasation of circulating tumor cells through endothelial cells, colonizing the PMN, is an important step in the metastatic process [80]. Many of the CTCs circulate as single cells, while others pass in groups. On the other hand, circulating clusters are much more prone to develop metastases [64]. Every day, a large amount of CTC, almost 4×10^6 cells /gram of tumour per day, can release into the bloodstream by a late-stage tumour [113]. Cluster formation is heavily influenced by neutrophils which inhibit leukocyte activation, thus raising the probability of CTC survival. In addition, the association of CTCs with platelets contributes to the creation of a platelet coating barrier over cancer cells that hinders CTC identification by immune cells while also providing the structural support needed to withstand the physical stresses of circulation [114 - 116]. Invasion, followed by intravasation, circulation, extravasation, and colonization, are all processes that lead to the creation of a secondary tumor in a single tumor cell. An event that can block any steps of cancer development can lower the likelihood of metastasis. Even after substantial research has been done for the treatment and therapeutic intervention for the development of cancer, the exact pathophysiology is still unknown. The dearth of clinical studies that can target metastasis, as well as a lack of understanding of the molecular underpinnings that control the metastatic phases, have been identified as key roadblocks in the development of therapeutic interventions [20, 61].

The purpose of successful metastasis-blocking strategies is to resolve dissemination processes and identify common bottlenecks. Despite the fact that metastatic spread is known to follow disease-specific patterns [117], a quantitative understanding of the metastatic dissemination process would improve our ability for better therapy and minimize overtreatment. At present, to target pathways in the metastatic cascade, many techniques have been investigated [118]. Intratumoral linkages, intercellular interaction through ECM adhesion molecules, protease. However, at the time of the diagnosis of metastasis, cancer cells may have already been seeded in the circulatory system. The most probable therapeutic approach, however, appears to be addressing metastatic colonization, as it coincides more with the clinical scene. Interactions between CTCs and the microenvironmental components of circulation determine CTC survival and the ability of CTCs to potentially extravagate at distant places. Metastatic cancer disease appears to be synonymous with a terminal mark today. In order to construct selective therapeutics for metastatic cancer cells, genetic and phenotypic differences between parental and metastatic/circulating cells must be taken into account. While there has been preclinical prevention of metastasis, medication development has been slowed by insufficient research design and therapeutic options [61, 119].

Dissemination of Cancer Cells from a Primary Tumour

The properties of the tumor vasculature and the function of the immune system determine the mechanism of tumor cell spread and transfer from diverse microenvironments and states. Cancer cells may encounter intact or partially lined vasculature at the original site, which can affect the intravasation mode. Micro emboli have shorter half-lives in circulation than single tumor cells and are more likely to bind with blood components. These interactions define the form of arrest in downstream vessels, such as rolling adhesion or vessel blockage, and organs, which finally affect extravasation and likely dormancy and/or extravascular growth.

The supporting clinical and pre-clinical evidence for tumor cell transition between states is depicted, respectively, by dashed or solid lines.

Quantitation of tumour cell dissemination is important and plays a significant role in elucidating mechanisms of cancer and strategies for therapeutic intervention [20]. A fundamental barrier to success in the field is the lack of quantitative understanding of dissemination. For example, it will provide useful insight into dissemination processes to increase understanding of CTCs in a time-dependent manner and CTMs in patients with various cancer types and in response to various treatments.

Advanced quantification methods would enable the development of mathematical models of dissemination, comparable to pharmacokinetic models, to aid in therapy and clinical management. For higher resolution, new *in vivo* approaches may allow real-time calculation and precise counting of CTCs and CTMs.

Similarly, novel methods for quantifying intravasation and extravasation levels may be helpful to researchers for better understanding the sources and sinks of disseminated tumor cells, as well as the effectiveness of the metastatic cascade phases [120]. We can conclude that intravasation, extravasation, and dissemination are the key steps in metastasis. It is complex to develop new therapies based on anti-intravasation. If tumor cell viability is not impaired by anti-intravasative therapy, then it can simply limit the tumor cells to the primary tumor. This could be effective for minimizing tumor cell dissemination caused by other treatments, as well as improving the combined therapy's killing efficacy. The effective strategies for blocking metastasis involve intervention in dissemination processes and the identification of common bottlenecks. It is difficult to treat metastatic cancer due to a lack of early diagnosis of primary tumors and limits in therapy. The development of early detection techniques will enhance strategies that target different metastasis measures, which can prevent secondary/tertiary cancers from spreading from dormant locations and prevent patients with early signs of recurrence from relapsing.

GROWTH FACTORS INDUCE EVASION FROM CYTOTOXIC THERAPIES: AS TARGETS FOR A NEW STRATEGY IN CANCER TREATMENT

Cytotoxic Therapy: An Alternative Approach to Treat Cancer Cells

Cytotoxic therapies are modern treatment approaches that can kill or delay the growth of cancer cells. This is the combination of two words "cyto" means to cell, and "toxic" to poison. Toxins, such as venom, can also be classified as cytotoxic agents. Cytotoxic T cells (CTL) are T cells in our immune system that can kill bacteria, viruses, and cancer cells [121].

T cells are activated by their T-cell receptor, which can bind to antigen peptides on major histocompatibility complex molecules (MHCs). TRAIL (TNF-related apoptosis-inducing ligand) or perforin/granzyme pathway execution following the identification of peptides presented by MHC class I molecules can be used by activated CD8+ cytotoxic T cells (CTLs) to effectively kill target cells [122, 123]. The CD4+ T cells, another fraction of T cells which could be important in adaptive anticancer immunity, recognizing the peptides presented by MHC class II molecules [124]. Recent advancements suggest that rapidly progressing fields of cancer science are now focusing on harnessing and enhancing our bodies' own cytotoxic cells to fight cancer [125]. Many hypotheses have been proposed to understand the mechanism of the cytotoxic effects of natural and artificial cytotoxic agents, but the exact mechanism of cell destruction is still unknown.

Cytotoxic agents affect the cells in such a way that the cell membrane is weakened, resulting in cell bursts, or they may obstruct cell division, causing the cell to stop growing and dividing [126]. The words cytotoxic and genotoxic are a bit confusing. In general, cytotoxic describes the condition in which substance's can cause cell damage however, genotoxic refers to a substance's ability to damage DNA in cells directly. In genotoxic cases, the cell may or may not die. Genetic mutation or damaged DNA is considered a major risk factor for the development of cancers.

Growth Factor-Mediated Evasion from Cytotoxicity

One of the main characteristics of human cancers is intrinsic or acquired resistance to apoptosis [127, 128]. Evasion of apoptosis can lead to tumor growth, progression, and also resistance to treatment, as chemotherapy and radio- and immunotherapy are most of the currently available anticancer therapies. The development of molecular targeted therapies is thus expected to result in a better understanding of the molecular mechanisms underlying tumor resistance to apoptotic cell death.

When the p53 tumour suppressor gene is mutated, apoptosis resistance is increased in cancer cells. Furthermore, the PI3K-AKT pathway, which transmits anti-apoptotic signals, that have been reported in the weakening of apoptosis in human tumors. The extensive involvement of GFs, such as IGF-1 and other EGF-like ligands, in the evasion of apoptosis, is likely to underlie this antiapoptotic survival pathway [12].

The inhibition of growth factor-mediated evasion of cell death has clinical implications. Tumour development above a few millimeters in size is important for the generation of new vessels. The mature endothelial cells may form new vessels, which is important for vasculogenesis [129]. VEGFs, fibroblast growth factors (FGFs), and TGF-β play a considerable role in vasculogenesis and angiogenesis [130]. There are three isoforms of TGF-β exists such as TGF-β1, TGF-β2, and TGF-β3. These cytokines are responsible to exert control over cell proliferation, differentiation, and programmed cell death [131]. TGF-β dimers bind to a type II receptor in the SMAD pathway that recruits and activates a type I receptor by phosphorylation. As a result, the type-I receptor recruits a receptor-regulated SMAD (R-SMAD) [132].

Targeted therapy intercepts signalling pathways, including its precursor, hormone therapy, by using highly selective drugs, for example, tyrosine kinase inhibitors and monoclonal antibodies. These medications are distinguished by their lower toxicity and optimal tolerable doses [133].

T-Cell-Mediated Cytotoxicity

In cancer immunotherapy therapies, T cell-mediated cytotoxicity can be used to destroy the cells. The majority of T-cells function is mediated through T-cell receptors (TCRs) which is a kind of antigen-specific receptors. This mechanism is accompanied by CD8 or CD4 glycoproteins. CTLs are able to kill target cells by subjecting them to programmed cell death. There are two prominent mechanisms that lead to cell death, namely phagocytosis and apoptosis. In phagocytosis, cells pick up and degrade the dead or necrotic tissue, which will gradually heal the wound and remove the damaged tissue. However, in programmed death or apoptosis, there is nuclear blebbing, and cell morphological alterations such as cell shrinkage, chromatin condensation, and DNA fragmentation all take place. The cell then kills itself from inside, shrinking and destroying until nothing is left by shedding membrane-bound vesicles [134]. The CTL programs usually kill their target by apoptosis mechanism. In this, CTLs were mixed with target cells first, then centrifuged to bring them into contact quickly and then to cause the death of the target cell within 5 minutes, but death could be fully evident after an hour. It releases several effector molecules, which activate an endogenous apoptotic pathway within the target cell. Although, CD4+ T cells alone have the ability to remove tumours effectively, CD4+ T cells mediate the destruction of tumours in collaboration with other immune cells. An array of effector molecules, including CD40L, IL2, IFN, and TNF, are produced once CD4+ T cells have been adequately activated, and they play a vital role in coordinating successful antitumor immune responses [135, 136]. Cytotoxic T cells may also react by producing cytokines such as IFN and TNF which are important in defense of the host. IFN blocks viral replication while also increasing the production of newly produced MHC-I proteins. This increase the possibility of the infected cells being identified as target cells for a cytotoxic attack. TNF-α or TNF-β interacts with IFN-γ to activate the macrophage for program cell death.

Several previous studies have shown that maximal antitumor effects are often achieved when CD4+ T cells operate in conjunction with tumour-reactive CD8+T cells, macrophages, or NK cells [137, 138]. A long-standing belief is that immunity to CD4 antitumor can play a significant role in treating only MHC-II+ tumours. Nevertheless, CD4+ T cells are reported for their active role in regulating both MHC-II+ and MHC-II- tumours due to their various mode of action. The effective CD4+ T-cell responses are one of the important therapeutic aspects and have wide clinical significance. Some studies have also shown that CD4+ effector T cells select activated CD8+ T cells through the action of IFN-γ, which can promote cytolytic activity and proliferation mediated by CTL cells through IL22. Beatty *et al.*, [139] revealed that in mice and humans with pancreatic cancer, CD40-activated macrophages become tumoricidal and enhance tumor stroma elimination. They used an agonist CD40 antibody to activate macrophages, it is tempting to speculate that similar effects can be achieved by CD40L-expressing CD4+ effector T cells. Thus, CTL cells function in a number of ways to restrict the spread of cytosolic pathogens by armed effectors. However, the relative importance of each of these mechanisms is still illusive [140].

TGF-β and its Role in Tumour Evasion of Immune Surveillance

Cancer cells often encounter resistance during their development due to the deep growth inhibitory activity of TGF-β. The immunosuppressive effect of TGF-β affects the immune system consisting of immune cell types and their functions [141, 142]. In contrast, TGF-β dysfunction enhances the tumor progression in three aspects: loss of growth inhibitory control, gain of metastagenicity, and evasion of immune surveillance. The functional mutation in the TGF-β receptors gene, the transducers of the Smad signal or by selective loss of cytostatic, differentiate or apoptotic gene responses downstream could be the possible reasons for the loss of growth inhibitory control. This may allow tumour cells to use TGF-β for evasion of immune surveillance. TGF-β regulates T cell homeostasis by specifically suppressing both the proliferation and activation of T cells. It may also prevent antigen presentation on antigen-presenting cells [141].

TGF has been proposed as an important immunosuppressive molecule in the tumor microenvironment, promoting neoplastic progression [143]. Cell engineering in murine xenograft models has resulted in increased expression of the dominant-negative TGF receptor, which could further enhance the potency of prostate-specific membrane antigen-specific CAR T-cells [144]. Further, TGF-β blockade with Mab, such as fresolimumab, indicates antitumor activity regardless of dose-dependent toxicity in advanced melanoma cases [145]. The TGF-β-receptor kinase inhibitors with Galunisertib and Vactosertib may be used against various types of cancer effectively; however, it needs further authentication by conducting clinical trials.

In an *in vivo* model of glioblastoma, the efficacy of SD-208 in the presence of TGF-β against immune cell effector has been explained [146]. TGF-β has shown a suppressing effect by activating CD8+ T cells. In a pre-clinical model, Stüber *et al.* [147], reported the suppressive effect of TGF-β on ROR1-CAR T-cells and destroyed $ROR1^+$ TNBC.

GROWTH FACTORS INDUCE ANGIOGENESIS

In early embryogenesis, a closed circulatory system develops through vasculogenesis and angiogenesis to give oxygen and nutrients to a different part of the body. These processes include a variety of signal transduction systems, including VEGFS and its receptors, angiopoietin/Tie receptors, and Platelet-derived growth factors (PDGFS)/PDGFRs. The VEGFS and VEGF receptors play a key role in regulating both angiogenesis and vasculogenesis.

Vasculogenesis is the *de novo* process to form new vessels from progenitor cells. This occurs in the mammalian embryo where initially angioblasts are recruited to distinct locations, and they differentiate to form endothelial cells setting up the early stage of a vascular network, then this primitive blood vessel is extended by the physiological process of formation of the new capillary from a pre-existing small vessel leading to develop a full flagged vascular network. This process is known as angiogenesis.

The vascular blood supply network is necessary during embryonic development and later stages of life. It's also important for wound healing and female reproductive tract development. Angiogenesis is as well involved in the pathogenesis of variable disorders, such as proliferative retinopathies may cause vision loss and chronic inflammation, such as rheumatoid arthritis, and in tumours [148].

Blood vessels provide a transport system for nutrients, oxygen, and immune and cancer cells throughout the body and may also be co-opted in cancer to feed and sustain tumor growth. Physiological angiogenesis processes are crucial during embryo development, wound healing, and collateral formation for improved organ perfusion.

Although angiogenesis plays a pivotal role in the various physiological processes of life, including embryonic development, pathological angiogenesis leading to causes many disorders, such as malignancies, cannot be ignored.

Angiogenesis is a multistep process regulated by a number of growth factors and inhibitors [149]. The basic steps include degradation of the basement membrane, endothelial cell proliferation and migration, tube formation, new basement membrane formation, pericyte stabilization, *etc.*

The pro-angiogenic factors that influence the new blood vessels formation and initiate angiogenesis changes are mainly VEGF, together with the transformation of extracellular matrix (ECM) that take place through the involvement of metalloproteinases. Angiogenic switches occur as a result of the advantage of paracrine secretion of pro-angiogenic GFs over the anti-angiogenic factors, and by this, the tumor passes from the avascular to the vascular phase.

The VEGFs, Fibroblast Growth Factor (FGFS), and TGF-β play a crucial role in both vasculogenesis and angiogenesis. On the contrary, VEGF role as an antagonist to limit angiogenesis has also been observed.

Endothelial progenitor cells (EPCs) may regulate the release of proangiogenic growth factors as well as direct luminal integration into sprouting budding capillaries to control angiogenesis switch [150, 151].

Furthermore, Kerbel *et al.*, described that the cancer treatment, including cytotoxic medication and also EPCs, should be mobilized to the tumor's viable edge [152]. Regulation of angiogenesis involves pro and anti-angiogenic factors; the balance of both determines the status of the "angiogenic switch". Only when a trigger commands the balance towards pro-angiogenic factors (as in the case of malignancy), then the switch is turned on, and the vascular-quiescent tissues will show the signs of angiogenesis. Proteolytic enzymes that destroy the perivascular matrix (ECM) and the basement membrane are formed once angiogenic stimuli have activated endothelial cells. The proliferation and migration of endothelial cells into the perivascular area result in the formation of primary sprouts. It is then followed by the lumenization of these primary sprouts, the formation of capillary loops, and the synthesis of new basement membranes and blood vessels, culminating in the formation of mature blood vessels [153].

Mechanism of Angiogenesis in Cancer

Tumour tissue warrants oxygen and nutrients to grow and metastasize locally, and these are provided by blood vessels that carry the oxygen. The presence of good oxygen profusion is utilized by endothelial cells to form a vascular network *in vivo* or sprouts *in vitro*. Oxygen is important for cancer cell growth, therefore tumour cells that have been deprived of oxygen will not divide. Hypoxia is the main trigger of angiogenesis initiation and vessel formation [154].

Endothelial cells (ECs) have several variable mechanisms of oxygen sensing (such as nitric oxide synthase, and NADPH oxidases), primarily those that interface with the family of hypoxia-inducible transcription factors (HIF). It can regulate oxygen hemostasis in angiogenesis. High levels of oxygen are needed to maintain the abnormal vasculature and cell proliferation during tumour growth [155]. Under hypoxic circumstances, HIF-1α (HIF-1 to 3 isoforms) is stabilized, allowing an increase in the level of protein's concentration & initiates an adaptive transcriptional response. The HIF heterodimer, along with transcriptional coactivators and CAMP response element-binding protein (CBP), binds to the hypoxic response elements to stimulate the production of gene transcription to cope and survive with hypoxia. These transcription products are involved in angiogenesis, erythropoiesis and glucose transport & in turning on the angiogenic switch as hypoxia is an important feature of tumours. Therefore the presence of high HIF levels in many cancers correlate with an unfavourable prognosis [156]. It has been observed that hypoxia is higher in a larger tumour. The study of human glioblastoma *in vitro*, showed that the degree of hypoxia increases about five times in 8 mm as compared with a 2 mm tumor, similarly, VEGF concentration is increased alongside the growth of tumour. Studies by Wang`s group has shown the importance of HIF-1 in the formation blood vessel. Other triggers for the angiogenic switch include metabolic rewiring of ECs, creating an acidic TME, gene alterations resulting in controlling the production of angiogenic regulators, and inflammatory cell infiltration [157]. It can be tumour specific and might alternate during various stages of tumor development. The most potent effector is the VEGF signaling pathway. Several VEGF-independent effectors exist, and they may work independently and compensatively for VEGF signaling.

VEGF is overexpressed in a multitude of malignancies regulated by HIF activity, and also directly by growth signaling also involved in proliferation, survival, migration, and differentiation, as well as vascular permeability mediation.

Vascular Endothelial Growth Factor (VEGF)

The angiogenesis is regulated by many factors, such as VEGFs, VEGFR angiopoietin, EphrinB2/EphB4 and Delta-Notch. Among them, VEGF-VEGFR is essential for angiogenesis (physiologically & pathologically) and vasculogenesis. VEGFs is a member of the Vascular Permeability Factor family proteins (VPF) & it is Platelet Derived Growth Factor, an endothelial-cell-specific mitogen, that promotes endothelial cell proliferation and migration while also increasing vascular permeability and causes the development of cancer of leaky blood vessels, which encourages the dissemination of neoplastic cells from the primary tumour [12]. There are several members in the VEGFs gene family, such as Placenta Growth Factor (PIGF), VEGF-A (VEGF), VEGF- VEGFC and VEGFD [158].

VEGF-A is the primary angiogenesis factor, binds to 2 receptors of tyrosine kinase, VEGFR-1 (Fit-1) & VEGFR-2 (Flk-1 or KDR) and is likely to present in vascular endothelial cells and hematopoietic stem cells consecutively & controls endothelial cells proliferation migration, secretion, vascular permeability. VEGFR-1 and 2 have been identified in the cells of solid tumour, and activation of VEGFR-1 in breast tumor promote its survival and growth [12]. VEGFRs signalling regulate angiogenesis by many intermediates where cell vasopermeability and proliferation are induced by the protein kinase C pathway, cell survival, proliferation *via* AKT and MAPK pathway and migration *via* SRC and Paxillin. Independently of vascular process, VEGF has an autocrine effect on the tumor cells activities, bone marrow progenitors recruitment and suppression of the immune system [12].

Soluble VEGFR-1 (sFit-1), an endogenous VEGF-inhibitor, is abnormally predominant in women with preeclampsia, leading to abnormal VEGF trapping of VEGFs and hence fatal disease. Many experimental studies have confirmed the role of VEGF in tumour neovascularisation, demonstrating that inhibition of VEGF activity *in vivo* decreases tumor growth through its effect on reducing tumour angiogenesis [159]. VEGF-mediated tumor angiogenesis depends on hypoxia, just parallel to normal angiogenesis.

Physiological and tumor angiogenesis are both similar, and VEGF plays a key role in stimulating the proliferation and migration of ECS though, VEGF, and other pro-angiogenic factors, may affect the tumour microenvironment. As documented, angiogenesis in the body is triggered for a short time and then shut off, but tumor angiogenesis is a continual process.

Degradation of basement membrane with a contribution of MMPS occurs prior to maturation and stabilization of a new vessel, and includes alterations of extracellular matrix transformation of the vessel basement membrane, modifications of ECS surface molecules, and also the release of pro-angiogenic agents from the ECM, primarily VEGF.

Fibroblast Growth Factor (FGF)

FGF is a transcription factor known to induce endothelial cell proliferation and neovascularization *in vivo*. Its angiogenic effect is mediated by its release by tumor and stromal cells, followed by paracrine signaling, or by its mobilization from the ECM. FGF has been shown to stimulate the expression of VEGF and angiopoietin-2, a key regulator of vascular networking and angiogenesis. Angiopoietin and basic FGF (bFGF) are both important in tumor angiogenesis because they increase endothelial cell proliferation and migration. It has been shown that bFGF works in synergy with VEGF to stimulate *in vitro* & *in vivo* vascularization. And it provokes the production of VEGF and VEGF receptors.

Many studies that suppress bFGF receptors have shown that the tumor tissues and their vascular supply have regressed.

Other Modes of Tumour Vascularization

There is a debate whether the term "angiogenesis" can include all forms of neo-vascularization, or it refers to the classic vascular sprouting. Angiogenesis is the process of sprouting, cell division, migration and assembly of ECS from pre-existing vessels. The process of sprouting, cell proliferation, migration, and assembly of ECS from pre-existing vessels is referred to as angiogenesis. Spouting angiogenesis is the proliferation of endothelial cells to form a spout from the margin of the present vessel, resulting in expanding the vascular tree. It is one of the most common mechanisms of tumour blood vessel formation.

The sprouting tumour vasculature varies from standard vasculature in addition to evasion. Leakiness is caused by dilated and tortuous vessels with ECs not forming typical monolayers and resting on a variable thickness basement membrane and pericytes forming abnormally loose connections with ECs. With the resultant areas of hypoxia and acidosis, the blood flow is chaotic; these stressful conditions have a variety of consequences, including potentiating angiogenesis, decreasing therapeutic efficacy and leading to resistance to clonal expansion.

On the other hand, "Splitting angiogenesis" or "Intussusceptive Microvascular Growth (IMG)" occurs when the number of existing blood vessels (splits into tiny daughter vessels in the earlier or form a septum in the second process) increases while there is no massive increase in the number of endothelial cells *via* rearranging the available cells and allows the capillary network to expand within itself. This ripening process might comprise myocytes & pericytes. IMG is reported in various tumour types as faster, less energy-consuming, and more permeable than sprouting angiogenesis. The shift to IMG could serve as an adaptive response to restore hemodynamic homeostasis to tumour vasculature or an escape mechanism from anti-angiogenic therapy. To date, no molecule has been directly linked to IMG, although shear stress and blood flow seem to play some role. There are many modes of non-angiogenic tumor vascularization although less attention is received, they may help to better understand the complex tumour vascularity and in the design of rational drugs.

Vascular co-option allows for the acquisition of the needed tumor blood supply by hijacking the existing vasculature. Angiogenesis and vascular co-option both play a distinctive role in the initiation of micro-tumours. Meanwhile, the rapid growth of the tumour is dependent on angiogenesis; vascular co-option is another indispensable way for tumour cell survival. The functional plasticity of destructive tumor cells in voicing a stem-cell-like phenotype forming *de-novo* vascular networks defines vasculogenic mimicry (VM), which is described in most main types of malignancies and is always associated with poor prognosis.

VM infers useful advantages that promote the survival of some phenotypes of an aggressive tumour. A significant driver for VM tends to be hypoxia (hypoxia is a significant trigger for VM) [160].

GROWTH FACTORS INVOLVED IN TUMOUR PROGRESSION

- Platelet-derived growth factor (PDGF) family
- Vascular endothelial growth factor (VEGF) family
- Neuregulins and the EGF family
  - Epidermal growth factor (EGF)
  - Hepatocyte growth factor (HGF)
  - Fibroblast growth factor (FGF) family
- Transforming growth factor-β (TGF-β)
- Insulin-like growth factor (IGF) family
- Neurotrophin family (NF)

Once the normal or premalignant cells acquire driver mutations, there may be an accumulation of additional oncogenic mutations, which could have a key role in tumor growth, invasion, and metastasis, as well as all of the hallmarks of cancer [161]. There are several different families of growth factors that may cause tumor progression. It includes PDGF, VEGF, EGF, TGF-β, FGF, the insulin family (IF), *etc.*

Platelet-Derived Growth Factor (PDGF) Family

PDGF is the most abundant of the growth factors present in the serum and is extremely heat-stable. The PDGF A, B, C and D and their receptors (PDGFR) α and β, which are structurally related tyrosine kinase receptors (TKRs), exist as either homo/hetero dimeric forms and their interactions result in activation of a signalling mechanism which has a number of physiological roles mainly associated with embryonic development of blood vessels. Most of the dimeric forms of PDGF interact with the isoforms of their receptors, and the signalling cascade begins first with the dimerization of the receptors, which makes it stable, followed by its rapid trans-autophosphorylation. The pathways activated by these receptors include many enzymatic proteins such as phosphatidylinositol 3′-kinase (PI3-K), phospholipase C (PLC)-γ, the Src family of tyrosine kinases, tyrosine phosphatase SHP-2, and GTPase-activating protein [162, 163]. In cancer, PDGFR mutations involving the TKRs lead to alterations in its dimerization and ligand binding, thus affecting the entire process of activation of these kinases [164]. There are many cancers in which there is over expression of PDGFs or PDGFRs, such as pancreatic, gastric, prostrate and oral cancer [165 - 168]. Co-overexpression of these two together suggests an autocrine loop that is activated to promote cancer growth and motility, which is in contrast with normal physiological actions of the pair, which are accomplished by paracrine stimulation [169, 170]. This autocrine activation of PDGFRs has been shown to promote tumor cell motility by causing epithelial-mesenchymal transition (EMT), which can lead to metastasis [171, 172]. TKRs have been found to have transactivated when ligands of other receptors, such as EGFR are bound to them. Thus, PDGF stimulation has been found to activate EGFR as well [173].

Vascular Endothelial Growth Factor (VEGF) Family

Angiogenesis has long been investigated for its function in tumor progression. The role of VEGF (VEGF-A) seems to be the most studied among all of the members of this family, like VEGF-B, VEGF-C, VEGF-D and PLGF [174]. The receptors that mediate the functions of these growth factors are the TKRs; VEGFR1, VEGFR2 and VEGFR3 [175]. Although angiogenesis and lymphangiogenesis in both normal and cancerous tissues seem to be the primary function of these growth factors, recent evidence also shows their other roles in the tumor microenvironment. For example: they have an immunosuppressive effect on T cells, resulting in increased regulatory T cells recruitment and myeloid-derived suppressor cells to be recruited, as well as preventing DC differentiation and activation [176]. In certain malignancies, they also appear to boost cancer cell proliferation and cancer cell survival [177]. Although the chief cells that produce VEGFs are the endothelial cells, other cells, such as tumour-associated macrophages and fibroblasts, also secrete them in a hypoxic environment which favours the progression of tumor [178].

Neuregulins and the EGF Family

Epidermal Growth Factor (EGF)

The receptors (EGFR) of epidermal growth factors are more studied in cancer compared to the EGF itself as the EGFR can be activated by multiple ligands, one of which is EGF. The others are TGF-α, HBE-GF, betacellulin (BTC), amphiregulin (AREG), EREG, and epigene (EPGN). Among all, EGF, TGF-α, HBE-GF, and BTC are considered high-affinity ligands however, AREG, EREG, and EPGN are low-affinity ligands [179]. As the name indicates, this receptor physiologically is mainly involved in epithelial tissue development and homeostasis. The receptor belongs to the ErB family of the TKRs and consists of the following; ErbB-1 (EGFR), ErbB-2 (HER2 or Neu), ErbB-3, and ErbB-4 [180]. EGFR can be abnormally active in the development of tumors by a variety of pathways, including receptor overexpression, mutation, ligand-dependent and independent activation.

As it is mainly involved in cell proliferation, overexpression of these in tumors contributes significantly to the progression of almost all carcinomas. Apart from the above-mentioned mechanisms of activation of these receptors, it has been found the presence of hypoxia can also increase the expression of EGFR. This seems to occur *via* gene amplification and increased mRNA translation [181]. Similarly, recent studies have shown there could be an association between immune evasion in EGFR-mutated lung cancers [182, 183].

Fibroblast Growth Factor (FGF) Family

The FGF is a kingpin in relation to being a mediator of cross-talks between various aspects of tumor progression involving angiogenesis and inflammation. The FGF and its receptors' (FGFR) signalling pathway is critical for tumor growth as it is involved in progression by affecting the stromal and tumor cells [184]. The FGF family includes 22 members which are divided into seven subfamilies based on evolutionary relationships, sequence similarities and biochemical functions. These proteins bind to tyrosine kinase-associated FGFRs, and heparan sulphate proteoglycans stabilise this. These ternary complexes are required for signal transduction [185, 186]. FGF19/21/23 subfamily is the hormone-like growth factor mainly involved in the metabolism of lipids, glucose and phosphates [187]. Intracrine FGFs, such as FGF11/12/13/14, work independently of FGFRs and play a role in neuronal and cardiac excitability [188]. Deregulation of the FGF/FGFR signalling occurs in many cancers, which results in aberrant signalling in a ligand-dependent/independent fashion. Gene amplification of FGF is the most common aberration that occurs and is seen in about 14% of cancers and that of FGFR in about 7.1% of about 4,85 solid tumours analysed by next-generation sequencing [189]. Although gene amplification seems to be the most common of the aberrations in the FGF/FGFR system, the chromosomal translocation and gene fusion of this system is also seen in tumors. Oncogenic activation occurs by this aberration and has been found in glioblastoma, bladder, triple-negative breast cancers, and head and neck cancer [190 - 193].

Hepatocyte Growth Factor (HGF)

HGF, also known as the scatter factor (SF), is a strong hepatocyte mitogen that is mostly released by fibroblasts. It has been found that it is mainly involved in promoting the motility of epithelial cells and in tumor progression [194]. HGF is the only ligand for HGFR, also known c-MET or MET, which is also a TKR [195, 196]. When this ligand binds to the receptor, it causes receptor dimerization, autophosphorylation of tyrosine residues and activation of Ras-Raf-MAPK and PI3K/AKT/mTOR signalling pathways [197]. Thus, the aberrant boost of the HGF/c-MET axis, which occurs in cancers, results in the progression of tumors. The aberrant activation of this axis mainly occurs *via* various types of mutations in the genes encoding MET and results in carcinogenesis, resistance to various forms of therapy & recurrence, thus contributing to cancer progression [198].

Transforming Growth Factor-β (TGF-β)

TGF is a well-studied cytokine superfamily that includes three TGFs (TGF1, TGF2, and TGF3), activins, inhibins, Glial-derived Neurotrophic Factors (GDNFs), Bone Morphogenic Proteins (BMPs), *etc.* There are three receptors for TGF-β; TGF-βRI, TGF-βRII, and TGF-βRIII. The first two are involved in signalling *via* the SMADs, whereas the third acts as a co-receptor which increases the ligand binding to TGF-βRII [184, 199]. TGF- β is a tumour suppressor and maintains tissue homeostasis by thwarting tissues from developing cancerous properties through regulation of their proliferative, differentiative, survival, and adhesive properties. But when there are inactivating mutations involving the genes of TGF-β receptors (*e.g.,* Head & neck cancer, ovarian cancer, gastrointestinal cancers) [200 - 202] and SMAD proteins (*e.g.,* Glioma, breast cancer) [203, 204], the cells become cancerous. The cells lose the ability to evade apoptosis when there is a defective receptor and attain various tumor progressive capabilities when the signalling mechanism activated by these receptors is disrupted [205]. Recently, the immunosuppressive and immune evasive activity of TGF-β has gained significant attention, especially in epithelial carcinomas, whereby the canonical pathways seem to play a crucial role in tumor progression [206].

Insulin-Like Growth Factor (IGF) Family

The sustained growth of tumors is a hallmark of any cancer, and like many other growth factors, IGF plays a crucial role in the proliferation, migration and invasion of both tumor and stromal cells, which contributes to the progression of cancers. The IGF family is made up of polypeptide growth factor ligands (IGF-I, IGF-II), two cell membrane receptors (IGF-IR and IGF-IIR) and six binding proteins (IGFBP 1 to 6). A large group of proteases also hydrolyse the IGFBP's, which results in the release of bound IGFs that again interact with their corresponding receptors [207]. Activation of this family of growth factors results in cytosolic signalling transduction of multiple pathways such as PI3K, MAPK and JAK/STAT [208]. All these pathways are involved in different aspects of tumor progression including but not limited to cell proliferation, anoikis, stemness and invasion & metastasis. Apart from these effects, overexpression of IGFR1 has been associated with neoadjuvant therapies such as chemo and endocrine therapy, which indicates its role in promoting drug resistance [209]. Studies have shown that these factors are also secreted by various cells in TME, such as tumour-associated macrophages (TAM's), which confer the tumors chemoresistance [210].

Neurotrophin Family (NF)

The neurotrophins consist of a group of growth factors that play a key role in the development of the central and peripheral nervous systems [211]. There are four neurotrophins: the prototypical nerve growth factor (NGF), brain-derived neurotrophic factor (BDNF), neurotrophin 3 (NT-3) and neurotrophin 4/5 (NT-4/5). They exist as homodimers and act as ligands for various TKRs and p75 neurotrophin receptors, which is a member of the TNF superfamily of receptors. p75NTR is activated by all of the neurotrophins, but the TKRs are selective. TrkA is activated by NGF and NT-3, TrkB by BDNF, NT-4/5, NT-3 and TrkC by just NT3 [212]. Once the ligands bind to the TKRs, they get dimerized, the tyrosine residues undergo autophosphorylation, and the following RAS signalling cascades are activated; extracellularly regulated kinases (ERK), phosphatidyl-inositol kinase 3 (PI3K) and phospholipase C (PLC) [212, 213]. Once these systems are activated, it leads predominantly to tumor cell survival by proliferation and/or differentiation. Alternatively, when the neurotrophins bind to p75NTR c-Jun N-terminal kinase (JNK) signalling cascade is activated. Nuclear factor-κB (NF-κB) signalling, which promotes cell survival, is also activated when either of the ligands associated with p75NTR is bound to these receptors [213]. For a long time, the autocrine stimulation of these receptors has been studied and found to be associated with different types of cancer, but recently the association of nerve dependence in cancer is also being studied. The fact that neurotransmitters and neurotrophins are involved in regeneration and embryonic development by activation of the stem cell compartments is undeniable; recent advancement recommended the role of these factors in activation of cancer cells that promotes tumour growth, metastasis and neo-angiogenesis & inflammation [214].

CANCER THERAPEUTICS TARGETING GROWTH FACTOR SIGNALING

Cancer treatment has been a challenge for decades, and this has been attempted by a number of different methods. Targeting the growth factor signalling seems to be an important approach as the growth factor/receptor axis is imperative for cancer progression. There have been several sites/mechanisms in the growth factor signaling cascade that has been targeted to halt tumour progression. They include the drugs and Mabs that target the receptors directly, tyrosine kinase inhibitors, drugs that act as ligand traps, and oligonucleotide-based therapeutics.

Drugs and Mab that Target Receptors

The ligands binding to the receptors activate the growth factors mediated signaling hence, the drugs that target these receptor sites are quite useful in preventing the progression of cancer. The drugs that have entered clinical use mainly target the epidermal growth factor receptors (EGFR). Of these, Mabs seem to be the most useful because of their distinct advantages over small molecule inhibitors. Mabs have increased specificity, longer half-lives and more predictable pharmacological behaviours. Cetuximab, panitumumab, necitumumab and nimotuzumab are FDA approved Mab that is commonly used as a monotherapy or combination chemotherapy. All these drugs act by binding to the extracellular domain III of the EGFR and thus avert ligand binding and further activation of oncogenic signalling arising from this receptor [215, 216]. Cetuximab and Panitumumab have been approved to be used for the treatment of colorectal cancer, whereas Cetuximab is for head & neck cancer, non-small cell lung cancer and non-melanoma skin cancers [217 - 220]. Nimotuzumab has also been granted approval for use in head and neck cancer [221 - 223]. Besides the above-approved drugs, the other Mabs candidates currently under preclinical testing and clinical trials are Mab A13, AMG595, depatuxizumab, mafodotin, duligotuzumab, futuximab, GC1118, imgatuzumab, matuzumab, anitumumab, zalutumumab, humMR1 and tomuzotuximab [224, 225]. HER2 receptors of the EGFR family have also been targeted for cancer therapy. HER2-positive breast cancer is given as a reference of malignancy that shows drugs targeting this receptor have a good effect on outcomes. FDA-approved HER2 inhibitors such as pertuzumab, trastuzumab, and trastuzumab emtansine have a profound effect on progression-free survival and overall survival of patients with breast cancer [226 - 228]. One of the challenges faced by clinical oncologists regarding the use of these drugs is the development of resistance. It is known that colorectal cancer patients might exhibit "primary" or "*de novo*" resistance to cetuximab or panitumumab or even refractory resistance after treatment with these drugs has been initiated [229, 230]. The mechanisms for this resistance are currently unknown, but several hypotheses have been postulated. One of them is that point mutations or gene amplifications of KRAS occur, and as a result, there is an activation of EGFR signalling. Similarly, BRAF and PI3KCA, or PTEN loss of function, might also result in persistent activation of EGFR signalling despite the use of inhibitors. Activation of alternate receptors such as HER2/MET or binding of ligands such as VEGF also seems to confer resistance [231].

Targeting of VEGF Signalling Pathways

Preclinical data established VEGF and its respective receptors are an important target for cancer therapy. In a xenograft animal model, the hypothesized mechanism includes the neutralization of anti-VEGF antibody [159] and suppression of a dominant negative form of VEGFR2 [232].

There are two major barriers which need to be resolved for cancer cells to acquire unrestricted proliferation anti-growth signaling, primarily regulated by tumour suppressor proteins, and immune surveillance.

Tumor suppressors are proteins that kill damaged or cancerous cells; effective cancer therapy is expected to activate them. Most cancer medications now in use, including newly developed targeted therapies, elicit antigrowth signaling in order to prevent cell multiplication. Resistance arises primarily because of alternate mechanisms for cell survival and multi-targeted approaches and high cost. Thus, after considering these variables, natural dietary compounds are highly desirable, and most are multi-targeted, affecting several cancer hallmarks. The production of natural substances, not only for prevention but also for therapy, should therefore be explored in the future.

Targeting TGF-β Signaling

TGF-β's function in cancer progression as tumor suppressive *via* inducing growth arrest and apoptosis at the early phase of the disease and as a promotor by inhibition of cancer cell migration and stimulation of epithelial to mesenchymal transition. Considering this dual action, the challenge is to use therapies that target only the tumor promoting component of TGF-signaling while minimizing the effect on the tumor suppressive signal. It is critical to identify patients who are most likely to respond to anti-TGF therapy [233].

Tyrosine Kinase Inhibitors

TKIs are the most studied of all the classes of drugs discussed in this chapter. Tyrosine kinase receptors (TKRs) play a significant role in regulating a variety of cellular functions, and their role in cancer progression is well documented. The structure of the receptors consists of a ligand-binding region in the extracellular domain, a single transmembrane helix, and a cytoplasmic region consisting of protein tyrosine kinase and additional carboxy-(C-) terminal. When ligands are bound to the receptors, there is phosphorylation of the kinases, which results in a cascade of events resulting in the activation of multiple oncogenic pathways [234]. As such aberrant activation of these kinases can also occur by mutations, translocations or amplifications, which can lead to cancer progression [235]. TKIs can influence various targets, including EGFR, HER2, ALK, MET, ROS1, NTRK, MEK, FGFR, PDGFR, and VEGFR. Some of these inhibitors target multiple sites, such as the ones associated with VEGFR [236, 237].

A number of inhibitors (first to the fourth generation) targeting tyrosine kinase cascade *via* the EGFR have been used or are under development, especially for non-small cell lung cancer patients (NSCLCs)with EGFR mutations [238]. The first-generation drugs in this category include gefitinib [239], icotinib [240] and erlotinib [241], whereas the second-generation drugs include afatinib [242] and dacomitinib [243]. For the patients who do not respond to the first and second-generation drugs due to mutations in EGFR T790M, third-generation drugs osimertinib [244], almonertinib [245], furmonertinib [246], lazertinib [247] and nazartinib [248] have been shown to be effective. Mutations in EGFR exon 20 C797S have shown resistance against the third-generation drugs, for which the fourth-generation drugs are under development, such as EAI045 [249] and TQB3804 [250]. HER2 is another receptor that is structurally similar to EGFR as it belongs to the ErbB family of drugs. HER2-targeted TKIs are fairly common for treatment in patients with HER2 positive metastatic breast cancers. The drugs that have been used in such patients include lapatinib, neratinib, pyrotinib, and tucatinib either alone or in combination with other drugs [251 - 254].

A subgroup of NSCLCs that have a rearrangement in the anaplastic lymphocyte kinase (ALK) has been treated with ALK-TKIs [255]. Crizotinib is the first generation of these inhibitors, which has been found to target ALK, ROS1, and c-MET and thus can be included under ROS1-TKIs and MET-TKIs as well [256, 257]. Second-generation inhibitors ceritinib [258], alectinib [259] and brigatinib [260] have a more selected target on ALK and drugs such as ensartinib are found to be effective on crizotinib-resistant tumors [261]. Tumors resistant to the above classes of drugs are being tested with a third-generation ALK-TKI, lorlatinib [262].

Some of the drugs, such as cabozantinib, merestinib, glesatinib, and sitravatinib, are multi-targeted TKIs that have shown significant anti-MET activity, particularly in NSCLC [263]. The similarity between ROS1 and ALK has prompted the use of crizotinib, ceritinib, and lorlatinib as targeted therapy for the subgroup of cancers that have rearrangements in both these genes [264].

The tropomyosin receptor kinase (TRK) family of receptor tyrosine kinases is of interest because the NTRK genes are members of this family. They have been targeted in many adult and paediatric solid tumours [265]. Larotrectinib, a selective inhibitor of TRKA/B/C, a first-generation inhibitor that has been approved for use and multiple other drugs that are still in pre-clinical testing [266 - 268]. Selitrectinib (LOXO-195) and repotrectinib (TPX0005) are second-generation TRK inhibitors, and they have been shown to be effective against Larotrectinib-resistant tumors [269, 270].

Inhibitors of MEK act mainly by preventing tyrosine and serine/threonine molecule phosphorylation and, thus, downstream ERK activation [271]. Trametinib, cobimetinib, binimetinib, and selumetinib are drugs that have been approved primarily for the treatment of melanoma [272]. FGFR inhibitors are mainly drugs that target multiple TKIs including mainly the ones associated with PDGFR and VEGFR (Sorafenib, Sunitinib, Regorafenib, Lenvatinib, Axitinib, Pazopanib, Anlotinib) [273]. Some of them are selective as well, such as Erdafitinib, which is a selective inhibitor of FGFR1–4 and is primarily used as a target for locally advanced or metastatic urothelial carcinoma [274]. Similarly, Pemigatinib, which is a selective inhibitor of FGFR1-3, has been successfully used for the treatment of cholangiocarcinoma [275]. Other drugs, such as Infigratinib and Futibatinib, are also under the testing phase for a variety of tumours, including cholangiocarcinoma [276, 277].

Ligand Traps of Growth Factors

Ligand traps are artificial binding molecules that bind to their corresponding growth factors with higher specificity and affinity [278]. By binding to them, they prevent the ligands from attaching to their receptors and further avoid activation of oncogenic signalling pathways. Until now, there is only one FDA-approved drug, Aflibercept which is a VEGF trap approved for use in metastatic colorectal cancer.

Monoclonal antibodies have gained popularity in recent years because they are a recombinant protein with high therapeutic value on the market [279]. It prevents the VEGF from binding to its receptors, thus preventing tumour angiogenesis and metastasis. Many of these molecules are currently still in the preclinical evaluation and seem to be promising approaches to arrest tumour growth. One of the methods used is related to the design of the trap containing a portion of an immunoglobulin. For example, it has been shown that the chimeric proteins which contain the ligand-interacting ectodomain of TGF-β fused with the Fc domain of IgG resulted in the decreased oncogenic ability of oral cancer cell lines [280]. Similarly, Chudzian *et al.*, reported that phage display selection of scFv antibody fragments could be used to target FGF1. These were transfected into osteosarcoma cell lines, and these *in vitro* studies too promising results indicating a possible future therapeutic agent in the form of ligand traps [281]. Bifunctional antibody-ligand traps, also known as 'Y traps,' have also been recently tested *in vitro*. These ligand traps bind to two proteins such as PD-L1 and TGF-β receptor. This resulted in the simultaneous disabling of autocrine/paracrine TGF-β signalling and thus acted as a potentially more effective immunotherapeutic strategy [282].

Oligonucleotide-Based Therapeutics

Oligonucleotide-based technologies are currently offering a rapidly expanding class of therapeutic options with which cellular biology can be influenced in novel ways. This is useful for cancer therapeutics as most of the currently approved drugs develop resistance at some point. The mechanism of action of these therapeutics involves the silencing of genes involved in cancer progression. The therapeutic target of non-coding RNA and structural nucleotides, such as antisense oligonucleotides (ASOs), small interfering RNAs (siRNAs), microRNAs (miRNAs), *etc*., are emerging approaches for treating various types of cancers. Of these, ASOs and siRNAs are the most developed technologies [283]. Although the technology of ASOs extends as far back as 1978 [284], targeting growth factors using ASOs is still in the developmental stage. Preclinical studies of ASOs targeting EGF in liver cancer [285] and TGF-β in glioblastoma [286] have shown promising results, and there are few studies in progress which are at the stage of clinical trials as summarised by Teixier *et al.* [287]. Similarly studies using siRNA have also progressed quite well but the challenges faced are mainly related to the delivery system. These days, approaches of chemical modifications of siRNA, lipid-based siRNA delivery systems, polymer-based siRNA delivery systems, conjugate siRNA delivery systems and co-delivery of siRNA and anticancer drugs have been adopted and good efficiency have been reported [288]. Currently, studies are mainly focussing on the use of nanoparticles, a field in which tremendous advances have been achieved. For example, preclinical studies using a functionalized nanohydrogel siRNA delivery system [289] or immune nanoparticles [288] targeting EGFR have shown good results. In the near future, it can be expected that these studies would reach the stages of clinical trials and finally reach the patients as an approved drug delivery system.

CONCLUSION

One of the main characteristics of human cancer is the development of evasion of apoptosis, which can lead to tumor growth, progression, and resistance to the currently available anticancer therapies. Therefore, a better understanding of the molecular mechanisms underlying tumor resistance to apoptotic cell death is the basic approach to the development of molecular targeted therapies.

CONSENT FOR PUBLICATION

Not applicable.

CONFLICT OF INTEREST

The author declares no conflict of interest, financial or otherwise.

ACKNOWLEDGEMENTS

I would like to thank professor Faeres Al Enazi for his guidance and persistence in making the dream to be real. Thanks to the great team that I have worked with writing this chapter. And a special word of appreciation for the real friends whom I consider as a member of my family, thanks for their presence in our life. My deepest appreciation and thanks to my mother, my paradise.

REFERENCES

[1] Jiang WG, Sanders AJ, Katoh M, *et al.* Tissue invasion and metastasis: Molecular, biological and clinical perspectives. Semin Cancer Biol 2015; 35 (Suppl.): S244-75. [PMID: 25865774]

[2] Acharyya S, Matrisian L, Welch DR, *et al.* 18 - Invasion and Metastasis The Molecular Basis of Cancer. 4th ed. Philadelphia: W.B. Saunders 2015; pp. 269-84.e2.

[3] Yilmaz M, Christofori G. EMT, the cytoskeleton, and cancer cell invasion. Cancer Metastasis Rev 2009; 28(1-2): 15-33. [PMID: 19169796]

[4] Seton-Rogers SE, Brugge JS. ErbB2 and TGF-beta: a cooperative role in mammary tumor progression? Cell Cycle 2004; 3(5): 597-600. [PMID: 15107620]

[5] Neal CL, Yao J, Yang W, *et al.* 14-3-3zeta overexpression defines high risk for breast cancer recurrence and promotes cancer cell survival. Cancer Res 2009; 69(8): 3425-32. [PMID: 19318578]

[6] Nieman MT, Prudoff RS, Johnson KR, Wheelock MJ. N-cadherin promotes motility in human breast cancer cells regardless of their E-cadherin expression. J Cell Biol 1999; 147(3): 631-44. [PMID: 10545506]

[7] Katz M, Amit I, Citri A, *et al.* A reciprocal tensin-3-cten switch mediates EGF-driven mammary cell migration. Nat Cell Biol 2007; 9(8): 961-9. [PMID: 17643115]

[8] Voudouri K, Berdiaki A, Tzardi M, Tzanakakis GN, Nikitovic D. Insulin-like growth factor and epidermal growth factor signaling in breast cancer cell growth: focus on endocrine resistant disease. Anal Cell Pathol (Amst) 2015; 2015: 975495. [PMID: 26258011]

[9] Gupta GP, Massagué J. Cancer metastasis: building a framework. Cell 2006; 127(4): 679-95.

[PMID: 17110329]

[10] O'Hayre M, Salanga CL, Handel TM, Allen SJ. Chemokines and cancer: migration, intracellular signalling and intercellular communication in the microenvironment. Biochem J 2008; 409(3): 635-49. [PMID: 18177271]

[11] van Zijl F, Krupitza G, Mikulits W. Initial steps of metastasis: cell invasion and endothelial transmigration. Mutat Res 2011; 728(1-2): 23-34. [PMID: 21605699]

[12] Witsch E, Sela M, Yarden Y. Roles for growth factors in cancer progression. Physiology (Bethesda) 2010; 25(2): 85-101. [PMID: 20430953]

[13] Wee P, Wang Z. Epidermal Growth Factor Receptor Cell Proliferation Signaling Pathways. Cancers (Basel) 2017; 9(5): E52. [PMID: 28513565]

[14] Hanahan D, Weinberg RA. Hallmarks of cancer: the next generation. Cell 2011; 144(5): 646-74. [PMID: 21376230]

[15] Ferguson LR, Chen H, Collins AR, *et al.* Genomic instability in human cancer: Molecular insights and opportunities for therapeutic attack and prevention through diet and nutrition. Semin Cancer Biol 2015; 35 Suppl(Suppl): S5-S24.

[16] Vogelstein B, Papadopoulos N, Velculescu VE, Zhou S, Diaz LA Jr, Kinzler KW. Cancer genome landscapes. Science 2013; 339(6127): 1546-58. [PMID: 23539594]

[17] Vogelstein B, Kinzler KW. The Path to Cancer -Three Strikes and You're Out. N Engl J Med 2015; 373(20): 1895-8. [PMID: 26559569]

[18] Chambers AF, Groom AC, MacDonald IC. Dissemination and growth of cancer cells in metastatic sites. Nat Rev Cancer 2002; 2(8): 563-72. [PMID: 12154349]

[19] Steeg PS. Tumor metastasis: mechanistic insights and clinical challenges. Nat Med 2006; 12(8): 895-904. [PMID: 16892035]

[20] Katt ME, Wong AD, Searson PC. Dissemination from a Solid Tumor: Examining the Multiple Parallel Pathways. Trends Cancer 2018; 4(1): 20-37. [PMID: 29413419]

[21] Chang YS, di Tomaso E, McDonald DM, Jones R, Jain RK, Munn LL. Mosaic blood vessels in tumors: frequency of cancer cells in contact with flowing blood. Proc Natl Acad Sci USA 2000; 97(26): 14608-13. [PMID: 11121063]

[22] Goswami S, Sahai E, Wyckoff JB, *et al.* Macrophages promote the invasion of breast carcinoma cells *via* a colony-stimulating factor-1/epidermal growth factor paracrine loop. Cancer Res 2005; 65(12): 5278-83. [PMID: 15958574]

[23] Padua D, Zhang XH, Wang Q, *et al.* TGFbeta primes breast tumors for lung metastasis seeding through angiopoietin-like 4. Cell 2008; 133(1): 66-77. [PMID: 18394990]

[24] Nierodzik ML, Karpatkin S. Thrombin induces tumor growth, metastasis, and angiogenesis: Evidence for a thrombin-regulated dormant tumor phenotype. Cancer Cell 2006; 10(5): 355-62. [PMID: 17097558]

[25] Ostman A, Augsten M. Cancer-associated fibroblasts and tumor growth-bystanders turning into key players. Curr Opin Genet Dev 2009; 19(1): 67-73.
[PMID: 19211240]

[26] Finak G, Bertos N, Pepin F, *et al.* Stromal gene expression predicts clinical outcome in breast cancer. Nat Med 2008; 14(5): 518-27.
[PMID: 18438415]

[27] Iozzo RV, Zoeller JJ, Nyström A. Basement membrane proteoglycans: modulators Par Excellence of cancer growth and angiogenesis. Mol Cells 2009; 27(5): 503-13.
[PMID: 19466598]

[28] Ewald AJ, Huebner RJ, Palsdottir H, *et al.* Mammary collective cell migration involves transient loss of epithelial features and individual cell migration within the epithelium. J Cell Sci 2012; 125(Pt 11): 2638-54.
[PMID: 22344263]

[29] Tanos B, Rodriguez-Boulan E. The epithelial polarity program: machineries involved and their hijacking by cancer. Oncogene 2008; 27(55): 6939-57.
[PMID: 19029936]

[30] Ozanne BW, Spence HJ, McGarry LC, Hennigan RF. Invasion is a genetic program regulated by transcription factors. Curr Opin Genet Dev 2006; 16(1): 65-70.
[PMID: 16377173]

[31] Joyce JA, Pollard JW. Microenvironmental regulation of metastasis. Nat Rev Cancer 2009; 9(4): 239-52.
[PMID: 19279573]

[32] Wiseman BS, Werb Z. Stromal effects on mammary gland development and breast cancer. Science 2002; 296(5570): 1046-9.
[PMID: 12004111]

[33] Nguyen-Ngoc K-V, Cheung KJ, Brenot A, *et al.* ECM microenvironment regulates collective migration and local dissemination in normal and malignant mammary epithelium. Proc Natl Acad Sci USA 2012; 109(39): E2595-604.
[PMID: 22923691]

[34] Gimona M, Buccione R, Courtneidge SA, Linder S. Assembly and biological role of podosomes and invadopodia. Curr Opin Cell Biol 2008; 20(2): 235-41.
[PMID: 18337078]

[35] Santiago-Medina M, Gregus KA, Nichol RH, O'Toole SM, Gomez TM. Regulation of ECM degradation and axon guidance by growth cone invadosomes. Development 2015; 142(3): 486-96.
[PMID: 25564649]

[36] Friedl P, Wolf K. Tumour-cell invasion and migration: diversity and escape mechanisms. Nat Rev Cancer 2003; 3(5): 362-74.
[PMID: 12724734]

[37] Tosios KI, Kapranos N, Papanicolaou SI. Loss of basement membrane components laminin and type IV collagen parallels the progression of oral epithelial neoplasia. Histopathology 1998; 33(3): 261-8.
[PMID: 9777393]

[38] Hanahan D, Weinberg RA. The hallmarks of cancer. Cell 2000; 100(1): 57-70.
[PMID: 10647931]

[39] Moustakas A, Heldin C-H. The regulation of TGFbeta signal transduction. Development 2009; 136(22): 3699-714.
[PMID: 19855013]

[40] Pickup M, Novitskiy S, Moses HL. The roles of TGFβ in the tumour microenvironment. Nat Rev

Cancer 2013; 13(11): 788-99.
[PMID: 24132110]

[41] Yang L, Moses HL. Transforming growth factor beta: tumor suppressor or promoter? Are host immune cells the answer? Cancer Res 2008; 68(22): 9107-11.
[PMID: 19010878]

[42] Massagué J. TGFβ signalling in context. Nat Rev Mol Cell Biol 2012; 13(10): 616-30.
[PMID: 22992590]

[43] Miyazono K. Transforming growth factor-beta signaling in epithelial-mesenchymal transition and progression of cancer. Proc Jpn Acad, Ser B, Phys Biol Sci 2009; 85(8): 314-23.
[PMID: 19838011]

[44] Moustakas A, Heldin CH. Signaling networks guiding epithelial-mesenchymal transitions during embryogenesis and cancer progression. Cancer Sci 2007; 98(10): 1512-20.
[PMID: 17645776]

[45] Xu J, Lamouille S, Derynck R. TGF-β-induced epithelial to mesenchymal transition. Cell Res 2009; 19(2): 156-72.
[PMID: 19153598]

[46] Welch DR, Fabra A, Nakajima M. Transforming growth factor beta stimulates mammary adenocarcinoma cell invasion and metastatic potential. Proc Natl Acad Sci USA 1990; 87(19): 7678-82.
[PMID: 2217201]

[47] Derynck R, Akhurst RJ, Balmain A. TGF-beta signaling in tumor suppression and cancer progression. Nat Genet 2001; 29(2): 117-29.
[PMID: 11586292]

[48] Cui W, Fowlis DJ, Bryson S, *et al.* TGFbeta1 inhibits the formation of benign skin tumors, but enhances progression to invasive spindle carcinomas in transgenic mice. Cell 1996; 86(4): 531-42.
[PMID: 8752208]

[49] Thiery JP, Chopin D. Epithelial cell plasticity in development and tumor progression. Cancer Metastasis Rev 1999; 18(1): 31-42.
[PMID: 10505544]

[50] Portella G, Cumming SA, Liddell J, *et al.* Transforming growth factor beta is essential for spindle cell conversion of mouse skin carcinoma *in vivo*: implications for tumor invasion. Cell Growth Differ 1998; 9(5): 393-404.
[PMID: 9607560]

[51] Janda E, Lehmann K, Killisch I, *et al.* Ras and TGF[beta] cooperatively regulate epithelial cell plasticity and metastasis: dissection of Ras signaling pathways. J Cell Biol 2002; 156(2): 299-313.
[PMID: 11790801]

[52] Lamouille S, Xu J, Derynck R. Molecular mechanisms of epithelial-mesenchymal transition. Nat Rev Mol Cell Biol 2014; 15(3): 178-96.
[PMID: 24556840]

[53] Akhurst RJ. TGF-beta antagonists: why suppress a tumor suppressor? J Clin Invest 2002; 109(12): 1533-6.
[PMID: 12070299]

[54] Huynh LK, Hipolito CJ, Ten Dijke P. A Perspective on the Development of TGF-β Inhibitors for Cancer Treatment. Biomolecules 2019; 9(11): E743.
[PMID: 31744193]

[55] Dawson MA, Kouzarides T. Cancer epigenetics: from mechanism to therapy. Cell 2012; 150(1): 12-27.
[PMID: 22770212]

[56] Jones PA, Baylin SB. The epigenomics of cancer. Cell 2007; 128(4): 683-92. [PMID: 17320506]

[57] Bedi U, Mishra VK, Wasilewski D, Scheel C, Johnsen SA. Epigenetic plasticity: a central regulator of epithelial-to-mesenchymal transition in cancer. Oncotarget 2014; 5(8): 2016-29. [PMID: 24840099]

[58] De Craene B, Berx G. Regulatory networks defining EMT during cancer initiation and progression. Nat Rev Cancer 2013; 13(2): 97-110. [PMID: 23344542]

[59] Cho M-H, Park J-H, Choi H-J, *et al.* DOT1L cooperates with the c-Myc-p300 complex to epigenetically derepress CDH1 transcription factors in breast cancer progression. Nat Commun 2015; 6(1): 7821. [PMID: 26199140]

[60] Choi HJ, Park JH, Park M, *et al.* UTX inhibits EMT-induced breast CSC properties by epigenetic repression of EMT genes in cooperation with LSD1 and HDAC1. EMBO Rep 2015; 16(10): 1288-98. [PMID: 26303947]

[61] Martin MD, Kremers GJ, Short KW, *et al.* Rapid extravasation and establishment of breast cancer micrometastases in the liver microenvironment. Mol Cancer Res 2010; 8(10): 1319-27. [PMID: 20724460]

[62] Chiang SPH, Cabrera RM, Segall JE. Tumor cell intravasation. Am J Physiol Cell Physiol 2016; 311(1): C1-C14. [PMID: 27076614]

[63] Micalizzi DS, Maheswaran S, Haber DA. A conduit to metastasis: circulating tumor cell biology. Genes Dev 2017; 31(18): 1827-40. [PMID: 29051388]

[64] Aceto N, Bardia A, Miyamoto DT, *et al.* Circulating tumor cell clusters are oligoclonal precursors of breast cancer metastasis. Cell 2014; 158(5): 1110-22. [PMID: 25171411]

[65] Cristofanilli M, Budd GT, Ellis MJ, *et al.* Circulating tumor cells, disease progression, and survival in metastatic breast cancer. N Engl J Med 2004; 351(8): 781-91. [PMID: 15317891]

[66] Stegner D, Dütting S, Nieswandt B. Mechanistic explanation for platelet contribution to cancer metastasis. Thromb Res 2014; 133 (Suppl. 2): S149-57. [PMID: 24862136]

[67] Spano D, Heck C, De Antonellis P, Christofori G, Zollo M. Molecular networks that regulate cancer metastasis. Semin Cancer Biol 2012; 22(3): 234-49. [PMID: 22484561]

[68] Friedl P, Alexander S. Cancer invasion and the microenvironment: plasticity and reciprocity. Cell 2011; 147(5): 992-1009. [PMID: 22118458]

[69] Yao L-C, Baluk P, Srinivasan RS, Oliver G, McDonald DM. Plasticity of button-like junctions in the endothelium of airway lymphatics in development and inflammation. Am J Pathol 2012; 180(6): 2561-75. [PMID: 22538088]

[70] Baluk P, Fuxe J, Hashizume H, *et al.* Functionally specialized junctions between endothelial cells of lymphatic vessels. J Exp Med 2007; 204(10): 2349-62. [PMID: 17846148]

[71] Sleeman JP, Nazarenko I, Thiele W. Do all roads lead to Rome? Routes to metastasis development. Int

J Cancer 2011; 128(11): 2511-26.
[PMID: 21365648]

[72] Han W, Chen S, Yuan W, *et al.* Oriented collagen fibers direct tumor cell intravasation. Proc Natl Acad Sci USA 2016; 113(40): 11208-13.
[PMID: 27663743]

[73] Pollard JW. Macrophages define the invasive microenvironment in breast cancer. J Leukoc Biol 2008; 84(3): 623-30.
[PMID: 18467655]

[74] Lin EY, Gouon-Evans V, Nguyen AV, Pollard JW. The macrophage growth factor CSF-1 in mammary gland development and tumor progression. J Mammary Gland Biol Neoplasia 2002; 7(2): 147-62.
[PMID: 12465600]

[75] Wyckoff J, Wang W, Lin EY, *et al.* A paracrine loop between tumor cells and macrophages is required for tumor cell migration in mammary tumors. Cancer Res 2004; 64(19): 7022-9.
[PMID: 15466195]

[76] Lustberg MB, Balasubramanian P, Miller B, *et al.* Heterogeneous atypical cell populations are present in blood of metastatic breast cancer patients. Breast Cancer Res 2014; 16(2): R23.
[PMID: 24602188]

[77] Akhter MZ, Sharawat SK, Kumar V, *et al.* Aggressive serous epithelial ovarian cancer is potentially propagated by EpCAM^{+}CD45^{+} phenotype. Oncogene 2018; 37(16): 2089-103.
[PMID: 29379166]

[78] Joly E, Hudrisier D. What is trogocytosis and what is its purpose? Nat Immunol 2003; 4(9): 815.
[PMID: 12942076]

[79] Zavyalova MV, Denisov EV, Tashireva LA, *et al.* Intravasation as a Key Step in Cancer Metastasis. Biochemistry (Mosc) 2019; 84(7): 762-72.
[PMID: 31509727]

[80] Strilic B, Offermanns S. Intravascular Survival and Extravasation of Tumor Cells. Cancer Cell 2017; 32(3): 282-93.
[PMID: 28898694]

[81] Kienast Y, von Baumgarten L, Fuhrmann M, *et al.* Real-time imaging reveals the single steps of brain metastasis formation. Nat Med 2010; 16(1): 116-22.
[PMID: 20023634]

[82] Al-Mehdi AB, Tozawa K, Fisher AB, Shientag L, Lee A, Muschel RJ. Intravascular origin of metastasis from the proliferation of endothelium-attached tumor cells: a new model for metastasis. Nat Med 2000; 6(1): 100-2.
[PMID: 10613833]

[83] Stoletov K, Kato H, Zardouzian E, *et al.* Visualizing extravasation dynamics of metastatic tumor cells. J Cell Sci 2010; 123(Pt 13): 2332-41.
[PMID: 20530574]

[84] Gassmann P, Haier J, Schlüter K, *et al.* CXCR4 regulates the early extravasation of metastatic tumor cells *in vivo.* Neoplasia 2009; 11(7): 651-61.
[PMID: 19568410]

[85] Schumacher D, Strilic B, Sivaraj KK, Wettschureck N, Offermanns S. Platelet-derived nucleotides promote tumor-cell transendothelial migration and metastasis *via* P2Y2 receptor. Cancer Cell 2013; 24(1): 130-7.
[PMID: 23810565]

[86] Leong HS, Robertson AE, Stoletov K, *et al.* Invadopodia are required for cancer cell extravasation and are a therapeutic target for metastasis. Cell Rep 2014; 8(5): 1558-70.

[PMID: 25176655]

[87] Khuon S, Liang L, Dettman RW, Sporn PH, Wysolmerski RB, Chew TL. Myosin light chain kinase mediates transcellular intravasation of breast cancer cells through the underlying endothelial cells: a three-dimensional FRET study. J Cell Sci 2010; 123(Pt 3): 431-40.
[PMID: 20067998]

[88] Tremblay PL, Huot J, Auger FA. Mechanisms by which E-selectin regulates diapedesis of colon cancer cells under flow conditions. Cancer Res 2008; 68(13): 5167-76.
[PMID: 18593916]

[89] Alix-Panabières C, Pantel K. Clinical Applications of Circulating Tumor Cells and Circulating Tumor DNA as Liquid Biopsy. Cancer Discov 2016; 6(5): 479-91.
[PMID: 26969689]

[90] Hamidi H, Ivaska J. Every step of the way: integrins in cancer progression and metastasis. Nat Rev Cancer 2018; 18(9): 533-48.
[PMID: 30002479]

[91] Labelle M, Hynes RO. The initial hours of metastasis: the importance of cooperative host-tumor cell interactions during hematogenous dissemination. Cancer Discov 2012; 2(12): 1091-9.
[PMID: 23166151]

[92] Reymond N, d'Água BB, Ridley AJ. Crossing the endothelial barrier during metastasis. Nat Rev Cancer 2013; 13(12): 858-70.
[PMID: 24263189]

[93] Strilic B, Yang L, Albarrán-Juárez J, *et al.* Tumour-cell-induced endothelial cell necroptosis *via* death receptor 6 promotes metastasis. Nature 2016; 536(7615): 215-8.
[PMID: 27487218]

[94] Huang RL, Teo Z, Chong HC, *et al.* ANGPTL4 modulates vascular junction integrity by integrin signaling and disruption of intercellular VE-cadherin and claudin-5 clusters. Blood 2011; 118(14): 3990-4002.
[PMID: 21841165]

[95] Tichet M, Prod'Homme V, Fenouille N, *et al.* Tumour-derived SPARC drives vascular permeability and extravasation through endothelial VCAM1 signalling to promote metastasis. Nat Commun 2015; 6(1): 6993.
[PMID: 25925867]

[96] Cools-Lartigue J, Spicer J, McDonald B, *et al.* Neutrophil extracellular traps sequester circulating tumor cells and promote metastasis. J Clin Invest 2013; 123(8): 3446-58.
[PMID: 23863628]

[97] Najmeh S, Cools-Lartigue J, Rayes RF, *et al.* Neutrophil extracellular traps sequester circulating tumor cells *via* β1-integrin mediated interactions. Int J Cancer 2017; 140(10): 2321-30.
[PMID: 28177522]

[98] Häuselmann I, Roblek M, Protsyuk D, *et al.* Monocyte Induction of E-Selectin-Mediated Endothelial Activation Releases VE-Cadherin Junctions to Promote Tumor Cell Extravasation in the Metastasis Cascade. Cancer Res 2016; 76(18): 5302-12.
[PMID: 27488527]

[99] Wolf MJ, Hoos A, Bauer J, *et al.* Endothelial CCR2 signaling induced by colon carcinoma cells enables extravasation *via* the JAK2-Stat5 and p38MAPK pathway. Cancer Cell 2012; 22(1): 91-105.
[PMID: 22789541]

[100] Qian B, Deng Y, Im JH, *et al.* A distinct macrophage population mediates metastatic breast cancer cell extravasation, establishment and growth. PLoS One 2009; 4(8): e6562.
[PMID: 19668347]

[101] Prager GW, Lackner E-M, Krauth M-T, *et al.* Targeting of VEGF-dependent transendothelial

migration of cancer cells by bevacizumab. Mol Oncol 2010; 4(2): 150-60.
[PMID: 20106729]

[102] Bendas G, Borsig L. Cancer cell adhesion and metastasis: selectins, integrins, and the inhibitory potential of heparins. Int J Cell Biol 2012; 2012: 676731.
[PMID: 22505933]

[103] Mackay CR. Moving targets: cell migration inhibitors as new anti-inflammatory therapies. Nat Immunol 2008; 9(9): 988-98.
[PMID: 18711436]

[104] Mammadova-Bach E, Mangin P, Lanza F, Gachet C. Platelets in cancer. From basic research to therapeutic implications. Hamostaseologie 2015; 35(4): 325-36.
[PMID: 26289826]

[105] Childs RW, Carlsten M. Therapeutic approaches to enhance natural killer cell cytotoxicity against cancer: the force awakens. Nat Rev Drug Discov 2015; 14(7): 487-98.
[PMID: 26000725]

[106] Rothwell PM, Wilson M, Price JF, Belch JF, Meade TW, Mehta Z. Effect of daily aspirin on risk of cancer metastasis: a study of incident cancers during randomised controlled trials. Lancet 2012; 379(9826): 1591-601.
[PMID: 22440947]

[107] Zhao X, Xu Z, Li H. NSAIDs Use and Reduced Metastasis in Cancer Patients: results from a meta-analysis. Sci Rep 2017; 7(1): 1875.
[PMID: 28500305]

[108] Connolly EM, Harmey JH, O'Grady T, *et al.* Cyclo-oxygenase inhibition reduces tumour growth and metastasis in an orthotopic model of breast cancer. Br J Cancer 2002; 87(2): 231-7.
[PMID: 12107848]

[109] Strell C, Entschladen F. Extravasation of leukocytes in comparison to tumor cells. Cell Commun Signal 2008; 6: 10.
[PMID: 19055814]

[110] Qi J, Chen N, Wang J, Siu CH. Transendothelial migration of melanoma cells involves N-cadheri--mediated adhesion and activation of the beta-catenin signaling pathway. Mol Biol Cell 2005; 16(9): 4386-97.
[PMID: 15987741]

[111] Sever R, Brugge JS. Signal transduction in cancer. Cold Spring Harb Perspect Med 2015; 5(4): a006098.
[PMID: 25833940]

[112] Vogelstein B, Kinzler KW. The Path to Cancer -Three Strikes and You're Out. N Engl J Med 2015; 373(20): 1895-8.
[PMID: 26559569]

[113] Kowalik A, Kowalewska M, Góźdź S. Current approaches for avoiding the limitations of circulating tumor cells detection methods-implications for diagnosis and treatment of patients with solid tumors. Transl Res 2017; 185: 58-84.e15.
[PMID: 28506696]

[114] Hu C, Chen R, Chen W, *et al.* Thrombocytosis is a significant indictor of hypercoagulability, prognosis and recurrence in gastric cancer. Exp Ther Med 2014; 8(1): 125-32.
[PMID: 24944610]

[115] Gay LJ, Felding-Habermann B. Contribution of platelets to tumour metastasis. Nat Rev Cancer 2011; 11(2): 123-34.
[PMID: 21258396]

[116] Placke T, Örgel M, Schaller M, *et al.* Platelet-derived MHC class I confers a pseudonormal phenotype

to cancer cells that subverts the antitumor reactivity of natural killer immune cells. Cancer Res 2012; 72(2): 440-8.
[PMID: 22127925]

[117] Fontebasso Y, Dubinett SM. Drug Development for Metastasis Prevention. Crit Rev Oncog 2015; 20(5-6): 449-73.
[PMID: 27279241]

[118] Victoria EJ, Mahan LC, Masouredis SP. The IgG binding function of the normal red cell plasma membrane: identification of integral polypeptides that bind IgG. Br J Haematol 1982; 50(1): 101-10.
[PMID: 7055530]

[119] Elgundi Z, Papanicolaou M, Major G, *et al.* Cancer Metastasis: The Role of the Extracellular Matrix and the Heparan Sulfate Proteoglycan Perlecan. Front Oncol 2020; 9(1482): 1482.
[PMID: 32010611]

[120] Castro-Giner F, Aceto N. Tracking cancer progression: from circulating tumor cells to metastasis. Genome Med 2020; 12(1): 31.
[PMID: 32192534]

[121] Andersen MH, Schrama D, Thor Straten P, Becker JC. Cytotoxic T cells. J Invest Dermatol 2006; 126(1): 32-41.
[PMID: 16417215]

[122] Kayagaki N, Yamaguchi N, Nakayama M, Eto H, Okumura K, Yagita H. Type I interferons (IFNs) regulate tumor necrosis factor-related apoptosis-inducing ligand (TRAIL) expression on human T cells: A novel mechanism for the antitumor effects of type I IFNs. J Exp Med 1999; 189(9): 1451-60.
[PMID: 10224285]

[123] Rousalova I, Krepela E. Granzyme B-induced apoptosis in cancer cells and its regulation (review). Int J Oncol 2010; 37(6): 1361-78.
[PMID: 21042704]

[124] Wang RF. The role of MHC class II-restricted tumor antigens and CD4+ T cells in antitumor immunity. Trends Immunol 2001; 22(5): 269-76.
[PMID: 11323286]

[125] Papaioannou NE, Beniata OV, Vitsos P, Tsitsilonis O, Samara P. Harnessing the immune system to improve cancer therapy. Ann Transl Med 2016; 4(14): 261.
[PMID: 27563648]

[126] Bracci L, Schiavoni G, Sistigu A, Belardelli F. Immune-based mechanisms of cytotoxic chemotherapy: implications for the design of novel and rationale-based combined treatments against cancer. Cell Death Differ 2014; 21(1): 15-25.
[PMID: 23787994]

[127] Ferguson LR, Baguley BC. Multidrug resistance and mutagenesis. Mutat Res 1993; 285(1): 79-90.
[PMID: 7678136]

[128] Baguley BC. Multidrug resistance in cancer. Methods Mol Biol 2010; 596: 1-14.
[PMID: 19949917]

[129] Asahara T, Murohara T, Sullivan A, *et al.* Isolation of putative progenitor endothelial cells for angiogenesis. Science 1997; 275(5302): 964-7.
[PMID: 9020076]

[130] Ferrari G, Cook BD, Terushkin V, Pintucci G, Mignatti P. Transforming growth factor-beta 1 (TGF-beta1) induces angiogenesis through vascular endothelial growth factor (VEGF)-mediated apoptosis. J Cell Physiol 2009; 219(2): 449-58.
[PMID: 19180561]

[131] Poniatowski ŁA, Wojdasiewicz P, Gasik R, Szukiewicz D. Transforming growth factor Beta family: insight into the role of growth factors in regulation of fracture healing biology and potential clinical

applications. Mediators Inflamm 2015; 2015: 137823.
[PMID: 25709154]

[132] Perlman R, Schiemann WP, Brooks MW, Lodish HF, Weinberg RA. TGF-beta-induced apoptosis is mediated by the adapter protein Daxx that facilitates JNK activation. Nat Cell Biol 2001; 3(8): 708-14.
[PMID: 11483955]

[133] Ben-Kasus T, Schechter B, Sela M, Yarden Y. Cancer therapeutic antibodies come of age: targeting minimal residual disease. Mol Oncol 2007; 1(1): 42-54.
[PMID: 19383286]

[134] Nowsheen S, Yang ES. The intersection between DNA damage response and cell death pathways. Exp Oncol 2012; 34(3): 243-54.
[PMID: 23070009]

[135] Bennett SRM, Carbone FR, Karamalis F, Flavell RA, Miller JFAP, Heath WR. Help for cytotoxic-T-cell responses is mediated by CD40 signalling. Nature 1998; 393(6684): 478-80.
[PMID: 9624004]

[136] Schoenberger SP, Toes RE, van der Voort EI, Offringa R, Melief CJ. T-cell help for cytotoxic T lymphocytes is mediated by CD40-CD40L interactions. Nature 1998; 393(6684): 480-3.
[PMID: 9624005]

[137] Malhotra A, Shanker A. NK cells: immune cross-talk and therapeutic implications. Immunotherapy 2011; 3(10): 1143-66.
[PMID: 21995569]

[138] Uzhachenko RV, Shanker A. $CD8^+$ T Lymphocyte and NK Cell Network: Circuitry in the Cytotoxic Domain of Immunity. Front Immunol 2019; 10: 1906.
[PMID: 31456803]

[139] Beatty GL, Chiorean EG, Fishman MP, *et al.* CD40 agonists alter tumor stroma and show efficacy against pancreatic carcinoma in mice and humans. Science 2011; 331(6024): 1612-6.
[PMID: 21436454]

[140] Tay NQ, Lee DCP, Chua YL, Prabhu N, Gascoigne NRJ, Kemeny DM. CD40L Expression Allows $CD8^+$ T Cells to Promote Their Own Expansion and Differentiation through Dendritic Cells. Front Immunol 2017; 8: 1484.
[PMID: 29163545]

[141] Gorelik L, Flavell RA. Abrogation of TGFbeta signaling in T cells leads to spontaneous T cell differentiation and autoimmune disease. Immunity 2000; 12(2): 171-81.
[PMID: 10714683]

[142] Letterio JJ. Murine models define the role of TGF-β as a master regulator of immune cell function. Cytokine Growth Factor Rev 2000; 11(1-2): 81-7.
[PMID: 10708955]

[143] Baselga J, Rothenberg ML, Tabernero J, *et al.* TGF-beta signalling-related markers in cancer patients with bone metastasis. Biomarkers 2008; 13(2): 217-36.
[PMID: 18270872]

[144] Kloss CC, Lee J, Zhang A, *et al.* Dominant-Negative TGF-β Receptor Enhances PSMA-Targeted Human CAR T Cell Proliferation And Augments Prostate Cancer Eradication. Mol Ther 2018; 26(7): 1855-66.
[PMID: 29807781]

[145] Morris JC, Tan AR, Olencki TE, *et al.* Phase I study of GC1008 (fresolimumab): a human anti-transforming growth factor-beta (TGFβ) monoclonal antibody in patients with advanced malignant melanoma or renal cell carcinoma. PLoS One 2014; 9(3): e90353.
[PMID: 24618589]

[146] Uhl M, Aulwurm S, Wischhusen J, *et al.* SD-208, a novel transforming growth factor beta receptor I

kinase inhibitor, inhibits growth and invasiveness and enhances immunogenicity of murine and human glioma cells *in vitro* and *in vivo.* Cancer Res 2004; 64(21): 7954-61.
[PMID: 15520202]

[147] Stüber T, Monjezi R, Wallstabe L, *et al.* Inhibition of TGF-β-receptor signaling augments the antitumor function of ROR1-specific CAR T-cells against triple-negative breast cancer. J Immunother Cancer 2020; 8(1): e000676.
[PMID: 32303620]

[148] Folkman J, Shing Y. Angiogenesis. J Biol Chem 1992; 267(16): 10931-4.
[PMID: 1375931]

[149] Maisonpierre PC, Suri C, Jones PF, *et al.* Angiopoietin-2, a natural antagonist for Tie2 that disrupts *in vivo* angiogenesis. Science 1997; 277(5322): 55-60.
[PMID: 9204896]

[150] Ribatti D. The involvement of endothelial progenitor cells in tumor angiogenesis. J Cell Mol Med 2004; 8(3): 294-300.
[PMID: 15491505]

[151] Lyden D, Hattori K, Dias S, *et al.* Impaired recruitment of bone-marrow-derived endothelial and hematopoietic precursor cells blocks tumor angiogenesis and growth. Nat Med 2001; 7(11): 1194-201.
[PMID: 11689883]

[152] Kerbel RS. Antiangiogenic therapy: a universal chemosensitization strategy for cancer? Science 2006; 312(5777): 1171-5.
[PMID: 16728631]

[153] Koh W, Stratman AN, Sacharidou A, Davis GE. *In vitro* three dimensional collagen matrix models of endothelial lumen formation during vasculogenesis and angiogenesis. Methods Enzymol 2008; 443: 83-101.
[PMID: 18772012]

[154] Rankin EB, Giaccia AJ. The role of hypoxia-inducible factors in tumorigenesis. Cell Death Differ 2008; 15(4): 678-85.
[PMID: 18259193]

[155] Lv X, Li J, Zhang C, *et al.* The role of hypoxia-inducible factors in tumor angiogenesis and cell metabolism. Genes Dis 2016; 4(1): 19-24.
[PMID: 30258904]

[156] Semenza GL. Defining the role of hypoxia-inducible factor 1 in cancer biology and therapeutics. Oncogene 2010; 29(5): 625-34.
[PMID: 19946328]

[157] Hanahan D, Weinberg RA. Hallmarks of cancer: the next generation. Cell 2011; 144(5): 646-74.
[PMID: 21376230]

[158] Ferrara N. VEGF and the quest for tumour angiogenesis factors. Nat Rev Cancer 2002; 2(10): 795-803.
[PMID: 12360282]

[159] Kim KJ, Li B, Winer J, *et al.* Inhibition of vascular endothelial growth factor-induced angiogenesis suppresses tumour growth *in vivo.* Nature 1993; 362(6423): 841-4.
[PMID: 7683111]

[160] Knopik-Skrocka A, Kręplewska P, Jarmołowska-Jurczyszyn D. Tumor Blood Vessels and Vasculogenic Mimicry – Current Knowledge and Searching for New Cellular/Molecular Targets of Anti-Angiogenic Therapy. Med J Cell Biol 2017; 5(1): 50-71.

[161] Witsch E, Sela M, Yarden Y. Roles for growth factors in cancer progression. Physiology (Bethesda) 2010; 25(2): 85-101.
[PMID: 20430953]

[162] Chen PH, Chen X, He X. Platelet-derived growth factors and their receptors: structural and functional perspectives. Biochim Biophys Acta 2013; 1834(10): 2176-86.
[PMID: 23137658]

[163] Andrae J, Gallini R, Betsholtz C. Role of platelet-derived growth factors in physiology and medicine. Genes Dev 2008; 22(10): 1276-312.
[PMID: 18483217]

[164] He L, Hristova K. Physical-chemical principles underlying RTK activation, and their implications for human disease. Biochim Biophys Acta 2012; 1818(4): 995-1005.
[PMID: 21840295]

[165] Lin LH, Lin JS, Yang CC, Cheng HW, Chang KW, Liu CJ. Overexpression of Platelet-Derived Growth Factor and Its Receptor Are Correlated with Oral Tumorigenesis and Poor Prognosis in Oral Squamous Cell Carcinoma. Int J Mol Sci 2020; 21(7): E2360.
[PMID: 32235327]

[166] Ogawa N, Inokuchi M, Takagi Y, *et al.* Clinical significance of platelet derived growth factor-C and -D in gastric cancer. Oncol Lett 2015; 10(6): 3495-501.
[PMID: 26788156]

[167] Kong D, Wang Z, Sarkar SH, *et al.* Platelet-derived growth factor-D overexpression contributes to epithelial-mesenchymal transition of PC3 prostate cancer cells. Stem Cells 2008; 26(6): 1425-35.
[PMID: 18403754]

[168] McCarty MF, Somcio RJ, Stoeltzing O, *et al.* Overexpression of PDGF-BB decreases colorectal and pancreatic cancer growth by increasing tumor pericyte content. J Clin Invest 2007; 117(8): 2114-22.
[PMID: 17641778]

[169] Heldin CH, Westermark B. Mechanism of action and *in vivo* role of platelet-derived growth factor. Physiol Rev 1999; 79(4): 1283-316.
[PMID: 10508235]

[170] Heldin CH. Autocrine PDGF stimulation in malignancies. Ups J Med Sci 2012; 117(2): 83-91.
[PMID: 22512244]

[171] Jechlinger M, Sommer A, Moriggl R, *et al.* Autocrine PDGFR signaling promotes mammary cancer metastasis. J Clin Invest 2006; 116(6): 1561-70.
[PMID: 16741576]

[172] Kong D, Wang Z, Sarkar SH, *et al.* Platelet-derived growth factor-D overexpression contributes to epithelial-mesenchymal transition of PC3 prostate cancer cells. Stem Cells 2008; 26(6): 1425-35.
[PMID: 18403754]

[173] Walker F, Burgess AW. Reconstitution of the high affinity epidermal growth factor receptor on cell-free membranes after transmodulation by platelet-derived growth factor. J Biol Chem 1991; 266(5): 2746-52.
[PMID: 1993654]

[174] Koch S, Claesson-Welsh L. Signal transduction by vascular endothelial growth factor receptors. Cold Spring Harb Perspect Med 2012; 2(7): a006502.
[PMID: 22762016]

[175] Kowanetz M, Ferrara N. Vascular endothelial growth factor signaling pathways: therapeutic perspective. Clin Cancer Res 2006; 12(17): 5018-22.
[PMID: 16951216]

[176] Yang J, Yan J, Liu B. Targeting VEGF/VEGFR to Modulate Antitumor Immunity. Front Immunol 2018; 9: 978.
[PMID: 29774034]

[177] Zhang L, Wang H, Li C, *et al.* VEGF-A/Neuropilin 1 Pathway Confers Cancer Stemness *via*

Activating Wnt/β-Catenin Axis in Breast Cancer Cells. Cell Physiol Biochem 2017; 44(3): 1251-62. [PMID: 29179185]

[178] Galdiero MR, Bonavita E, Barajon I, Garlanda C, Mantovani A, Jaillon S. Tumor associated macrophages and neutrophils in cancer. Immunobiology 2013; 218(11): 1402-10. [PMID: 23891329]

[179] Singh B, Carpenter G, Coffey RJ. EGF receptor ligands: recent advances. F1000Res. 2016; 5 F1000 Faculty Rev-2270. [PMID: 27635238]

[180] van der Geer P, Hunter T, Lindberg RA. Receptor protein-tyrosine kinases and their signal transduction pathways. Annu Rev Cell Biol 1994; 10: 251-337. [PMID: 7888178]

[181] Franovic A, Gunaratnam L, Smith K, Robert I, Patten D, Lee S. Translational up-regulation of the EGFR by tumor hypoxia provides a nonmutational explanation for its overexpression in human cancer. Proc Natl Acad Sci USA 2007; 104(32): 13092-7. [PMID: 17670948]

[182] Santaniello A, Napolitano F, Servetto A, *et al.* Tumour Microenvironment and Immune Evasion in EGFR Addicted NSCLC: Hurdles and Possibilities. Cancers (Basel) 2019; 11(10): 1419. [PMID: 31554160]

[183] Matsumoto Y, Koh Y. Tumor immune microenvironment of *EGFR*-mutant non-small-cell lung cancer and its impact on therapeutic efficacy. Immunotherapy 2020; 12(7): 431-7. [PMID: 32316809]

[184] Giacomini A, Chiodelli P, Matarazzo S, Rusnati M, Presta M, Ronca R. Blocking the FGF/FGFR system as a “two-compartment” antiangiogenic/antitumor approach in cancer therapy. Pharmacol Res 2016; 107: 172-85. [PMID: 27013279]

[185] Itoh N, Ornitz DM. Functional evolutionary history of the mouse Fgf gene family. Dev Dyn 2008; 237(1): 18-27. [PMID: 18058912]

[186] Ornitz DM. FGFs, heparan sulfate and FGFRs: complex interactions essential for development. BioEssays 2000; 22(2): 108-12. [PMID: 10655030]

[187] Itoh N, Ohta H, Konishi M. Endocrine FGFs: evolution, physiology, pathophysiology, and pharmacotherapy. Front Endocrinol (Lausanne) 2015; 6: 154. [PMID: 26483756]

[188] Olsen SK, Garbi M, Zampieri N, *et al.* Fibroblast growth factor (FGF) homologous factors share structural but not functional homology with FGFs. J Biol Chem 2003; 278(36): 34226-36. [PMID: 12815063]

[189] Helsten T, Elkin S, Arthur E, Tomson BN, Carter J, Kurzrock R. The FGFR landscape in cancer: analysis of 4,853 tumors by next-generation sequencing. Clin Cancer Res 2016; 22(1): 259-67. [PMID: 26373574]

[190] Singh D, Chan JM, Zoppoli P, *et al.* Transforming fusions of FGFR and TACC genes in human glioblastoma. Science 2012; 337(6099): 1231-5. [PMID: 22837387]

[191] Williams SV, Hurst CD, Knowles MA. Oncogenic FGFR3 gene fusions in bladder cancer. Hum Mol Genet 2013; 22(4): 795-803. [PMID: 23175443]

[192] Shaver TM, Lehmann BD, Beeler JS, *et al.* Diverse, biologically relevant, and targetable gene rearrangements in triple-negative breast cancer and other malignancies. Cancer Res 2016; 76(16):

4850-60.
[PMID: 27231203]

[193] Daly C, Castanaro C, Zhang W, *et al.* FGFR3-TACC3 fusion proteins act as naturally occurring drivers of tumor resistance by functionally substituting for EGFR/ERK signaling. Oncogene 2017; 36(4): 471-81.
[PMID: 27345413]

[194] Weidner KM, Arakaki N, Hartmann G, *et al.* Evidence for the identity of human scatter factor and human hepatocyte growth factor. Proc Natl Acad Sci USA 1991; 88(16): 7001-5.
[PMID: 1831266]

[195] Trusolino L, Bertotti A, Comoglio PM. MET signalling: principles and functions in development, organ regeneration and cancer. Nat Rev Mol Cell Biol 2010; 11(12): 834-48.
[PMID: 21102609]

[196] Li W, Dick A, Lu F, Zhang H, Sun H. Induction of MET Receptor Tyrosine Kinase Down-regulation through Antibody-mediated Receptor Clustering. Sci Rep 2019; 9(1): 1988.
[PMID: 30760737]

[197] Zhang Y, Xia M, Jin K, *et al.* Function of the c-Met receptor tyrosine kinase in carcinogenesis and associated therapeutic opportunities. Mol Cancer 2018; 17(1): 45.
[PMID: 29455668]

[198] Tovar EA, Graveel CR. MET in human cancer: germline and somatic mutations. Ann Transl Med 2017; 5(10): 205.
[PMID: 28603720]

[199] Massagué J. TGFβ signalling in context. Nat Rev Mol Cell Biol 2012; 13(10): 616-30.
[PMID: 22992590]

[200] Luo J, Chen X-Q, Li P. The Role of TGF-β and Its Receptors in Gastrointestinal Cancers. Transl Oncol 2019; 12(3): 475-84.
[PMID: 30594036]

[201] Alsina-Sanchís E, Figueras A, Lahiguera A, *et al.* TGFβ Controls Ovarian Cancer Cell Proliferation. Int J Mol Sci 2017; 18(8): 1658.
[http://dx.doi.org/10.3390/ijms18081658] [PMID: 28758950]

[202] Pang X, Tang YL, Liang XH. Transforming growth factor-β signaling in head and neck squamous cell carcinoma: Insights into cellular responses. Oncol Lett 2018; 16(4): 4799-806.
[PMID: 30250544]

[203] Han J, Alvarez-Breckenridge CA, Wang Q-E, Yu J. TGF-β signaling and its targeting for glioma treatment. Am J Cancer Res 2015; 5(3): 945-55.
[PMID: 26045979]

[204] Kretzschmar M. Transforming growth factor-β and breast cancer: Transforming growth factor-β/SMAD signaling defects and cancer. Breast Cancer Res 2000; 2(2): 107-15.
[PMID: 11250700]

[205] Massagué J. TGFbeta in Cancer. Cell 2008; 134(2): 215-30.
[PMID: 18662538]

[206] Smith PM, Means AL, Beauchamp RD. Immunomodulatory Effects of TGF-β Family Signaling within Intestinal Epithelial Cells and Carcinomas. Gastrointestinal Disorders 2019; 1(2): 290-300.
[PMID: 33834163]

[207] Yu H, Rohan T. Role of the insulin-like growth factor family in cancer development and progression. J Natl Cancer Inst 2000; 92(18): 1472-89.
[PMID: 10995803]

[208] Hua H, Kong Q, Yin J, Zhang J, Jiang Y. Insulin-like growth factor receptor signaling in

tumorigenesis and drug resistance: a challenge for cancer therapy. J Hematol Oncol 2020; 13(1): 64. [PMID: 32493414]

[209] Heskamp S, Boerman OC, Molkenboer-Kuenen JDM, *et al.* Upregulation of IGF-1R expression during neoadjuvant therapy predicts poor outcome in breast cancer patients. PloS one 2015; 10(2): e0117745.

[210] Ireland L, Santos A, Ahmed MS, *et al.* Chemoresistance in Pancreatic Cancer Is Driven by Stroma-Derived Insulin-Like Growth Factors. Cancer Res 2016; 76(23): 6851-63. [PMID: 27742686]

[211] Skaper SD. The Neurotrophin Family of Neurotrophic Factors: An Overview Neurotrophic Factors: Methods and Protocols. Totowa, NJ: Humana Press 2012; pp. 1-12.

[212] Bothwell M. Recent advances in understanding neurotrophin signaling. F1000 Res 2016; 5: 5. [PMID: 27540475]

[213] Chao MV. Neurotrophins and their receptors: a convergence point for many signalling pathways. Nat Rev Neurosci 2003; 4(4): 299-309. [PMID: 12671646]

[214] Boilly B, Faulkner S, Jobling P, Hondermarck H. Nerve Dependence: From Regeneration to Cancer. Cancer Cell 2017; 31(3): 342-54. [PMID: 28292437]

[215] Harding J, Burtness B. Cetuximab: an epidermal growth factor receptor chemeric human-murine monoclonal antibody. Drugs Today (Barc) 2005; 41(2): 107-27. [PMID: 15821783]

[216] Messersmith WA, Hidalgo M. Panitumumab, a monoclonal anti epidermal growth factor receptor antibody in colorectal cancer: another one or the one? Clin Cancer Res 2007; 13(16): 4664-6. [PMID: 17699842]

[217] García-Foncillas J, Sunakawa Y, Aderka D, *et al.* Distinguishing Features of Cetuximab and Panitumumab in Colorectal Cancer and Other Solid Tumors. Front Oncol 2019; 9(849): 849. [PMID: 31616627]

[218] Kabolizadeh P, Kubicek GJ, Heron DE, Ferris RL, Gibson MK. The role of cetuximab in the management of head and neck cancers. Expert Opin Biol Ther 2012; 12(4): 517-28. [PMID: 22413826]

[219] Mazzarella L, Guida A, Curigliano G. Cetuximab for treating non-small cell lung cancer. Expert Opin Biol Ther 2018; 18(4): 483-93. [PMID: 29534625]

[220] Wollina U. Update of cetuximab for non-melanoma skin cancer. Expert Opin Biol Ther 2014; 14(2): 271-6. [PMID: 24387664]

[221] Solomon MT, Miranda N, Jorrín E, *et al.* Nimotuzumab in combination with radiotherapy in high grade glioma patients: a single institution experience. Cancer Biol Ther 2014; 15(5): 504-9. [PMID: 24521695]

[222] Ramos TC, Fernández BM, Herrera ZM, Escobar NEI. Nimotuzumab for Patients With Inoperable Cancer of the Head and Neck. Front Oncol 2020; 10: 817. [PMID: 32537431]

[223] Lu Y, Chen D, Liang J, *et al.* Administration of nimotuzumab combined with cisplatin plus 5-fluorouracil as induction therapy improves treatment response and tolerance in patients with locally advanced nasopharyngeal carcinoma receiving concurrent radiochemotherapy: a multicenter randomized controlled study. BMC Cancer 2019; 19(1): 1262. [PMID: 31888551]

[224] Fala L. Portrazza (Necitumumab), an IgG1 Monoclonal Antibody, FDA Approved for Advanced Squamous Non-Small-Cell Lung Cancer. Am Health Drug Benefits. 2016; 9(Spec Feature): 119-22. [PMID: 27668058]

[225] Cai W-Q, Zeng L-S, Wang L-F, *et al.* The Latest Battles Between EGFR Monoclonal Antibodies and Resistant Tumor Cells. Front Oncol 2020; 10(1249): 1249. [PMID: 32793499]

[226] Slamon DJ, Leyland-Jones B, Shak S, *et al.* Use of chemotherapy plus a monoclonal antibody against HER2 for metastatic breast cancer that overexpresses HER2. N Engl J Med 2001; 344(11): 783-92. [PMID: 11248153]

[227] Oostra DR, Macrae ER. Role of trastuzumab emtansine in the treatment of HER2-positive breast cancer. Breast Cancer (Dove Med Press) 2014; 6: 103-13. [PMID: 25114588]

[228] Swain SM, Miles D, Kim S-B, *et al.* Pertuzumab, trastuzumab, and docetaxel for HER2-positive metastatic breast cancer (CLEOPATRA): end-of-study results from a double-blind, randomised, placebo-controlled, phase 3 study. Lancet Oncol 2020; 21(4): 519-30. [PMID: 32171426]

[229] Saltz LB, Meropol NJ, Loehrer PJ Sr, *et al.* Phase II trial of cetuximab in patients with refractory colorectal cancer that expresses the epidermal growth factor receptor. J Clin Oncol 2004; 22(7): 1201-8. [PMID: 14993230]

[230] Cunningham D, Humblet Y, Siena S, *et al.* Cetuximab monotherapy and cetuximab plus irinotecan in irinotecan-refractory metastatic colorectal cancer. N Engl J Med 2004; 351(4): 337-45. [PMID: 15269313]

[231] Leto SM, Trusolino L. Primary and acquired resistance to EGFR-targeted therapies in colorectal cancer: impact on future treatment strategies. J Mol Med (Berl) 2014; 92(7): 709-22. [PMID: 24811491]

[232] Millauer B, Shawver LK, Plate KH, Risau W, Ullrich A. Glioblastoma growth inhibited *in vivo* by a dominant-negative Flk-1 mutant. Nature 1994; 367(6463): 576-9. [PMID: 8107827]

[233] Colak.S, Ten Dijke. P. Targeting TGF-B signaling in cancer. Trends Cancer 2017; 3(1): 56-71. [PMID: 28718426]

[234] Lemmon MA, Schlessinger J. Cell signaling by receptor tyrosine kinases. Cell 2010; 141(7): 1117-34. [PMID: 20602996]

[235] Drake JM, Lee JK, Witte ON. Clinical targeting of mutated and wild-type protein tyrosine kinases in cancer. Mol Cell Biol 2014; 34(10): 1722-32. [PMID: 24567371]

[236] Krug M, Hilgeroth A. Recent advances in the development of multi-kinase inhibitors. Mini Rev Med Chem 2008; 8(13): 1312-27. [PMID: 18991750]

[237] Broekman F, Giovannetti E, Peters GJ. Tyrosine kinase inhibitors: Multi-targeted or single-targeted? World J Clin Oncol 2011; 2(2): 80-93. [PMID: 21603317]

[238] Zhang C, Leighl NB, Wu YL, Zhong WZ. Emerging therapies for non-small cell lung cancer. J Hematol Oncol 2019; 12(1): 45. [PMID: 31023335]

[239] Sim EH, Yang IA, Wood-Baker R, Bowman RV, Fong KM. Gefitinib for advanced non-small cell lung cancer. Cochrane Database Syst Rev 2018; 1(1): CD006847.

[PMID: 29336009]

[240] Song Z, Yu X, Cai J, *et al.* Efficacy of icotinib for advanced non-small cell lung cancer patients with EGFR status identified. Zhongguo Fei Ai Za Zhi 2013; 16(3): 138-43.
[PMID: 23514942]

[241] Piperdi B, Perez-Soler R. Role of erlotinib in the treatment of non-small cell lung cancer: clinical outcomes in wild-type epidermal growth factor receptor patients. Drugs 2012; 72 Suppl 1(0 1): 11-9.

[242] Deeks ED, Keating GM. Afatinib in advanced NSCLC: a profile of its use. Drugs Ther Perspect 2018; 34(3): 89-98.
[PMID: 29540977]

[243] Lau SCM, Batra U, Mok TSK, Loong HH. Dacomitinib in the Management of Advanced Non-Smal--Cell Lung Cancer. Drugs 2019; 79(8): 823-31.
[PMID: 31069718]

[244] Mok TS, Wu YL, Ahn MJ, *et al.* Osimertinib or Platinum-Pemetrexed in EGFR T790M-Positive Lung Cancer. N Engl J Med 2017; 376(7): 629-40.
[PMID: 27959700]

[245] Lu S, Wang Q-m, Zhang G, *et al.* Abstract CT190: A multicenter, open-label, single-arm, phase II study: The third generation EGFR tyrosine kinase inhibitor almonertinib for pretreated EGFR T790M-positive locally advanced or metastatic non-small cell lung cancer (APOLLO). Cancer Res 2020; 80.

[246] Shi Y, Hu X, Zhang S, *et al.* Efficacy and safety of alflutinib (AST2818) in patients with T790M mutation-positive NSCLC: A phase IIb multicenter single-arm study. J Clin Oncol 2020; 38(15) (Suppl.): 9602.

[247] Ahn MJ, Han JY, Lee KH, *et al.* Lazertinib in patients with EGFR mutation-positive advanced non-small-cell lung cancer: results from the dose escalation and dose expansion parts of a first-in-human, open-label, multicentre, phase 1-2 study. Lancet Oncol 2019; 20(12): 1681-90.
[PMID: 31587882]

[248] Tan DS, Leighl NB, Riely GJ, *et al.* Safety and efficacy of nazartinib (EGF816) in adults with EGFR-mutant non-small-cell lung carcinoma: a multicentre, open-label, phase 1 study. Lancet Respir Med 2020; 8(6): 561-72.
[PMID: 31954624]

[249] Wang S, Song Y, Liu D. EAI045: The fourth-generation EGFR inhibitor overcoming T790M and C797S resistance. Cancer Lett 2017; 385: 51-4.
[PMID: 27840244]

[250] Liu X, Zhang X, Yang L, *et al.* Preclinical evaluation of TQB3804, a potent EGFR C797S inhibitor. AACR 2019.

[251] Yang F, Huang X, Sun C, *et al.* Lapatinib in combination with capecitabine *versus* continued use of trastuzumab in breast cancer patients with trastuzumab-resistance: a retrospective study of a Chinese population. BMC Cancer 2020; 20(1): 255.
[PMID: 32223744]

[252] Martin M, Holmes FA, Ejlertsen B, *et al.* Neratinib after trastuzumab-based adjuvant therapy in HER2-positive breast cancer (ExteNET): 5-year analysis of a randomised, double-blind, placebo-controlled, phase 3 trial. Lancet Oncol 2017; 18(12): 1688-700.
[PMID: 29146401]

[253] Ma F, Li Q, Chen S, *et al.* Phase I Study and Biomarker Analysis of Pyrotinib, a Novel Irreversible Pan-ErbB Receptor Tyrosine Kinase Inhibitor, in Patients With Human Epidermal Growth Factor Receptor 2-Positive Metastatic Breast Cancer. J Clin Oncol 2017; 35(27): 3105-12.
[PMID: 28498781]

[254] Murthy RK, Loi S, Okines A, *et al.* Tucatinib, Trastuzumab, and Capecitabine for HER2-Positive Metastatic Breast Cancer. N Engl J Med 2020; 382(7): 597-609.

[PMID: 31825569]

[255] McCusker MG, Russo A, Scilla KA, Mehra R, Rolfo C. How I treat ALK-positive non-small cell lung cancer. ESMO Open 2019; 4 (Suppl. 2): e000524.
[PMID: 31423342]

[256] Camidge DR, Otterson GA, Clark JW, *et al.* Crizotinib in patients (pts) with MET-amplified non-small cell lung cancer (NSCLC): Updated safety and efficacy findings from a phase 1 trial. American Society of Clinical Oncology 2018.

[257] Jorge SE, Schulman S, Freed JA, *et al.* Responses to the multitargeted MET/ALK/ROS1 inhibitor crizotinib and co-occurring mutations in lung adenocarcinomas with MET amplification or MET exon 14 skipping mutation. Lung Cancer 2015; 90(3): 369-74.
[PMID: 26791794]

[258] Shaw AT, Kim D-W, Mehra R, *et al.* Ceritinib in ALK-rearranged non-small-cell lung cancer. N Engl J Med 2014; 370(13): 1189-97.
[PMID: 24670165]

[259] Tomasini P, Egea J, Souquet-Bressand M, Greillier L, Barlesi F. Alectinib in the treatment of ALK-positive metastatic non-small cell lung cancer: clinical trial evidence and experience with a focus on brain metastases. Ther Adv Respir Dis 2019; 13: 1753466619831906.
[PMID: 30786826]

[260] Camidge DR, Kim HR, Ahn MJ, *et al.* Brigatinib *Versus* Crizotinib in Advanced ALK Inhibitor-Naive ALK-Positive Non-Small Cell Lung Cancer: Second Interim Analysis of the Phase III ALTA-1L Trial. J Clin Oncol 2020; 38(31): 3592-603.
[PMID: 32780660]

[261] Yang Y, Zhou J, Zhou J, *et al.* Efficacy, safety, and biomarker analysis of ensartinib in crizotinib-resistant, ALK-positive non-small-cell lung cancer: a multicentre, phase 2 trial. Lancet Respir Med 2020; 8(1): 45-53.
[PMID: 31628085]

[262] Solomon BJ, Besse B, Bauer TM, *et al.* Lorlatinib in patients with ALK-positive non-small-cell lung cancer: results from a global phase 2 study. Lancet Oncol 2018; 19(12): 1654-67.
[PMID: 30413378]

[263] Rehman S, Dy GK. MET inhibition in non-small cell lung cancer. EMJ Respir 2018; 6(1): 100-11.

[264] Shaw AT, Ou SH, Bang YJ, *et al.* Crizotinib in ROS1-rearranged non-small-cell lung cancer. N Engl J Med 2014; 371(21): 1963-71.
[PMID: 25264305]

[265] Drilon A, Laetsch TW, Kummar S, *et al.* Efficacy of Larotrectinib in TRK Fusion-Positive Cancers in Adults and Children. N Engl J Med 2018; 378(8): 731-9.
[PMID: 29466156]

[266] Farago AF, Demetri GD. Larotrectinib, a selective tropomyosin receptor kinase inhibitor for adult and pediatric tropomyosin receptor kinase fusion cancers. Future Oncol 2020; 16(9): 417-25.
[PMID: 32129093]

[267] Drilon A. TRK inhibitors in TRK fusion-positive cancers. Ann Oncol. 2019; 30 Suppl 8: viii23-viii30.

[268] Cocco E, Scaltriti M, Drilon A. NTRK fusion-positive cancers and TRK inhibitor therapy. Nat Rev Clin Oncol 2018; 15(12): 731-47.
[PMID: 30333516]

[269] Drilon A, Nagasubramanian R, Blake JF, *et al.* A Next-Generation TRK Kinase Inhibitor Overcomes Acquired Resistance to Prior TRK Kinase Inhibition in Patients with TRK Fusion-Positive Solid Tumors. Cancer Discov 2017; 7(9): 963-72.
[PMID: 28578312]

[270] Drilon A, Ou SI, Cho BC, *et al.* Repotrectinib (TPX-0005) Is a Next-Generation ROS1/TRK/ALK Inhibitor That Potently Inhibits ROS1/TRK/ALK Solvent- Front Mutations. Cancer Discov 2018; 8(10): 1227-36.
[PMID: 30093503]

[271] Roskoski R Jr. ERK1/2 MAP kinases: structure, function, and regulation. Pharmacol Res 2012; 66(2): 105-43.
[PMID: 22569528]

[272] Grimaldi AM, Simeone E, Festino L, Vanella V, Strudel M, Ascierto PA. MEK Inhibitors in the Treatment of Metastatic Melanoma and Solid Tumors. Am J Clin Dermatol 2017; 18(6): 745-54.
[PMID: 28537004]

[273] Huang L, Jiang S, Shi Y. Tyrosine kinase inhibitors for solid tumors in the past 20 years (2001-2020). J Hematol Oncol 2020; 13(1): 143.
[PMID: 33109256]

[274] Loriot Y, Necchi A, Park SH, *et al.* Erdafitinib in Locally Advanced or Metastatic Urothelial Carcinoma. N Engl J Med 2019; 381(4): 338-48.
[PMID: 31340094]

[275] Abou-Alfa GK, Sahai V, Hollebecque A, *et al.* Pemigatinib for previously treated, locally advanced or metastatic cholangiocarcinoma: a multicentre, open-label, phase 2 study. Lancet Oncol 2020; 21(5): 671-84.
[PMID: 32203698]

[276] Sootome H, Fujita H, Ito K, *et al.* Futibatinib Is a Novel Irreversible FGFR 1-4 Inhibitor That Shows Selective Antitumor Activity against FGFR-Deregulated Tumors. Cancer Res 2020; 80(22): 4986-97.
[PMID: 32973082]

[277] Javle M, Kelley RK, Roychowdhury S, *et al.* AB051. P-19. A phase II study of infigratinib (BGJ398) in previously-treated advanced cholangiocarcinoma containing FGFR2 fusions. Hepatobiliary Surg Nutr 2019; AB051.

[278] Assenmacher M, Avraham HK, Avraham S, *et al.* Ligand Traps Encyclopedic Reference of Immunotoxicology. Berlin, Heidelberg: Springer Berlin Heidelberg 2005; p. 385.

[279] Wang T-F, Lockhart AC. Aflibercept in the treatment of metastatic colorectal cancer. Clin Med Insights Oncol 2012; 6: 19-30.
[PMID: 22253552]

[280] Takahashi K, Akatsu Y, Podyma-Inoue KA, *et al.* Targeting all transforming growth factor-β isoforms with an Fc chimeric receptor impairs tumor growth and angiogenesis of oral squamous cell cancer. J Biol Chem 2020; 295(36): 12559-72.
[PMID: 32631954]

[281] Chudzian J, Szlachcic A, Zakrzewska M, *et al.* Specific Antibody Fragment Ligand Traps Blocking FGF1 Activity. Int J Mol Sci 2018; 19(9): 2470.
[PMID: 30134556]

[282] Ravi R, Noonan KA, Pham V, *et al.* Bifunctional immune checkpoint-targeted antibody-ligand traps that simultaneously disable TGFβ enhance the efficacy of cancer immunotherapy. Nat Commun 2018; 9(1): 741.
[PMID: 29467463]

[283] Takakura K, Kawamura A, Torisu Y, Koido S, Yahagi N, Saruta M. The Clinical Potential of Oligonucleotide Therapeutics against Pancreatic Cancer. Int J Mol Sci 2019; 20(13): 3331.
[PMID: 31284594]

[284] Zamecnik PC, Stephenson ML. Inhibition of Rous sarcoma virus replication and cell transformation by a specific oligodeoxynucleotide. Proc Natl Acad Sci USA 1978; 75(1): 280-4.
[PMID: 75545]

[285] Harada T, Matsumoto S, Hirota S, *et al.* Chemically Modified Antisense Oligonucleotide Against ARL4C Inhibits Primary and Metastatic Liver Tumor Growth. Mol Cancer Ther 2019; 18(3): 602-12. [PMID: 30647122]

[286] Papachristodoulou A, Silginer M, Weller M, *et al.* Therapeutic Targeting of TGFβ Ligands in Glioblastoma Using Novel Antisense Oligonucleotides Reduces the Growth of Experimental Gliomas. Clin Cancer Res 2019; 25(23): 7189-201. [PMID: 31530630]

[287] Teixeira AF, Ten Dijke P, Zhu H-J. On-Target Anti-TGF-β Therapies Are Not Succeeding in Clinical Cancer Treatments: What Are Remaining Challenges? Front Cell Dev Biol 2020; 8(605): 605. [PMID: 32733895]

[288] Singh A, Trivedi P, Jain NK. Advances in siRNA delivery in cancer therapy. Artif Cells Nanomed Biotechnol 2018; 46(2): 274-83. [PMID: 28423924]

[289] Satpathy M, Mezencev R, Wang L, McDonald JF. Targeted *in vivo* delivery of EGFR siRNA inhibits ovarian cancer growth and enhances drug sensitivity. Sci Rep 2016; 6(1): 36518. [PMID: 27819259]

CHAPTER 6

Cell Signaling Pathways in Cancer

Hajir A. Al-Saihati[1,*], Mashael Al-Toub[2], Hanaa I. Sharaf[3], Manjari Singh[4], Mohd. Nazam Ansari[5] and **Abdulaziz Bin Saeedan[5]**

[1] *Department of Clinical Laboratory Sciences, College of Applied Medical Sciences, University of Hafr Al-Batin, Hafr Al-Batin, Saudi Arabia*

[2] *Department of Clinical Laboratory Sciences, College of Applied Medical Sciences, King Saud University, Riyadh, Saudi Arabia*

[3] *King Saud Medical City, Riyadh, Saudi Arabia*

[4] *Department of Pharmaceutical Sciences, College of Pharmacy, Assam University, Silchar (Assam), India*

[5] *College of Pharmacy, Prince Sattam Bin Abdulaziz University, Alkharj, Saudi Arabia*

Abstract: Cancer is characterized by atypical cell proliferation that has the possibility of dissemination to different body parts. Tumor formation is influenced by genetic mutations and environmental pollutants. The formation and progression of malignancies have been linked to a diversity of molecular paths. The JAK/STAT, NOTCH, PI3K/AKT pathway, mitogen-activated protein kinase (MAPK), transforming growth factor-beta (TGF-beta) (TGF-), NF-B, and Wnt signaling pathways will be highlighted in this chapter. Cancer development has been linked to various changes to the signaling pathways' components. As a result, various initiatives to target signaling pathways in order to build distinct treatment lines have been approved. In this chapter, we discuss the role of signal transduction in cancer-associated processes and how their targets influence the behavior of the tumor cells.

Keywords: Cancer, JAK/STAT, Map Kinase/Erk, NFκB, Notch, PI3K/AKT/mTOR, TGF-β, Wnt/β catenin.

INTRODUCTION

Malignance is a widespread disease described by genetic modifications in signaling pathways, for instance, cell division, death, and proliferation. Mutations in proto-oncogenes can alter cell formation and homeostasis by regulating signaling pathways such as NFB, TGF-β, PI3K/AKT/mTOR, MAP Kinase/ERK,

* **Corresponding author Hajir A Al-Saihati:** Department of Clinical Laboratory Sciences, College of Applied Medical Sciences, University of Hafr Al-Batin, Hafr Al-Batin, Saudi Arabia; E-mail: hajirsh@uhb.edu.sa

Faris Q.B. Alenzi (Ed.)

Notch, JAK/STAT, and Wnt/catenin. These pathways will give crucial information for the proper identification of cancer biomarkers in the future, which will aid in the treatment and prevention of cancer. During cancer formation, genetic and epigenetic changes cause cells to break free from homeostatic control, multiply, expand, and spread to other organs [1].

Liver, Lung, breast, skin, and pancreatic cancers arise in epithelial cells. Sarcomas in fibroblasts, myocytes, adipocytes, and osteoblasts are thought to originate in the mesenchymal tissues. Non-epithelial tumors, on the other hand, develop in nervous system cells such as glioma cells and hematopoietic tissues such as leukemia and lymphoma [2]. In solid tumors, such cellular changes drive the evolution of benign tumors into proliferative malignancies [1]. The tumor cell loses access to oxygen and other nutrients during tumor excursion, causing the development of angiogenesis, which restores cell's access to oxygen and nutrients [3]. Consequently, the tumor cells gain the potential to travel beyond their normal bounds to surrounding organs, enter circulation, and start metastasis, indicating that the tumor is malignant [4].

This design illustrates how complicated cancer-related events occur in a linear sequence in a varied manner in which cancers differ from one another and between tumour locations. This sequence also offers a useful foundation for various signaling pathways tangled during cancer onset and course [5]. The major reason for malignancy, as stated above, is epigenetics or genetic abnormalities in tumor cells. Tumor cells also have a variety of distinct characteristics. These factors include resistance to apoptosis and other kinds of cell death, metabolic changes, genetic instability, angiogenesis activation, and other factors with greater travelling potential, in addition to cell proliferation [6]. The majority of these features are caused by the dysregulation of various cellular signal transduction pathways [7, 8].

JAK/STAT Signaling Pathway

General Features of the JAK/STAT Pathway

JAK-STAT signaling pathways are based on traditional signaling models in which a ligand binds to the transmembrane receptor's extracellular side and initiates a cascade of phosphorylation events [9]. Phosphorylation of JAK kinases, the receptor cytoplasmic tail and STAT transcription factors are among these processes. STAT phosphorylation leads to nuclear localization, DNA binding, and gene regulation [10]. Combining a variety of ligands and receptors with four JAK proteins (JAK1, TYK2, JAK2 and JAK3), 7STAT members (STAT1, STAT2, STAT3, STAT4, STAT5a, STAT5b, and STAT6) are cytokine signaling suppressors. Proteins (SOCS), and multiple STAT-dependent operons allow for fine control of expression (Fig. **6.1**) [11].

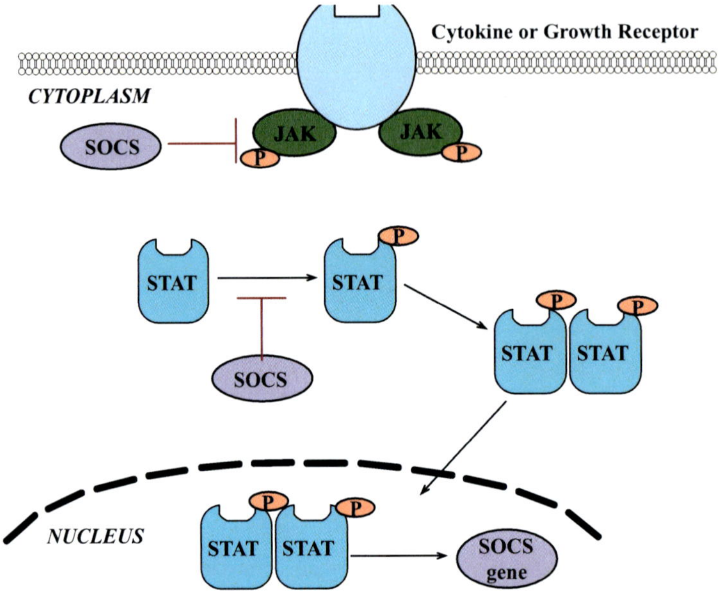

Fig. (6.1). JAK/STAT signaling pathway. The JAK/STAT signaling pathway is a signaling system that involves the proteins JAK and STAT proteins. JAK is phosphorylated by cytokines and growth receptors, and it recruits signal transducers and transcription activators (STAT). Dimer phosphorylated STAT enters the nucleus and stimulates gene transcription, where it attaches to DNA, regulates immunity, and promotes cell growth and survival.

JH1 encompasses the kinase domain, JH2 encompasses the inhibitory pseudo kinase domain, JH3-5 contains the SH2 receptor interaction domains, and JH6-7 contains the FERM domain [12]. In the most basic paradigm, ligand-receptor interaction modifies the shape of receptor-JAK complexes, permitting the phosphorylation of certain tyrosine residues in JH1. This causes additional conformational shifts in JAK proteins, resulting in receptor phosphorylation and the creation of STAT protein binding sites [13].

The JAK/STAT signaling system can be triggered by external stimuli, for instance, cytokines. JAK and STAT are intracellular proteins that work with the transmembrane receptor to deliver signals to the nucleus, allowing DNA transcription and gene expression to occur [14]. STAT acts as a JAK substrate, phosphorylating and transporting to the nucleus to stimulate gene transcription.

The JAK/STAT signaling system is involved in stem cell maintenance, hematopoiesis, and the immune response [15].

The Role of the JAK/STAT Pathway in Cancer

JAK-STAT signaling is one of the critical components of malignancy development, either as a tumor-specific driver of cancer development and spread or a regulator of immune surveillance. This distinct concern emphasizes recent study results that link JAK-STAT signaling to a variety of cancer forms, as well as providing up-to-date assessments from experts in the field. A multitude of causes, including increased cytokine production, can trigger constitutive activation of JAK-STAT signaling (Fig. **6.1**). As a result of the Signal transducer and activator of transcription (STAT)3 activation mediated by Janus kinase (JAK) has increased, oncogenic transcription factor, an activator of transcription and signal transducer (STAT)3, is produced [16]. Otherwise, IL-6 "trans-signaling," facilitated *via* IL-6 binding to an IL-6R, can activate JAK-STAT signaling in any cell [17].

The disinterring and metalloproteinase 17 (ADAM17) is now revealed to be accountable for the protease-driven shedding of IL-6R [17], exposing a hitherto underappreciated possibility to therapeutically modify IL-6 mediated signaling. The importance of IL-6/IL-6R/GP130 in hepatocellular carcinoma and lung cancer is discussed in depth in this issue [16, 17]. In many tumors, STAT3 functions throughout. Multiple novel research examining the role of STAT3 signaling in solid tumors (medulloblastoma, cervical, bladder, breast, and colon cancers) in addition to blood cancers are included in this issue (including leukemia). Activated STAT3 has been linked to urothelial bladder malignancy cell viability and invasion [18]. PAK1 (p21-activated kinase) was discovered to show a new role in breast cancer stem cells, interacting with JAK2 and STAT3, and regulating STAT3 signaling [19]. Furthermore, they discovered that IL-6 boosts gene regulation by SHH in a STAT3-dependent manner way [20]. STAT3 activation has been recognized as a possible biomarker for people with colorectal cancer; it was found that peripheral blood T cells get STAT3 hyperactivation in response to IL-10 [21]. Furthermore, active STAT3 was discovered in most individuals with chronic lymphocytic leukemia, and when IL-6 or BM-MSCs were added to the mix, the amount of activation increased [22]. JAK2 inhibition reduced STAT3 activation in cervical cancer cells, which was linked to decreased cell expansion and augmented cisplatin insensitivity [23], showing that blocking this signaling cascade has therapeutic potential.

Notch Signaling Pathway

General Features of the Notch Signaling Pathway

Cell propagation, differentiation and homeostasis are all aided by the Notch signaling pathway [24]. T-cell leukemia, prostate malignancy, breast cancer, colorectal malignancy, and nervous system malignancies all have deregulated Notch signaling [25]. Notch signaling has been associated with cancers of the oesophagus, breast and cancer stem cells in several studies [26]. Once a ligand interacts with the Notch receptor, Notch signaling is initiated (Fig. **6.2**). NOTCH1, NOTCH2, NOTCH3, and NOTCH4 are transcription factors. the four types of Notch receptors found in mammals [27]. Five ligands are also present: DLL1, DLL3, DLL4, Jagged 1 (JAG1), and Jagged 2 (JAG2) are examples of delta-similar ligands (JAG2) [28].

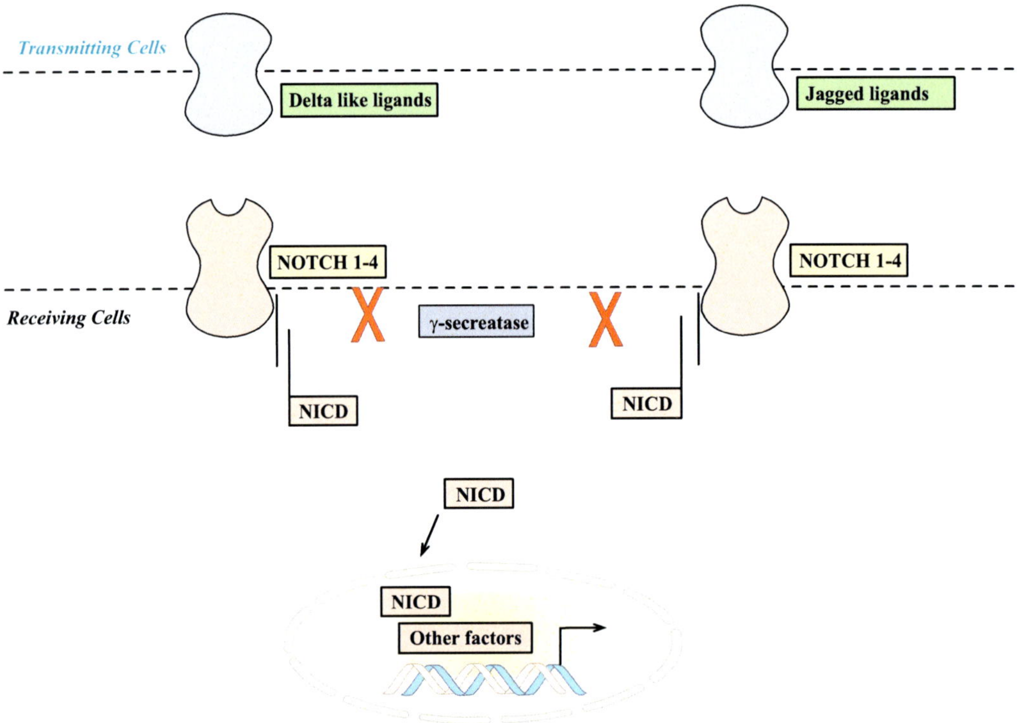

Fig. (6.2). Notch signaling pathway. This diagram depicts the Notch signaling pathway. Jagged ligands and delta-like ligands interact with Notch receptors in receiving and transmitting cells. The enzyme secretase is in charge of this activation. NICD is released by secretase when intracellular activation occurs, and subsequently, NICD enters the nucleus to control the transcription process. They translocate to the nucleus.

On the surface of the brain, there are Notch receptors cell membrane's surface can be cleaved by members of the metalloproteinase and disinterring family of proteases (ADAM10 and ADAM17), as well as a presenilin-1 -dependent gamma-secretase-like protease mediates [29]. The Notch Intracellular Domain is a protein that helps cells communicate with one another. NICD is then liberated and translocated to the nucleus as a result [30]. This pathway is a highly conserved intracellular process that is necessary for normal embryonic development in all metazoan organisms. Several studies in primary human breast cancer have discovered that tumors with great amounts of Jag1 or Notch mRNA had a bad prognosis [31].

The Role of the Notch Signaling Pathway in Cancer

The Notch signaling pathway controls a diversity of cellular activities, including apoptosis, expansion, and differentiation (Fig. **6.2**). The consequences of disrupting or changing these functions could be disastrous. Surprisingly, the function of the Notch signaling system is extremely reliant on the cellular environment [32]. Notch is a gene that can perform as equally as an oncogene and a suppressor [32]. We have focused on the most recent study on the oncogene and anti-oncogene roles of the Notch signaling pathway in different malignancies. Human T-cell lymphoblastic leukemia/lymphomas (T-ALL) was the first disease linked to Notch malfunction in 1991. Hence it deserves special consideration when considering Notch-related malignancy [33]. T-ALL, a malignant tumor, affects both children and teenagers. In human T-ALL, the intercellular domain of the Notch 1 receptor has been discovered to be the most commonly changed region [34, 35]. According to a recent study, mutations in the Notch 1 receptor were discovered in 50% of all T-ALL cases [36]. Based on these data, we believe that the Notch 1 receptor has a strong connection to T-ALL genesis, but additional research is needed to identify exactly how the Notch 1 receptor contributes to T-ALL genesis.

The Notch 1 receptor has been verified to be significant in T-cell generation and cell fate [37, 38], so its dysfunction negatively impacts T-cell activity. Another notion is that T-ALL is caused by a frameshift or nonsense mutation in the PEST domain, which has been discovered in 20–25% of all T-ALL cases [32].

The PEST domain regulates intercellular Notch 1 (ICN1) stability, and this mutation increases ICN1 concentration [36]. A mutation in the juxtamembrane expansion makes the Notch 1 receptor more active [39]. T-ALL patients with Notch 1 receptor mutations have a better prognosis, according to recent research [40 - 42]. These findings imply that the Notch signaling system may be a potential therapeutic target for T-ALL and that the mechanism of action in T-ALL should be further studied.

Furthermore, in T-ALL, the Notch signaling pathway is dysregulated in a variety of hematological malignancies. Chronic lymphocytic leukemia (CLL) is an incurable blood malignancy with abnormal B cells. The Notch signaling pathway has been linked to CLL in recent studies, with the Notch 1 receptor mutant being expressed in 10–20% of the patients with CLL [32, 43]. According to genetic studies, the bulk of Notch 1 is found in the PEST domain receptor mutations [44, 45]. In contrast to T-ALL, the Notch 1 receptor mutations are associated with a poor prognosis in CLL patients [46, 47], and a higher frequency of mutation is also reported in chemo-resistant CLL patients [43].

Other Notch family members, besides the Notch 1 receptor, play a significant role in hematological cancer. Since the Notch 2 receptor is crucial in B cell development, mutations in this gene are likely to cause aberrant B cell production and additional pathologic alterations [48]. A growing body of evidence suggests that a Notch 2 receptor mutation can be found in B-cell malignancies [49, 50].

MAP Kinase, ERK, Ras, and Raf Pathways

General Features of the Map Pathway

Pathways involving MAPK, which have evolved over time, govern gene expression, proliferation, growth, differentiation, apoptosis and migration [51]. MAPK is a signaling pathway in eukaryotes, which ranges from yeast to humans, that connects extracellular signals to the machinery that monitors key cellular processes, such as cell propagation, differentiation, and death. MAPK is made up of three active protein kinases, which are crucial components of signal transduction cascades that regulate its activity [52 - 54].

Subsequently, in sequential stimulation, MAPKKK is activated by interactions with a small GTPase and/or activation by protein kinases downstream of cell surface receptors, causing the stimulation of a specific MAPK [55]. The MAPKKK phosphorylates the MAPKK, then stimulate the MAPK through dual phosphorylation of the preserved tripeptide TxY motif in the initiation region. The MAPK phosphorylates different substrates in the cytosol once activated, triggering the necessary biological response [56]. The reason for this is the changes in protein function and gene expression profiles (Fig. **6.3**).

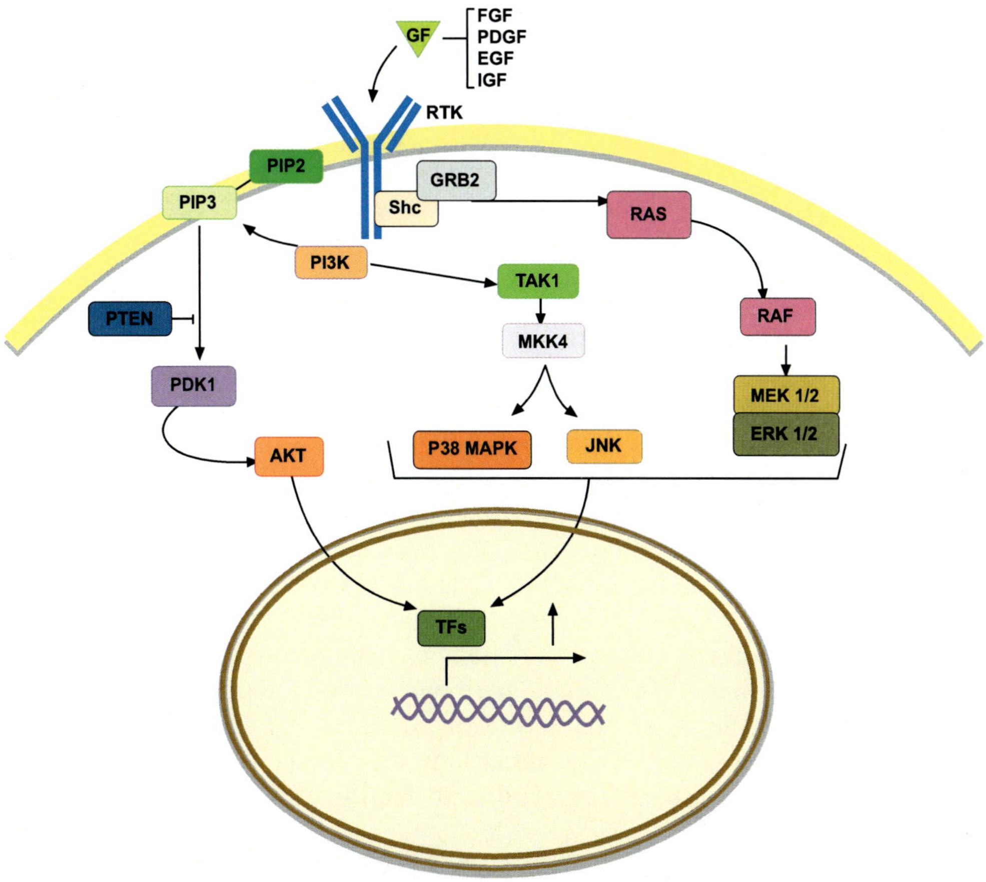

Fig. (6.3). Receptor tyrosine kinase pathways (RTKs) in cancer. Many growth factors can activate RTKs. After which, RAS, PI3K, P38 MAPK, and JNK are some of the signaling pathways that can be activated. These signaling pathways cause transcription factors to bind to promoters, causing the genes involved in cancer progression to be induced or repressed. In cancer cells, PTEN is a phosphatase that suppresses the PI3K and Wnt signaling pathways [60].

Three families of MAPKs have been identified. Jun amino-terminal kinases (JNKs) and extracellular signal-regulated kinases (ERKs) are two types of JNKs, and p38/ stress-activated protein kinases are extracellular-signal-regulated kinases. The initiation fragment of ERK family members has a TEY motif, and they may be distributed into two groups: classic ERKs (ERK1 and ERK2), which largely comprise a kinase domain, and bigger ERKs (such as ERK5), which feature an extended stretch carboxy-terminal in their kinase domain (Fig. **6.3**) [57].

The classic ERK1/2 module reacts predominantly to mitogens and growth stimuli and drives cell growth and differentiation. Upstream regulators of this module comprise G-protein-coupled receptors, receptor tyrosine kinases (RTKs), and integrins. There are cell surface receptors in addition to the small GTPasesRas and Rap. MEK1 and MEK2 are ERK1/2 MAPKKs modules, whereas MAPKKKs include Raf family members, Mos, and Tpl2 [58, 59].

General Features of the ERK Pathway

The ERK pathway is disrupted in roughly 30% of all human malignancies. Although ERK signaling has long been linked to cell proliferation, it is now obvious that its dysregulation is associated with a variety of other tumor phenotypic characteristics. ERK (ERK1 and ERK2) is triggered ERK-MAPK, a module in the ERK MAPK pathway when MEK (MEK1 and MEK2) is phosphorylated, and Raf phosphorylates MEK (MEK1 and MEK2) (Raf-1, B-Raf, and A-Raf) (Fig. **6.3**). A multitude of extrinsic triggers can activate ERK signaling. In cancer signaling, the process by which mitogens and growth factors promote ERK signaling is important [61]. The Ras-GTPase loads GTP after the activation of RTKs by ligands, allowing Raf kinases to be recruited to the plasma membrane for activation. The most prevalent cancer-related disorders that lead to constitutive activation of ERK signaling are overexpression of RTKs, stimulating mutations in RTKs, persistent paracrine or autocrine production of activating ligands, Ras mutations, and B-Raf mutations. Cancer cells may also alter the extracellular matrix receptors they express to facilitate the transmission of pro-growth signals.

Consequently, this system being dysregulated at multiple levels in cancer underscores its importance (Table **6.1**). The Ras–Raf axis has a high frequency of activating mutations, indicating that it is the pathway's regulatory hotspot [62]. According to mathematical modeling, Raf and Ras stimulation are identical sensitive regulatory sites, which affects the overall stimulation profile [63]. Furthermore, the rare coexistence of B-Raf and Rasmutations in identical tumor cells implies that Raf is a key Ras-effector pathway in human cancer. Nevertheless, there is evidence that co-expression of mutant B-Raf with mutant N-Ras induces senescence, suggesting synthetic fatal mutations in B-Raf and Ras [64].

Tumorigenesis necessitates the disruption of at least six cellular procedures as well as cancer cells while acquiring the following capabilities: proliferation signal independence, anti-growth signal insensitivity, apoptosis evasion, unrestricted replicative potential, the capability to infiltrate and metastasize, and the capacity to appeal and stand with the angiogenesis for nut. As a result, alterations in

MAPK signaling influence the majority, if not all, of these systems and show a significant role in cancer creation and progression [65].

Table 6.1. Cancer-associated lesions in the ERK-signaling pathway in cancer.

EGFR Overexpression	*RAS* Mutation	*ERBB2* Overexpression	*BRAF* Mutation
Most carcinomas (>50%)	• Pancreas (90%) • Lung adenocarcinoma (35%) (non-small cell) • Thyroid; follicular (55%) • Thyroid; undifferentiated papillary (60%) • Seminoma (45%) • Melanoma (15%) • Bladder (10%) • Liver (30%) • Kidney (10%) • Myelodysplastic syndrome (40%) • Acutemyelogenous leukemia (30%)	Breast (30%)	• Melanoma (66%) • Colorectal (12%)

General Features of Ras Signaling Pathway

Ras GTPase performs as molecular switches that regulate the activation of numerous signaling pathways. Stimulating mutations in the N-Ras and K-Rasgenes have been discovered in a variety of cancers. These mutations, invariably found at codons 12, 13, or 61, prevent Ras from efficiently hydrolyzing GTP. Consequently, Ras remains stimulated and GTP-bound. In this structure, Ras oncogenes can interact and stimulate their effectors, including Raf [66, 67]. While isoform-specific Ras signaling is assumed to happen largely at the plasma membrane, accumulated proof shows that it can also occur at other cellular locations and within distinct sections of the plasma membrane.

Endogenous Ras oncogenes, which show a vital character in regulating downstream signaling cascades and are implicated in cancer (Fig. **6.3**), require greater investigation into their compartmentalization and trafficking. Drugs can be developed to selectively target Ras proteins' carcinogenic activity by modifying their subcellular positions, see [68 - 74]. Ras proteins' involvement in diverse cancers suggests that they could be effective therapeutic targets. Ras must be closer to the plasma membrane than the plasma membrane to function properly as a signal transducer. Isoprenylation (geranylation or farnesylation) is performed near the Ras C-terminus. Isoprenylation inhibitors are then used to target Ras. Nonetheless, these inhibitors have performed poorly in clinical trials [75, 76].

The reason for this is not immediately apparent. It could partly be explained by certain findings implying that farnesylation inhibitors' anti-tumor activities owe to special effects on Rho rather than Ras suppression. Furthermore, because farnesylation inhibitors cannot be differentiated between normal and mutant Ras and normal Ras can stabilize mutant Ras's transforming functions, they may disable the simultaneous use of both the accelerator and the brakes. As a result, current attempts have concentrated on the problematic signaling downstream of Ras [77].

Raf Regulation

The key effectors of Ras are Raf kinases, which are situated at the top of the ERK pathway's kinase module. While the architectures of the three Raf proteins are identical, the methods with which they are activated are rather different [78, 79]. Although the three mammalian Raf isoforms are structurally identical, their tissue distributions, modes of regulation, and ability to activate MEK differ significantly [80]. *In vivo* genetic ablation of the several Raf isoforms in mice demonstrates that they are mostly utilized for non-redundant tasks [81].

Raf kinases are triggered by a complex set of events involving phosphorylation as well as protein–protein and protein–lipid interactions after binding to Ras. By neutralizing auto-inhibition and increasing kinase domain activation, these actions improve Raf's catalytic activity (Fig. **6.3**) [82 - 84].

B-Raf mutations have also caught researchers' interest because they are found in 66% of malignant melanomas [85], as well as at a lower level in many other human malignancies, such as colon cancer, papillary thyroid cancer, and serous ovarian cancer. Ras proteins are required for the growth of a variety of cancers; therefore, they could be useful therapeutic targets [86].

PI3/AKT Signaling Pathway

General Features of the PI3/AKT Signaling Pathway

PI3K/AKT is a collection of intracellular pathways that control the cell cycle, propagation, growth, motility, and survival and are targets of rapamycin (mTOR) (Fig. **6.4**). The character of this signaling pathway has been investigated since 1980, and studies have proven that human cancer implicates downstream molecular pathways, attracting researchers to target this signaling pathway for anticancer therapy. The PI3K/AKT/mTOR signaling pathways have also been found to be the most commonly mutated genes in cancer [87, 88].

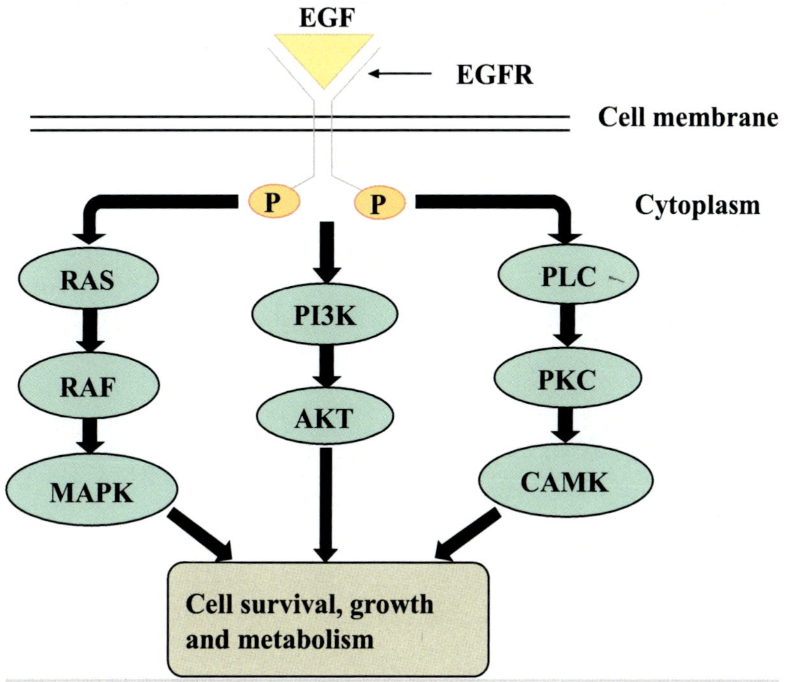

Fig. (6.4). PI3K/AKT pathway. The PI3K/AKT pathway shows how extracellular EGF and EGFR activate PI3K and AKT under functioning conditions, resulting in cell survival, proliferation, and metabolism.

PI3/AKT is a lipid kinase stimulated in the plasma membrane by phosphatidylinositol's inositol ring's 3-hydroxyl group is phosphorylated. The PI3/AKT signaling pathway is made up of two parts: phosphatidylinositol3-serine/threonine protein kinase B (PI3K) and its downstream molecule (AKT). The first part, phosphatidylinositol-3-kinases (PI3), is divided into three subunits based on their different class I, class II, and class III structures and substrate specificities The most significant of themis class I, which has a significant impact on malignancies and possesses a mechanism that allows cell surface receptors to directly stimulate it. The second half, AKT, is one of PI3 primary K's downstream effectors, and it was first discovered as a vital constituent of insulin receptor intracellular signaling [89]. Furthermore, AKT performs a key function in the PI3K pathway as one of the most active downstream effectors in the oncogenic landscape [90].

The Role of the PI3/AKT Signaling Pathway in Cancer

The platelet-derived growth factor receptor and the epidermal growth factor receptor (EGFR) are two types of growth factor receptors that determine the propagation of cancer. Insulin-like growth factor receptor, which promotes growth and survival, as well as insulin receptor, which controls metabolic homeostasis and has ectopic expression, are downstream effects of the PI3/AKT signaling pathway (Fig. **6.4**). In normal functioning conditions, extracellular signals activate PI3/AKT.

Furthermore, PI3/AKT is involved in metabolic programs that yield the energy and macromolecular synthesis essential for mitotic cell division and growth. PI3K signaling is involved in malignancy, neurological disorders, diabetes, cardiovascular disease, immunological disorders and localized tissue overgrowth [91].

Association Between PI3/AKT and Different Types of Cancer

The PI3/AKT signaling pathway shows a vital role in oncogenesis, and this has been widely investigated in recent years. It has been discovered that changed expressions or mutations of numerouseffectors of this pathway, such as PTEN, have been linked to a diversity of human malignancies, counting endometrium, skin, and brain cancers. Prostate cancer and breast cancer are two types of cancer [92 - 94].

PTEN, as well as mutations in the phosphoinositide-3-kinase, catalytic, alpha polypeptide (PIK3CA) gene, inactivation of PTEN, and missense alleles of PIK3CA, have all been linked to constitutive activation of AKT and a variety of cancer types, making PIK3CA the most studied gene (Fig. **6.5**) [95].

Activation of AKT has been associated with a variety of advanced diseases and/or poor prognosis in a diversity of malignancies. In cancer cells, mutations in some types of PI3 subunit genes, such as (PIK3R1 or PIK3R2), produce an increase in PI3K activity [96, 97].

Researchers have discovered a clear link between certain types of cancer and somatic changes that influence the PI3/AKT signaling pathway *via* either oncogene activation or tumor suppressor inactivation, disrupting a signaling pathway that can lead to cellular transformation by increasing matrix metalloproteinase secretion. Driving the AKT1 has been implicated in the epithelial-to-mesenchymal transition (EMT) related to tumor invasion and metastasis. Overexpression of another subtype of the AKT signaling pathway (AKTII) in breast and ovarian cancers has been associated with higher invasion, though the AKTIII subtype in breast and ovarian cancers has also been associated with higher invasion [98].

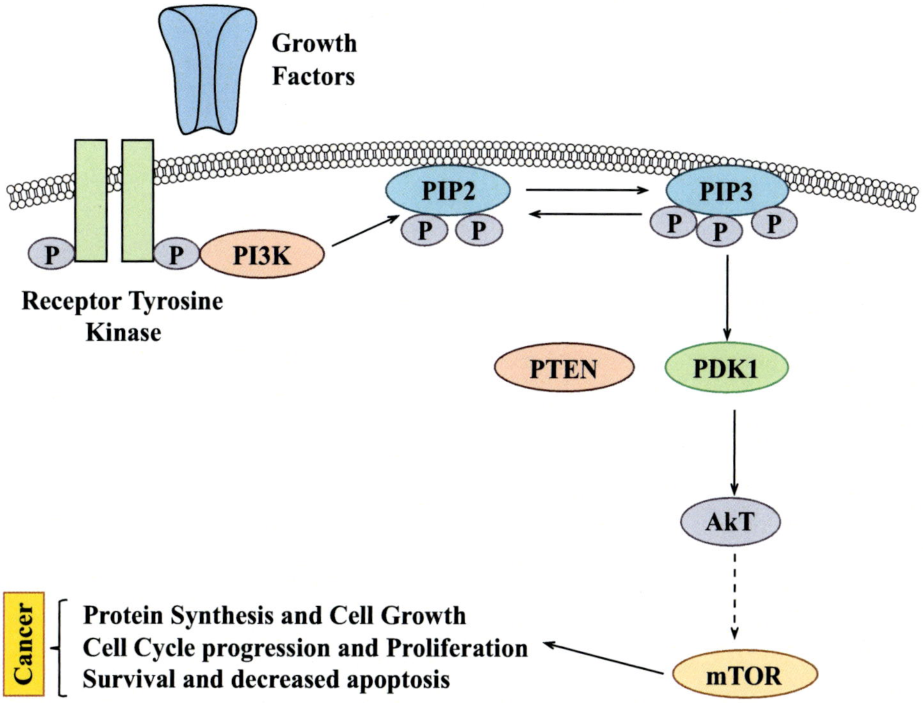

Fig. (6.5). PI3K/AKT/mTOR signaling pathway. Phosphorylated tyrosine receptors and growth factor kinases activate the PI3K/AKT/mTOR signaling pathway. These receptors activate PI3K, which then converts to PIP2 and PIP3. PTEN prevents the conversion of PIP2 to PIP3. PDK1 is then activated, which, in turn, stimulates AKT and mTOR. Protein synthesis and cell proliferation and cycle advancement, cell survival and cell growth, and reduced apoptosis are all regulated by mTOR in cancer cells.

Treatment for the PI3K/AKT Signaling Pathway

As hyperactivity of PI3/AKT signaling is highly connected with human malignant tumor advancement, increased tumor microvascular concentration, and greater chemotaxis, PI3/AKT signaling is considered vital for cancer treatment. As a result, many drugs targeting both PI3/AKT and mTOR have been developed to improve cancer treatment, and more than 50 PI3/AKT/mTOR drugs are currently in development [99]. For example, LY294002, a PI3K inhibitor, targets Pan-class I PI3K and is used to treat advanced solid tumors that lead to the arrest of the cell cycle and cell proliferation blockage [100]. Perifosine reduces the phosphorylation of AKT and improves the radiosensitivity of cancer cells [101].

The rational design of the signaling pathway in PI3K/AKT/mTOR molecular targets is also an important option for the treatment of numerous kinds of malignancies, and it is crucial to identify the implicated biomarkers that can help patients find the right treatment, as well as figure out which cancers and genetic profiles may benefit from PI3K/AKT/mTOR inhibitors (Fig. **6.5**). Furthermore, the major clinical utility of the combination of both PI3K and mTOR has been demonstrated by their influence on cell promotion of growth and apoptosis, as well as the strong effect of the duel PI3K/mTOR inhibitor (PI-103) on human ovarian cells *in vivo* [102].

Nuclear Factor Kappa B (NFκB) Signaling Pathway

General Features of the NFκB Signaling Pathway

NFκB is a group of inducible transcription factors that control gene expression and many inflammation-related genes [103]. The NFB family comprises five members: NFB1 (p50), NFB2 (p52), RelB, RelA (p65), and c-Rel. All of them facilitate the transcription of target genes *via* the union of specific DNA sites [104]. Two types of signaling pathways exist: canonical and non-canonical (Fig. **6.6**) [105]. Despite their differing communication mechanisms, both pathways are critical in the ruling of immunological and inflammatory responses [106, 107].

Various stimuli, including the TNF receptor (TNFR) superfamily, pattern recognition receptors (PRRs), cytokine receptors, and the canonical TCR, are activated by B cell receptors and TCR pathways [103]. The inducible degradation of IB, which is induced by its site-specific phosphorylation through a multi-subunit IB kinase (IKK) complex, is the mechanism behind canonical pathways [108]. IKK comprises two catalytic IKK and IKK subunits, as well as an NFB vital modulator or IKK as a monitoring subunit [109]. IKK may be triggered by a variety of circumstances, including growth factors and cytokines, stress agents, and microbial components [110]. After activation, IKK phosphorylates IB at two N terminal serines, causing ubiquitin-dependent IB breakdown in the proteasome and quick and temporary nuclear translocation of canonical NFB components, such as p50/RelA and p50/c-Rel, which are two different types of p50/Reldimers (Fig. **6.6**) [111 - 113].

Non-canonical pathways, on the other hand, respond to a limited set of stimuli, including ligands from TNFR superfamily members, such as LTR, BAFFR, CD40, and RANK [114]. Furthermore, rather than IB breakdown, the treatment of non-canonical activation is required in the NFB2 precursor protein, p100 [115]. A major signaling molecule in this pathway is NFB involving kinase (NIK), which stimulates and functionally collaborates with IKK to initiate p100 phosphorylation processing [116]. The creation of mature NFB2 p52 originates from the degradation of p100's C terminal IB-like structure, which is tracked by the non-canonical NFB complex p52/RelB's translocation to the nucleus (Fig. **6.6**) [103].

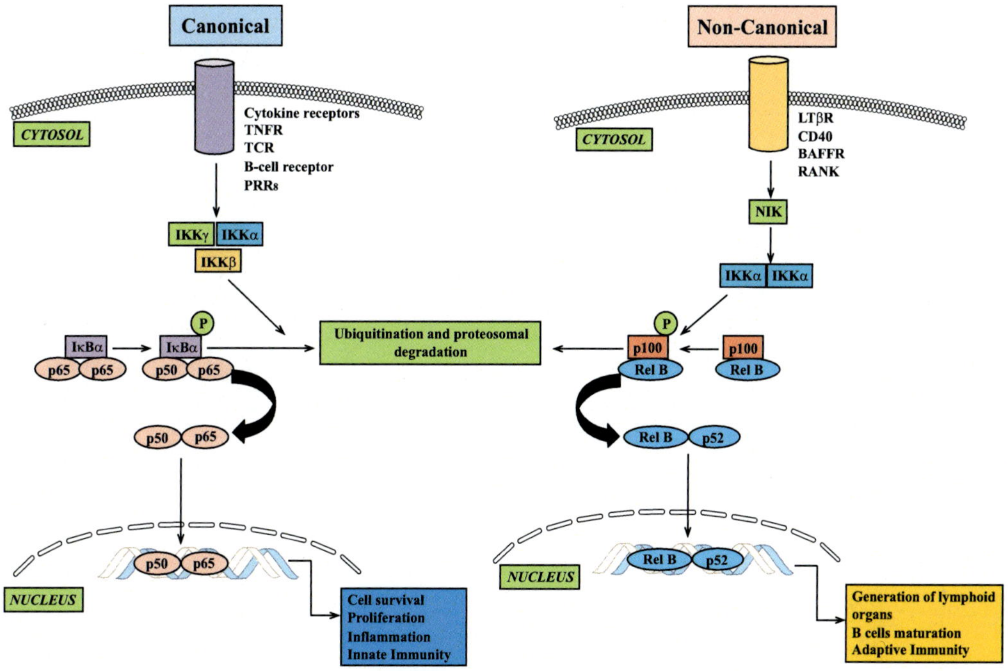

Fig. (6.6). NFκB signaling pathway. There are canonical and non-canonical routes in the NfκB signaling pathway. External stimuli, such as cytokine receptors, TNFR, TCR, B cell receptors, and PRRs, trigger the canonical pathway. When the cascade is activated, IB is phosphorylated, culminating in its ubiquitination and proteasomal destruction. This causes p50 and p65 to translocate into the nucleus, which governs cell survival, proliferation, inflammation, and other activities, such as innate immunity. The non-canonical pathway, on the other hand, is triggered by LTR, CD40, BAFFR, and RANK. When this route is activated, IKK is phosphorylated, and RelB and p52 are released. This complex travels to the nucleus and controls processes such as adaptive immunity, lymphoid organ growth, and B cell maturation.

NFB is activated in malignancies because of the maturation of the genes [117]. In the literature, it has been observed that some tumor cells release substances that activate NFB [118]. By inhibiting NFB, tumor cells may cease proliferating, perish, or become more sensitive to anticancer treatments [119]. NFB is also a programmed cell death inhibitor, and it also plays a role in the expansion of malignancies of epithelial organs, such as breast cancer [120, 121].

The Role of the NFκB Signaling Pathway in Cancer

NFκB has a complicated effect on malignancies, with mutually negative and positive effects on cancer origination and development. The activation of the NF-B signaling pathway occurs as a result of host defense for pathogen clearance, which leads and contributes to cancer growth as well as progression in certain malignancies, such as the hepatitis B virus. Furthermore, activation of NF-B stimulates the expression of cytokines, such as IL-1, TNF, and IL-6, which support the proliferation of tumor stroma cells and malignant cells and increase mutation rates primarily in a ROS- despite NF-B promoting the production of chemokines in an RNI-dependent and RNI-independent way, which operate more immune cells, such as DCs as well as macrophages [122].

By attaching to a definite DNA, the B enhancer subunit, like different homo- or hetero-dimers, mediates the transcription of target genes. IB is the IB family's most significant member. Although the NF-B1 and NF-B2 precursor proteins, p100 and p105, work as IB-like proteins for their C-terminal portion and contain NF-B inhibitory capabilities, they are not IB-like proteins [123 - 125]. The decreased immunity, inflammation and regulation of cell differentiation, propagation and apoptosis are all linked to NF-B signaling. The NF-B pathway is important in alternating hematopoietic and solid malignancies, as it promotes tumor cell propagation in addition to cell persistence. A recent study suggests that NF-B suppresses tumor growth in certain malignancies by activating the Fas ligand through transcriptional activation [126].

The active NF-B signaling system protects cells against apoptosis by regulating the genes that govern and progress the cell cycle. NF-B is stimulated in tumor cells due to mutations in the genes that code for the NF-B transcription factors or in the genes that control NF-B activity. Furthermore, certain cancer cells experience increases in the number of molecules that activate the NF-B signaling pathway [127].

A connection between the NFκB signaling pathway and inflammation in malignancies has been discovered. NF-kB activation in cancer might be triggered by pro-inflammatory stimuli in the malignancy microenvironment or mutational stimulation of upstream components in the IKK and NF-kB signaling pathways during the early days of RelA/p65 cloning and sequencing [128, 129].

Some IKK subunits (such as IKKa) can show NFκB autonomous characters in malignancies, for example, multiple myeloma [130, 131]. NFκB activation has been associated with further lymphoid cancers due to DNA or RNA tumor virus infections. Epstein-Barr virus, for example, promotes NFκB by producing latent membrane protein 1, a protein linked to lymphomas [132, 133]. NFκB protein has been established to mutate in a diversity of malignancies, involving several non-B-cell Hodgkin's lymphomas having v-Rel, the avian reticuloendothelios is virus's transforming gene, as well as certain NF-B mutant protein amplified and c-Rel rearrangements and NF-B2/p100, which is frequently activated through chromosomal alteration. On the other hand, antagonistic mutations in the EGFR, Ras, PI3K, and p53 signaling pathways have been discovered to be linked to NF-B stimulation in tumor cells, particularly in pancreatic, colorectal, and lung malignancies [134 - 136].

The Role of the NFκB Signaling Pathway in Cancer Therapy

The effect of the NFκB signaling pathway on malignancies and the potential of NFκB inhibitors as therapies have been widely researched in the latest years. Certain medicinal drugs have an indirect inhibitory effect by aggregating the expression of the malignant tumor suppressor p53, which stimulates apoptosis. Downregulation of genes occurs when NF-kB is inhibited, which inhibits cancer cell angiogenesis and metastasis. Furthermore, inhibiting the NF-kB signaling pathway may make malignant cells more susceptible to TNF-induced apoptosis [137].

Blocking NFκB on its own is not always enough to get cancer to go away. Both NFκB inhibitors and common treatments, such as radiotherapy and chemotherapy, may be more useful; nevertheless, it was discovered that using NF-kB inhibitors for a long time might result in immunodeficiency. Therefore, cancer therapy should be utilized for a limited length of time. There are no additional signaling pathways besides the NFκB pathway. The effectiveness, specificity, and adverse effects of NFκB inhibitors are still a big issue to be resolved. Anti-inflammatory medications like inhibition of NFκB activation, have also been seen with sodium salicylate, aspirin, and dexamethasone [138].

Wnt/β-Catenin Signaling Pathway

General Features of the Wnt/β-Catenin Signaling Pathway

Wnt/β-catenin signaling is crucial for growing processes such as cell fate determination and patterning. Porcupine secretes palmitoylated Wnt, which binds to both low-density lipoprotein receptor-related protein 5 and low-density lipoprotein receptor-related protein 6, two low-density lipoprotein receptor-related frizzled proteins [139]. Axin and disheveled proteins are attracted to the cell membrane when Wnt receptors interact, and the GSK-3 protein is inhibited [140].

GSK-3 is a phosphorylation-dependent negative regulator. Wnt/β-catenin is a signaling pathway that leads to proteasomal degradation. When GSK-3 is inhibited, catenin gathers in the cytoplasm, migrates to the nucleus, and performs the role of a transcriptional co-activator, with the T-cell factor and cAMP response element binding protein being transcription factors and lymphoid enhancing factors (TCF/LEF) (Fig. **6.7**) [141, 142].

Furthermore, the Wnt/β-catenin signaling pathway interrelates with other signaling pathways, such as EGFR, Hippo/YAP, NFB, Notch, and PI3K/AKT, all of which donate to the molecular mechanism of cell formation [143]. EGFR forms a compound with catenin and promotes cancer cell infiltration and progression [144]. Furthermore, in glioblastoma cells, stimulation of the Wnt and PI3K/AKT/GSK-3 pathways interacts with the catenin pathway, providing a molecular foundation for treatment resistance to multiple medications [145]. Consequently, the crosstalk Wnt/β-catenin and the PI3K/AKT signaling pathways have been proven to enhance carcinogenesis and cancer therapy resistance (Fig. **6.7**) [146].

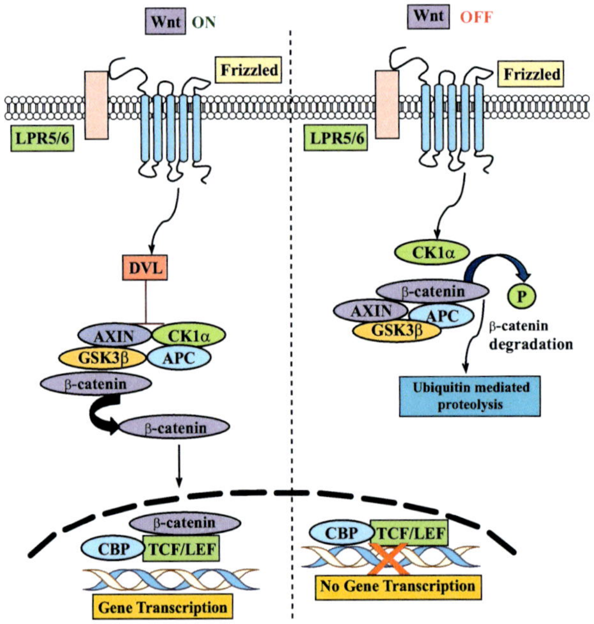

Fig. (6.7). Wnt/β-catenin signaling pathway. WNT ON and WNT OFF are the two states of this route. When WNT is turned on, ligands bind to the Wnt receptor, which is made up of lipoprotein receptorrelated protein 5/6 and frizzled proteins. GSK is decreased after the cytoplasmic protein DVL is activated. The antagonizing -catenin then translocates to the nucleus, where it interacts with TCF/LEF transcription factors to cause gene transcription. AXIN, CK1, and GSK3 create a ternary complex that phosphorylates -catenin. After that, the β-catenin undergoes ubiquitin proteasomal degradation, and no gene transcription occurs.

The Role of the Wnt/β-Catenin Pathway in Cancer

Various cancer signaling pathways are described and summarized in this chapter. These signaling pathways could be used as possible cancer treatment and preventive targets in the future. To date, many pharmacological elements have been produced to specifically target each of these signaling pathways in the treatment of cancer. It has also been observed that signaling channels can interact with one another in a well-coordinated network. Understanding the interactions between diverse signaling pathways is, therefore, vital for the expansion of tailored pharmacological treatment [147].

TGF-β

General Features of TGF-β

Among numerous transforming growth factors (TGFs) is a kind of growth factor and cytokine- (TGF-β) superfamily of proteins well-known for its character in controlling various physiological and pathological processes in the human body. TGF-β regulates a range of key actions in proper expansion and physiology, involving cell proliferation, cell differentiation, cell stemness, wound healing, and the immune system. These multifunctional ligands, which are highly dependent on the cellular environment, have revealed a diversity of often opposing reactions to TGF-β (Fig. **6.8**) [148].

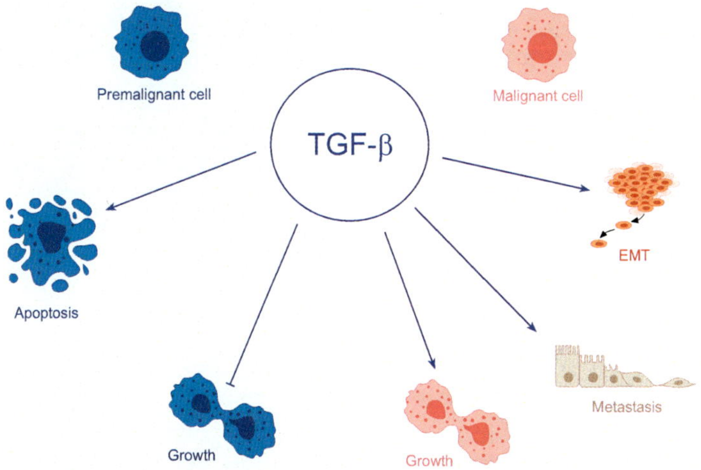

Fig. (6.8). Pleiotropic role of TGF-β in carcinogenesis. The TGF-β-signaling pathway can inhibit the carcinogenesis process by inducing apoptosis (programmed cell death) and suppressing the growth of the premalignant cell (blue side of the picture). In contrast, the TGF-β-signaling pathway can promote the carcinogenesis process by inducing growth, metastasis and EMT; epithelial-mesenchymal transition of the malignant cell in a welldeveloped tumour (pink side of the picture).

The TGF superfamily is a broad and rapidly expanding family of regulatory polypeptides that includes the archetypal and traditional TGF subfamily (which includes the three isoforms TGF-1, TGF-2, and TGF-3) as well as various subfamilies [149]. These subfamilies are the broad bone morphogenetic protein (BMP) subfamily (approximately 20 proteins), the growth and differentiation factor subfamily (approximately 9 proteins), activins (comprising activins A, B, and AB), and Glial-derived neurotrophic factors (GDNFs) and inhibins (INHs) (comprising GDNF and artemin) [150, 151].

Despite the diversity of ligand proteins, the majority of TGFs, except INHs and GDNF, and members of the superfamily subfamilies, utilize their influence and target cells by tying two kinds of Ser/Thr kinase receptors on the cell surface and building hetero-tetrameric complexes with them, which activate downstream intracellular SMAD transcription factors. TGF-signaling pathway mutations have been linked to a variety of human malignancies and developmental disorders [152, 153].

Role of TGF-β in Carcinogenesis

TGF signaling dysfunction has been connected to illnesses' etiology-like connective tissue disorders and malignancies. TGF-β shows a pleiotropic effect in the carcinogenesis procedure. In premalignant cells, it acts as a tumor suppressor, while in malignant cells, it acts as a tumor promoter, establishing malignancy [154 - 156]. TGF-β suppresses the immune system, which helps to reduce self-reactivity [68, 83]. Cancer cells can take advantage of this to hasten their progression [157, 158]. TGF levels have been found to be elevated in malignancy, which inhibits NK cell responses. TGF has been shown to suppress NK cells by antagonizing IL-15, through Inhibition of the pro-apoptotic transcription factors' exclusion by IL-15 FoxP3 from the nucleus, and by inhibiting stimulation of gene expression and proliferation associated with NK cell activation. TNF-mediated IL-15 suppression results in a lower expression of the NK cell surface protein NKG2D, according to *in vitro* experiments [159, 160].

Cancer-associated fibroblasts have been demonstrated to stimulate tumor growth by releasing ECM components in response to TGF-β growth and help tumors elude the host immune system, according to a recent study. This unique gene signature linked to the ECM and cancer-associated fibroblasts can be utilized to predict immune checkpoint blockade resistance.

The TGF-signaling pathway's suppressive effect in premalignant cells can be described by the following conceptual notions [161]:

1. TGF-β inhibits the transition of premalignant cells into a more malignant phenotype while also causing apoptosis.

2. There is an ontological basis for mutual TGF sensitivity.

3. The components of TGF signaling are insufficient for tumor development.

On the other hand, cells with oncogenic alterations may develop into aggressive cancer [162]. Moreover, in a recent study, TGF-β has been shown to have another noteworthy property: the propensity to promote carcinogenesis. TGF-β may promote tumor growth. The EMT is triggered by cell motility, resulting in a more chemo-resistant phenotype. TGF-β also indirectly promotes carcinogenesis by increasing extracellular matrix synthesis and primary tumor metastatic development by acting on the cancer microenvironment [163, 164].

TGF signaling pathways (*e.g.,* TGF-1 and TGF-3) inside the TME negatively regulate tumor reprogramming activation of MSCs at both cellular and molecular levels, a pro-inflammatory phenotype, which is consistent with this. As a result, blocking the tumor-derived pro-inflammatory mediator IL1's action on MSCs increases cancer growth [165]. TGF-1 downregulation, on the other hand, stops triple-negative breast cancer from migrating and invading [166]. Table **6.2** summarizes several examples of the TGF-signaling pathway's mutual significance in carcinogenesis.

Table 6.2. The involvement of the TGF signaling pathway in various cancer.

TGF-β-Family Member	Cell Context	The Roles in Carcinogenesis	Effect
TGF-β1	TNBC	Metastasis and invasion	Promotes [109]
	MCF-7	EMT	Promotes [110]
	NSCLC	Stemness	Promotes [111]
	Prostate cancer cells	EMT and invasion	Promotes [112]
	Colorectal cell lines	Recurrence	Promotes [113]
	Colorectal carcinoma	Metastasis and progression	Promotes [114]
BMP2	CSCs in HCC	EMT, proliferation, and invasion	Promotes [115]
BMP7	Colorectal tumors	Metastasis and progression	Promotes [116]
TGF-β1, TGF-β2, TGF-β3	Caco-2	Tumor growth	Suppresses [117]
TGF-β1	MCF-7	Tumor formation	Suppresses [118]

Abbreviations: TNBC (triple-negative breast cancer), MCF-7 (adenocarcinoma human breast cancer), EMT (epithelial-mesenchymal transition), NSCLC (non-small cell lung cancer), Caco-2 (human colon adenocarcinoma cell line), HCC (hepatocellular carcinoma), Cancer stem cells (CSCs).

CONCLUSION

This chapter tries to convey some of the current enthusiasm for cancer signaling pathway research. There are a lot of fresh discoveries in this field for further expansion. We hope that the chapter will serve as an up-to-date resource for recent advances in cancer signaling pathway research as well as the most promising treatment innovations based on these pathways. These novel discoveries and therapeutic breakthroughs have the potential to greatly enhance clinical cancer therapy.

CONSENT FOR PUBLICATION

Not applicable.

CONFLICT OF INTEREST

The authors declare that there are no conflicts of interest.

ACKNOWLEDGEMENTS

We thank Professor Faris Q.B. Alenzi, who encouraged and supported all the authors, especially the junior ones, of this chapter to experience and gain skills in writing and publishing a valuable book like this.

REFERENCES

[1] Sever R, Brugge JS. Signal transduction in cancer. Cold Spring Harb Perspect Med 2015; 5(4): a006098.

[2] Sung S-Y, Hsieh C-L, Wu D, *et al.* Tumor microenvironment promotes cancer progression, metastasis, and therapeutic resistance. Curr Probl Cancer 2007; 31(2): 36-100.

[3] Carmeliet P, Jain RK. Angiogenesis in cancer and other diseases. Nature 2000; 407(6801): 249-57.

[4] Martin TA, Ye L, Sanders AJ, *et al.* Cancer invasion and metastasis: molecular and cellular perspective Madame Curie Bioscience Database. Landes Bioscience 2013.

[5] Reisfeld RA. The tumor microenvironment: a target for combination therapy of breast cancer 2013: 18(1-2).

[6] Liou G-Y, Storz P. Reactive oxygen species in cancer. Free Radic Res 2010; 44(5): 479-96.

[7] Rawat JK, Roy S, Singh M, *et al.* Transcutaneous vagus nerve stimulation regulates the cholinergic anti-inflammatory pathway to counteract 1, 2-dimethylhydrazine induced colon carcinogenesis in albino wistar rats. Front Pharmacol 2019; 10: 353.

[8] Sammi SR, Rawat JK, Raghav N, *et al.* Galantamine attenuates N, N-dimethyl hydrazine induced neoplastic colon damage by inhibiting acetylcholinesterase and bimodal regulation of nicotinic cholinergic neurotransmission. Eur J Pharmacol 2018; 818: 174-83.

[9] Babon JJ, Lucet IS, Murphy JM, *et al.* The molecular regulation of Janus kinase (JAK) activation. Biochem J 2014; 462(1): 1-13.

[10] Seif F, Khoshmirsafa M, Aazami H, *et al.* The role of JAK-STAT signaling pathway and its regulators in the fate of T helper cells. Cell Commun Signal 2017; 15(1): 1-13.

[11] Yamaoka K, Saharinen P, Pesu M, *et al.* The janus kinases (jaks). Genome Biol 2004; 5(12): 1-6.

[12] Thomas S, Snowden J, Zeidler M, *et al.* The role of JAK/STAT signaling in the pathogenesis, prognosis and treatment of solid tumors. Br J Cancer 2015; 113(3): 365-71.

[13] Stark GR, Darnell JE Jr. The JAK-STAT pathway at twenty. Immunity 2012; 36(4): 503-14.

[14] Bousoik E. MontazeriAliabadi H. "Do we know jack" about JAK? A closer look at JAK/STAT signaling pathway. Front Oncol 2018; 8: 287.

[15] Stamos JL, Weis WI. The β-catenin destruction complex. Cold Spring Harb Perspect Biol 2013; 5(1): a007898.

[16] Lokau J, Schoeder V, Haybaeck J, Garbers C. Jak-Stat Signaling Induced by Interleukin-6 Family Cytokines in Hepatocellular Carcinoma. Cancers (Basel) 2019; 11: 1704.

[17] Saad MI, Rose-John S, Jenkins BJ. ADAM17: An Emerging Therapeutic Target for Lung Cancer. Cancers (Basel) 2019; 11: 1218.

[18] Gatta LB, Melocchi L, Bugatti M, *et al.* Hyper-Activation of STAT3 Sustains Progression of Non-Papillary Basal-Type Bladder Cancer *via* FOSL1 Regulome. Cancers (Basel) 2019; 11: 1219.

[19] Kim JH, Choi HS, Kim SL, Lee DS. The PAK1-Stat3 Signaling Pathway Activates IL-6 Gene Transcription and Human Breast Cancer Stem Cell Formation. Cancers (Basel) 2019; 11: 1527.

[20] White CL, Jayasekara WSN, Picard D, *et al.* A Sexually Dimorphic Role for STAT3 in Sonic Hedgehog Medulloblastoma. Cancers (Basel) 2019; 11: 1702.

[21] Yun JW, Lee S, Kim HM, *et al.* A Novel Type of Blood Biomarker: Distinct Changes of Cytokine-Induced STAT Phosphorylation in Blood T Cells Between Colorectal Cancer Patients and Healthy Individuals. Cancers (Basel) 2019; 11: 1157.

[22] Severin F, Frezzato F, Visentin A, *et al.* In Chronic Lymphocytic Leukemia the JAK2/STAT3 Pathway Is Constitutively Activated and Its Inhibition Leads to CLL Cell Death Unaffected by the Protective Bone Marrow Microenvironment. Cancers (Basel) 2019; 11: 1939.

[23] Morgan EL, Macdonald A. JAK2 Inhibition Impairs Proliferation and Sensitises Cervical Cancer Cells to Cisplatin-Induced Cell Death. Cancers (Basel) 2019; 11: 1934.

[24] Siebel C, Lendahl U. Notch signaling in development, tissue homeostasis, and disease. Physiol Rev 2017; 97(4): 1235-94.

[25] Yuan X, Wu H, Xu H, *et al.* Notch signaling: an emerging therapeutic target for cancer treatment. Cancer Lett 2015; 369(1): 20-7.

[26] Meisel CT, Porcheri C, Mitsiadis TA. Cancer Stem Cells, Quo Vadis? The notch signaling pathway in tumor initiation and progression. Cells 2020; 9(8): 1879.

[27] Kopan R. Notch signaling. Cold Spring Harb Perspect Biol 2012; 4(10): a011213.

[28] Murata A, Okuyama K, Sakano S, *et al.* A Notch ligand, Delta-like 1 functions as an adhesion molecule for mast cells. J Immunol 2010; 185(7): 3905-12.

[29] Groot AJ, Vooijs MA. The role of Adams in Notch signaling. Notch Signaling in Embryology and Cancer 2012; pp. 15-36.

[30] Wang Z, Li Y. H Sarkar F. Notch signaling proteins: legitimate targets for cancer therapy. Curr Protein Pept Sci 2010; 11(6): 398-408.

[31] Guruharsha K, Kankel MW. Artavanis-TsakonasS.The Notch signaling system: recent insights into the complexity of a conserved pathway. Nat Rev Genet 2012; 13(9): 654-66.

[32] South AP, Cho RJ, Aster JC. The double-edged sword of Notch signaling in cancer. Semin Cell Dev Biol 2012; 23: 458-64.

[33] Ellisen LW, Bird J, West DC, *et al.* TAN-1, the human homolog of the Drosophila notch gene, is

broken by chromosomal translocations in T lymphoblastic neoplasms. Cell 1999; 66: 649-61.

[34] Capobianco AJ, Zagouras P, Blaumueller CM, Artavanis-Tsakonas S, Bishop JM. Neoplastic transformation by truncated alleles of human NOTCH1/TAN1 and NOTCH2. Mol Cell Biol 1997; 17: 6265-73.

[35] Girard L, Hanna Z, Beaulieu N, *et al.* Frequent provirus insertional mutagenesis of Notch1 in thymomas of MMTVD/myc transgenic mice suggests a collaboration of c-myc and Notch1 for oncogenesis. Genes Dev 1996; 10: 1930-44.

[36] Weng AP, Ferrando AA, Lee W, *et al.* Activating mutations of NOTCH1 in human T cell acute lymphoblastic leukemia. Science 2004; 306: 269-71.

[37] Radtke F, Wilson A, Mancini SJ, MacDonald HR. Notch regulation of lymphocyte development and function. Nat Immunol 2004; 5: 247-53.

[38] Hoyne GF. Notch signaling in the immune system. J Leukoc Biol 2003; 74: 971-81.

[39] Sulis ML, Williams O, Palomero T, *et al.* NOTCH1 extracellular juxtamembrane expansion mutations in T-ALL. Blood 2008; 112: 733-40.

[40] Breit S, Stanulla M, Flohr T, *et al.* Activating NOTCH1 mutations predict favorable early treatment response and long-term outcome in childhood precursor T-cell lymphoblastic leukemia. Blood 2006; 108: 1151-7.

[41] Park MJ, Taki T, Oda M, *et al.* FBXW7 and NOTCH1 mutations in childhood T cell acute lymphoblastic leukaemia and T cell non-Hodgkin lymphoma. Br J Haematol 2009; 145: 198-206.

[42] Clappier E, Collette S, Grardel N, *et al.* EORTC-CLG. NOTCH1 and FBXW7 mutations have a favorable impact on early response to treatment, but not on outcome, in children with T-cell acute lymphoblastic leukemia (T-ALL) treated on EORTC trials 58881 and 58951. Leukemia 2010; 24: 2023-31.

[43] Weissmann S, Roller A, Jeromin S, *et al.* Prognostic impact and landscape of NOTCH1 mutations in chronic lymphocytic leukemia (CLL): A study on 852 patients. Leukemia 2013; 27: 2393–6.

[44] Di Ianni M, Baldoni S, Rosati E, *et al.* A new genetic lesion in B-CLL: A NOTCH1 PEST domain mutation. Br J Haematol 2009; 146: 689-91.

[45] Sportoletti P, Baldoni S, Cavalli L, *et al.* NOTCH1 PEST domain mutation is an adverse prognostic factor in B-CLL. Br J Haematol 2010; 151: 404-6.

[46] Wickremasinghe RG, Prentice AG, Steele AJ. p53 and Notch signaling in chronic lymphocytic leukemia: Clues to identifying novel therapeutic strategies. Leukemia 2011; 25: 1400-7.

[47] Rossi D, Rasi S, Fabbri G, *et al.* Mutations of NOTCH1 are an independent predictor of survival in chronic lymphocytic leukemia. Blood 2012; 119: 521-9.

[48] Kiel MJ, Velusamy T, Betz BL, *et al.* Whole-genome sequencing identifies recurrent somatic NOTCH2 mutations in splenic marginal zone lymphoma. J Exp Med 2012; 209: 1553-65.

[49] Lee SY, Kumano K, Nakazaki K, *et al.* Gainof-function mutations and copy number increases of Notch2 in diffuse large B-cell lymphoma. Cancer Sci 2009; 100: 920-6.

[50] Rossi D, Trifonov V, Fangazio M, *et al.* The coding genome of splenic marginal zone lymphoma: Activation of NOTCH2 and other pathways regulating marginal zone development. J Exp Med 2012; 209: 1537-51.

[51] Qi M, Elion EA. MAP kinase pathways. J Cell Sci 2005; 118: 3569-72.

[52] Raman M, Chen W, Cobb MH. Differential regulation and properties of MAPKs. Oncogene 2007; 26: 3100-12.

[53] Keshet Y, Seger R. The MAP kinase signaling cascades: A system of hundreds of components regulates a diverse array of physiological functions. Methods Mol Biol 2010; 661: 3-38.

[54] Cuevas BD, Abell AN, Johnson GL. Role of mitogen-activated protein kinase kinase kinases in signal integration. Oncogene 2007; 26: 3159-71.

[55] Tanoue T, Nishida E. Molecular recognitions in MAP kinase cascades. Cell Signal 2003; 15: 455-62.

[56] Zhang Y, Dong C. Regulatory mechanisms of mitogen-activated kinase signaling. Cell Mol Life Sci 2007; 64: 2771-89.

[57] McKay MM, Morrison DK. Integrating signals from RTKs to ERK/MAPK. Oncogene 2007; 26: 3113-21.

[58] Shaul YD, Seger R. The MEK/ERK cascade: From signaling specificity to diverse functions. Biochim Biophys Acta 2007; 1773: 1213-26.

[59] Giancotti FG, Ruoslahti E. Integrin signaling. Science 1999; 285: 1028-32.

[60] Orton RJ, Sturm OE, Vyshemirsky V, Calder M, Gilbert DR, Kolch W. Computational modelling of the receptortyrosine- kinase-activated MAPK pathway. Biochem J 2005; 392: 249-61.

[61] Petti C, Molla A, Vegetti C, Ferrone S, Anichini A, Sensi M. Coexpression of NRASQ61R and BRAFV600E in human melanoma cells activates senescence and increases susceptibility to cell-mediated cytotoxicity. Cancer Res 2006; 66: 6503-11.

[62] Hanahan D, Weinberg RA. The hallmarks of cancer. Cell 2000; 100: 57-70.

[63] Downward J. Targeting RAS signaling pathways in cancer therapy. Nat Rev Cancer 2003; 3: 11-22.

[64] Sebolt-Leopold JS, Herrera R. Targeting the mitogenactivated protein kinase cascade to treat cancer. Nat Rev Cancer 2004; 4: 937-47.

[65] Hancock JF. Ras proteins: different signals from different locations. Nat Rev Mol Cell Biol 2003; 4: 373-84.

[66] Hancock JF, Parton RG. Ras plasma membrane signaling platforms. Biochem J 2005; 389: 1-11.

[67] Philips MR. Compartmentalized signaling of Ras. BiochemSoc. Trans 2005; 33: 657-61.

[68] Mor A, Philips MR. Compartmentalized Ras/MAPK signaling. Annu Rev Immunol 2006; 24: 771-800.

[69] Sebolt-Leopold JS, Herrera R. Targeting the mitogenactivated protein kinase cascade to treat cancer. Nat Rev Cancer 2004; 4: 937-47.

[70] Beeram M, Patnaik A, Rowinsky EK. Regulation of c-Raf-1: therapeutic implications. Clin Adv Hematol Oncol 2003; 1: 476-81.

[71] Zhu K, Hamilton AD, Sebti SM. Farnesyltransferase inhibitors as anticancer agents: current status. Curr Opin Investig Drugs 2003; 4: 1428-35.

[72] To MD, Perez-Losada J, Mao JH, Hsu J, Jacks T, Balmain A. A functional switch from lung cancer resistance to susceptibility at the Pas1 locus in Kras2LA2 mice. Nat Genet 2006; 38: 926-30.

[73] O'Neill E, Kolch W. Conferring specificity on the ubiquitous Raf/MEK signaling pathway. Br J Cancer 2004; 2004(90): 283-8.

[74] Wellbrock C, Karasarides M, Marais R. The RAF proteins take centre stage. Nat Rev Mol Cell Biol 2004; 5: 875-85.

[75] Galabova-Kovacs G, Kolbus A, Matzen D, *et al.* ERK and beyond: insights from B-Raf and Raf-1 conditional knockouts. Cell Cycle 2006; 5: 1514-8.

[76] Dhillon AS, Kolch W. Untying the regulation of the Raf-1 kinase. Arch Biochem Biophys 2002; 404: 3-9.

[77] Chong H, Vikis HG, Guan KL. Mechanisms of regulating the Raf kinase family. Cell Signal 2003; 15: 463-9.

[78] Wellbrock C, Karasarides M, Marais R. The RAF proteins take centre stage. Nat Rev Mol Cell Biol 2004; 5: 875-85.

[79] Davies H, Bignell GR, Cox C, *et al.* Mutations of the BRAF gene in human cancer. Nature 2002; 417: 949-54.

[80] Sebolt-Leopold JS, Herrera R. Targeting the mitogenactivated protein kinase cascade to treat cancer. Nat Rev Cancer 2004; 4: 937-47.

[81] Javelaud D, Besancon F. NF-kappa B activation results in rapid inactivation of JNK in TNF alpha-treated Ewing sarcoma cells: a mechanism for the anti-apoptotic effect of NF-kappa B. Oncogene 2001; 20: 4365-72.

[82] Kim HL, Vander Griend DJ, Yang X, *et al.* Mitogen-activated protein kinase kinase 4 metastasis suppressor gene expression is inversely related to histological pattern in advancing human prostatic cancers. Cancer Res 2001; 61: 2833-7.

[83] Rojas JM, Oliva JL, Santos E. Mammalian son of sevenless Guanine nucleotide exchange factors: old concepts and new perspectives. Genes Cancer 2011; 2(3): 298-305.

[84] Braicu C, Buse M, Busuioc C, *et al.* A comprehensive review on MAPK: a promising therapeutic target in cancer. Cancers (Basel) 2019; 11(10): 1618.

[85] Monje P, Hernández-Losa J, Lyons RJ, *et al.* Regulation of the transcriptional activity of c-Fos by ERK: a novel role for the prolyl isomerase PIN1. J Biol Chem 2005; 280(42): 35081-4.

[86] Kiu H, Nicholson SE. Biology and significance of the JAK/STAT signaling pathways. Growth Factors 2012; 30(2): 88-106.

[87] Brian A. Hemmings and David F Restuccia. PI3K-PKB/Akt Pathway. Cold Spring Harb Perspect Biol 2012; 4: a011189.

[88] Vivanco I, Sawyers CL. The phosphatidylinositol 3-Kinase AKT pathway in human cancer. Nat Rev Cancer 2002; 2: 489-501.

[89] Burgering BM, Coffer PJ. Protein kinase B (c-Akt) in phosphatidylinositol-3-OH kinase signal transduction. Nature 1995; 376: 599-602.

[90] Manning BD, Cantley LC. AKT/PKB signaling: navigating downstream. Cell 2007; 129: 1261-74.

[91] Cantley LC, Songyang Z. Specificity in recognition of phosphopeptides by src-homology 2 domains. J Cell Sci Suppl 1994; 18: 121-6.

[92] Vivanco I, Sawyers CL. The phosphatidylinositol 3-Kinase AKT pathway in human cancer. Nat Rev Cancer 2002; 2: 489-501.

[93] Li J, Yen C, Liaw D, *et al.* PTEN, a putative protein tyrosine phosphatase gene mutated in human brain, breast, and prostate cancer. Science 1997; 275: 1943-7.

[94] Ali IU, Schriml LM, Dean M. Mutational spectra of PTEN/MMAC1 gene: a tumor suppressor with lipid phosphatase activity. J Natl Cancer Inst 1999; 91: 1922-32.

[95] Gabelli SB, Mandelker D, Schmidt-Kittler O, *et al.* Somatic mutations in PI3Kα: structural basis for the enzyme activation and drug design. Biochim Biophys Acta 2010; 1804: 533-40.

[96] Jaiswal BS, Janakiraman V, Kljavin NM, *et al.* Somatic mutations in p85alpha promote tumorigenesis through class IA PI3K activation. Cancer Cell 2009; 16: 463-74.

[97] Sun M, Hillmann P, Hofmann BT, *et al.* Cancer-derived mutations in the regulatory subunit p85alpha of phosphoinositide 3-kinase function through the catalytic subunit p110alpha. Proc Natl Acad Sci USA 2010; 107: 15547-52.

[98] Dillon RL, White DE, Muller WJ. The phosphatidyl inositol 3-kinase signaling network: implications for human breast cancer. Oncogene 2007; 26(9): 1338-45.

[99] Rodon J, Dienstmann R, Serra V, *et al.* Development of PI3K Inhibitors: Lessons Learned from early clinical trials. Nat Rev Clin Oncol 2013; 10(3): 143-53.

[100] Mokhtar AH, Malik IA, Abd Aziz NAA, *et al.* LY294002, a PI3K pathway inhibitor, prevents leptin-induced adverse effects on spermatozoa in Sprague-Dawley rats. Andrologia 2019; 51: e13196.

[101] Kaley TJ, Panageas KS, Mellinghof IK, *et al.* Phase II trial of an AKT inhibitor (perifosine) for recurrent glioblastoma. J Neurooncol 2019; 144: 403-7.

[102] Naing A, Aghajanian C, Raymond E, *et al.* Safety, tolerability, pharmacokinetics, and pharmacodynamics of AZD8055 in advanced solid tumors and lymphoma. Br J Cancer 2012; 107(7): 1093-9.

[103] Liu T, Zhang L, Joo D, *et al.* NF-κB signaling in inflammation. Signal Transduct Target Ther 2017; 2(1): 1-9.

[104] Oeckinghaus A, Ghosh S. The NF-κB family of transcription factors and its regulation. Cold Spring Harb Perspect Biol 2009; 1(4): a000034.

[105] Hayden MS. Ghosh S NF-κB in immunobiology. Cell Res 2011; 21(2): 223-44.

[106] Roy S, Singh M, Rawat A, *et al.* Mitochondrial apoptosis and curtailment of hypoxia-inducible factor-1α/fatty acid synthase: A dual edge perspective of gamma linolenic acid in ER+ mammary gland cancer. Cell Biochem Funct 2020; 38(5): 591-603.

[107] Singh M, Devi U, Roy S, *et al.* Chemical activation of prolyl hydroxylase-2 by BBAP-1 down regulates hypoxia inducible factor-1α and fatty acid synthase for mammary gland chemoprevention. RSC Advances 2018; 8(23): 12848-60.

[108] Gamble C, McIntosh K, Scott R, *et al.* Inhibitory kappa B Kinases as targets for pharmacological regulation. Br J Pharmacol 2012; 165(4): 802-19.

[109] Israël A. The IKK complex, a central regulator of NF-κB activation. Cold Spring Harb Perspect Biol 2010; 2(3): a000158.

[110] Karin M, Delhase M, Eds. The IκB kinase (IKK) and NF-κB: key elements of proinflammatory signaling. Seminars in immunology; 2000: 85-98.

[111] Hayden MS, Ghosh S. NF-κB, the first quarter-century: remarkable progress and outstanding questions. Genes Dev 2012; 26(3): 203-34.

[112] Manral C, Roy S, Singh M, *et al.* Effect of β-sitosterol against methyl nitrosourea-induced mammary gland carcinoma in albino rats. BMC Complement Altern Med 2016; 16(1): 1-10.

[113] Rani A, Roy S, Singh M, *et al.* α-Chymotrypsin regulates free fatty acids and UCHL-1 to ameliorate N-methyl nitrosourea induced mammary gland carcinoma in albino wistar rats. Inflammopharmacology 2016; 24(5): 277-86.

[114] Sun SC. The noncanonical NF-κB pathway. Immunol Rev 2012; 246(1): 125-40.

[115] Sun S-C. Non-canonical NF-κB signaling pathway. Cell Res 2011; 21(1): 71-85.

[116] Sun S-C. The non-canonical NF-κB pathway in immunity and inflammation. Nat Rev Immunol 2017; 17(9): 545.

[117] Mulero MC, Wang VY-F, Huxford T, *et al.* Genome reading by the NF-κB transcription factors. Nucleic Acids Res 2019; 47(19): 9967-89.

[118] Xia Y, Shen S, Verma IM. NF-κB, an active player in human cancers. Cancer Immunol Res 2014; 2(9): 823-30.

[119] Zeligs KP, Neuman MK, Annunziata CM. Molecular pathways: the balance between cancer and the immune system challenges the therapeutic specificity of targeting nuclear factor-κB signaling for cancer treatment. Clin Cancer Res 2016; 22(17): 4302-8.

[120] Brücher BL, Lang F, Jamall IS. NF-κB signaling and crosstalk during carcinogenesis. Open 2019; 2: 13.

[121] Wang W, Nag SA, Zhang R. Targeting the NFκB signaling pathways for breast cancer prevention and therapy. Curr Med Chem 2015; 22(2): 264-89.

[122] Karin M. Nuclear factor-kappaB in cancer development and progression. Nature 2006; 441: 431-6.

[123] Kim JS, Kim EJ, Kim HS, *et al.* MKK4 activates non-canonical NFκB signaling by promoting NFκB2-p100 processing. Biochem Biophys Res Commun 2017; 491(2): 337-42.

[124] Baud V, Karin M. Is NF-κB a good target for cancer therapy? Hopes and pitfalls. Nat Rev Drug Discov 2009; 8(1): 33-40.

[125] Prasad S, Ravindran J, Aggarwal BB. NF-κB and cancer: How intimate is this relationship. Mol Cell Biochem 2010; 336: 25-37.

[126] Gupta SC, Kim JH, Prasad S, *et al.* Regulation of survival, proliferation, invasion, angiogenesis, and metastasis of tumor cells through modulation of inflammatory pathways by nutraceuticals. Cancer Metastasis Rev 2010; 29: 405-34.

[127] Ben-Neriah Y, Karin M. Inflammation meets cancer, with NF-κB as the matchmaker. Nat Immunol 2011; 12: 715-23.

[128] Gilmore TD. The Rel/NF-k B/I k B signal transduction pathway and cancer. Cancer Treat Res 2003; 115: 241-65.

[129] Karin M, Cao Y, Greten FR, *et al.* NF-kB in cancer: From innocent bystander to major culprit. Nat Rev Cancer 2002; 2: 301-10.

[130] Annunziata CM, Davis RE, Demchenko Y, *et al.* Frequent engagement of the classical and alternative NF-kB pathways by diverse genetic abnormalities in multiple myeloma. Cancer Cell 2007; 12: 115-30.

[131] Keats JJ, Fonseca R, Chesi M, *et al.* Promiscuous mutations activate the noncanonical NF-kB pathway in multiple myeloma. Cancer Cell 2007; 12: 131-44.

[132] Eliopoulos AG, Young LS. LMP1 structure and signal transduction. Semin Cancer Biol 2001; 11: 435-44.

[133] Thornburg NJ, Kulwichit W, Edwards RH, *et al.* LMP1 signaling and activation of NF-kB in LMP1 transgenic mice. Oncogene 2006; 25: 288-97.

[134] Neri A, Chang CC, Lombardi L, *et al.* B cell lymphoma-associated chromosomal translocation involves candidate oncogene lyt-10, homologous to NF-kappa B p50. Cell 1991; 67: 1075-87.

[135] Gilmore TD. Multiple mutations contribute to the oncogenicity of the retroviral oncoprotein v-Rel. Oncogene 1999; 18: 6925-37.

[136] Meylan E, Dooley AL, Feldser DM, *et al.* Requirement for NF-kappaBsignaling in a mouse model of lung adenocarcinoma. Nature 2009; 462: 104-7.

[137] Yoshida S, Ono M, Shono T, *et al.* Involvement of interleukin-8, vascular endothelial growth factor, and basic fibroblast growth factor in tumor necrosis factor alpha-dependent angiogenesis. Mol Cell Biol 1997; 17(7): 4015-23.

[138] Li F, Zhang J, Arfuso F, *et al.* NF-κB in cancer therapy. Arch Toxicol 2015; 89: 711-31.

[139] MacDonald BT, Tamai K, He X. Wnt/β-catenin signaling: components, mechanisms, and diseases. Dev Cell 2009; 17(1): 9-26.

[140] Stamos JL, Weis WI. The β-catenin destruction complex. Cold Spring Harb Perspect Biol 2013; 5(1): a007898.

[141] Kim JG, Kim MJ, Choi WJ, *et al.* Wnt3A Induces GSK-3β Phosphorylation and β-Catenin Accumulation Through RhoA/ROCK. J Cell Physiol 2017; 232(5): 1104-13.

[142] Shang S, Hua F, Hu Z-W. The regulation of β-catenin activity and function in cancer: therapeutic opportunities. Oncotarget 2017; 8(20): 33972.

[143] Zhang Y, Wang X. Targeting the Wnt/β-catenin signaling pathway in cancer. J Hematol Oncol 2020; 13(1): 1-16.

[144] Paul I, Bhattacharya S, Chatterjee A, *et al.* Current understanding on EGFR and Wnt/β-catenin signaling in glioma and their possible crosstalk. Genes Cancer 2013; 4(11-12): 427-46.

[145] McCubrey JA, Steelman LS, Bertrand FE, *et al.* GSK-3 as potential target for therapeutic intervention in cancer. Oncotarget 2014; 5(10): 2881.

[146] Song Y, Li Z-x, Liu X, *et al.* The Wnt/β-catenin and PI3K/Akt signaling pathways promote EMT in gastric cancer by epigenetic regulation *via* H3 lysine 27 acetylation. Tumour Biol 2017; 39(7)

[147] Handy DE, Castro R, Loscalzo J. Epigenetic modifications: basic mechanisms and role in cardiovascular disease. Circulation 2011; 123(19): 2145-56.

[148] Morikawa M, Derynck R, Miyazono K. TGF- β and the TGF-β family: Context-dependent roles in cell and tissue physiology;(2015; Vol. 8, Cold Spring Harbor Perspectives in Biology. Cold Spring Harbor Laboratory Press. https://pubmed.ncbi.nlm.nih.gov/27141051/

[149] Morikawa M, Derynck R, Miyazono K. TGF- β and the TGF-β family: Context-dependent roles in cell and tissue physiology. 2016; Vol. 8, Cold Spring Harbor Perspectives in Biology. Cold Spring Harbor Laboratory Press. pmc/articles/PMC4852

[150] Javelaud D, Mauviel A. Mammalian transforming growth factor-βs: Smad signaling and physiopathological roles. Int J Biochem Cell Biol 2004; 36: 1161–5.

[151] Poniatowski LA, Wojdasiewicz P, Gasik R, *et al.* Transforming growth factor beta family: Insight into the role of growth factors in regulation of fracture healing biology and potential clinical applications; 2015: Mediators of Inflammation. Hindawi Limited. pmc/articles/PMC4325469

[152] Massagué J. TGF-β signal transduction. Annu Rev Biochem 1998; 67: 753–91.

[153] David CJ, Massagué J. Contextual determinants of TGFβ action in development, immunity and cancer. Nature Reviews Molecular Cell Biology. Nature Publishing Group 2018; Vol. 19: pp. 419-35.

[154] Colak S, ten Dijke P. Targeting TGF-β Signaling in Cancer. Trends in Cancer. Cell Press; 2017; Vol. 3: pp. 56–71.

[155] Pasche B. Role of transforming growth factor beta in cancer. J Cell Physiol 2001; 186(2): 153-68. [Internet].

[156] Al-Toub M, Almusa A, Almajed M, *et al.* Pleiotropic effects of cancer cells' secreted factors on human stromal (mesenchymal) stem cells. Stem Cell Res Ther 2013; 4(5): 114. [Internet].

[157] Flavell RA, Sanjabi S, Wrzesinski SH, Licona-Limón P. The Polarization of Immune Cells in the Tumour Environment by Tgfβ. Nat Rev Immunol 2010; 10(8): 554-67.

[158] Ikushima H, Miyazono K. Tgfbeta Signalling: A Complex Web in Cancer Progression. Nat Rev Cancer 2010; 10(6): 415-24.
[http://dx.doi.org/10.1038/nrc2853]

[159] Ikushima H, Miyazono K. Tgfβ Signalling: A Complex Web in Cancer Progression. Nat Rev Cancer 2010; 10(6): 415-24.

[160] Lee J-C, Lee K-M, Kim D-W, Heo DS. Elevated Tgf-B1 Secretion and Down-Modulation of Nkg2d Underlies Impaired Nk Cytotoxicity in Cancer Patients. J Immunol 2004; 172(12): 7335-40.

[161] Wang J, Xi C, Yang X, *et al.* LncRNA WT1-AS Inhibits Triple-Negative Breast Cancer Cell Migration and Invasion by Downregulating Transforming Growth Factor β1. Cancer Biother Radiopharm 2019; 34(10): 671-5. [Internet].

[162] Kim S, Lee J, Jeon M, *et al.* Zerumbone suppresses the motility and tumorigenecity of triple negative

breast cancer cells *via* the inhibition of TGF-β1 signaling pathway. Oncotarget 2016; 7(2): 1544-58. [Internet].

[163] Zuo XX, Yang Y, Zhang Y, *et al.* Platelets promote breast cancer cell MCF-7 metastasis by direct interaction: Surface integrin α2β1-contacting-mediated activation of Wnt-β-catenin pathway. Cell Commun Signal 2019; 17(1): 142.

[164] Jiang X, Wang J, Fang L. LncRNA WT1-AS over-expression inhibits non-small cell lung cancer cell stemness by down-regulating TGF-β1. BMC Pulm Med 2020; 20(1): 113.

[165] Lee MS, Lee J, Kim YM, *et al.* The metastasis suppressor CD82/KAI1 represses the TGF-β 1 and Wntsignalings inducing epithelial-to-mesenchymal transition linked to invasiveness of prostate cancer cells. Prostate 2019; 79(12): 1400-11. [Internet].

[166] Cargnello M, Roux PP. Activation and function of the MAPKs and their substrates, the MAPK-activated protein kinases. Microbiol Mol Biol Rev 2011; 75(1): 50-83.

CHAPTER 7

Transcription Factors in Cancer

Rawiah A. Alsiary[1,*], **Talat Abdullah Albukhari**[2] and **Waheed A. Filimban**[3]

[1] *King Abdullah International Medical Research Center (KAIMRC), WR King Saud Bin Abdulaziz University for Health Sciences (KSAU-HS), P.O. Box 9515, Jeddah, Saudi Arabia*

[2] *Haematology and Immunology Department, Faculty of Medicine, Um Al Qura University, Makkah, Saudi Arabia*

[3] *Pathology Department, Faculty of Medicine, Um Al Qura University, Makkah, Saudi Arabia*

Abstract: Different types of signalling pathways have been approved to be involved in cancer imitation and progression. These signalling pathways include the JAK-STAT signalling, NF-κB signalling, Wnt, Notch and Hedgehog. STAT (Signal Transducer and Activator of Transcription) transports signals between proteins from the cell membrane into the nucleus to contribute to cancer progression. NF-κB signalling is essential for the survival of the B cell tumor types. The Wnt, Notch, and Hedgehog signalling pathways play a significant role in carcinogenesis by upregulating the genes associated with these pathways. Hence, pharmacological inhibitors of WNT, NOTCH, and HH pathways are required in clinical studies. Such inhibitors have features that make them important during the clinical trial since they offer great potential as novel therapeutics for cancer. They also have an antitumor response which should be taken into consideration. The three signalling pathways are also known to shape cell fate determination and differentiation. In case of depletion of a single molecular component within the three pathways, embryonic lethality will form.

Keywords: HH signalling pathways, Hedgehog, NF-κB, NOTCH, Signaling, STAT, Transcription, Wnt (β)-Catenin.

TRANSCRIPTION FACTORS IN CANCER

A transcription factor is a sequence-based DNA-binding protein that regulates the transcription of genetic material from DNA to messenger RNA *via* binding to specific DNA sequences in molecular biology and genetics. There are three types of transcription factors that are believed to play a role in human cancer.

* **Corresponding author Rawiah A. Alsiary:** King Abdullah International Medical Research Center (KAIMRC), WR King Saud bin Abdulaziz University for Health Sciences (KSAU-HS), P.O. Box 9515, Jeddah, Saudi Arabia; E-mail: alsiaryra@ngha.med.sa

Faris Q.B. Alenzi (Ed.)

1- Steroid receptors, such as oestrogen receptors and androgen receptors, in breast cancer and prostate cancer, respectively. Anti-oestrogen and anti-androgen agents have been in clinical use for several years, such as tamoxifen and bicalutamide. Activated glucocorticoids have also been extensively used due to their ability to promote apoptosis, at least in lymphoid cells [1].

2- Resident nuclear proteins, which are activated by serine kinase cascades, are also transcription factors linked to cancer [2]. For example, JUN was identified as an oncogene in 1987, first as the viral Jun (v-Jun), then as the cellular Jun (c-Jun), and then as a transcription factor shortly after.

3- Latent cytoplasmic factor is the third and most recently identified group of transcription factors with oncogenic potential, whose function is usually activated by receptor-ligand interaction at the cell surface [2]. These transcription factors are triggered by serine or tyrosine kinases at the cell surface, or by a variety of cytoplasmic biochemical events that include kinases (some of which are regulated by Ca^{2+} flux) or precisely controlled proteolysis.

After synthesis, several transcription factors reach the nucleus spontaneously [2]. The bZip proteins include JUNB, c-JUN, c-FOS, JUND, ATFs, FRA, and the CREB-CREM family, the ETS proteins, the cEBP family, and the MAD box family, are among the main classes of structurally related proteins. In mammals, these classes comprise at least several hundred different proteins, only a few of which have been widely considered [3]. A general picture of the activities that regulate the resident nuclear-transcription factors' maximal transcriptional activity has arisen. While no JUN mutations have been identified in human cancers, upstream activators of JUN3 have been identified in a large number of mutations.

There are a variety of resident nuclear transcription factors that are overexpressed or presented as hyperactive fusion proteins in cancers. MYC, which is widely enhanced in cancer, is the most common of all [4]. MYC does not govern transcription by itself; instead, it forms a dimer with another protein called MAX [5]. E2F proteins are usually free in the tumor due to the common lack of RB. E2F is required for cell-cycle development, according to studies in cultured cells, though depletion of E2F prevents S-phase entry the most [6]. E2F dysfunction has been documented in cancer, despite the fact that most cancers have normal levels of E2F protein production. E2F level was significantly higher in 90% of small-cell lung cancer patients, but not in adenocarcinoma or squamous-cell lung carcinoma [7].

Signal Transducer and Activator of Transcription (STAT)

Definition

"STAT (Signal Transducer and Activator of Transcription) factors are proteins that have the ability to transduce signals from the cell membrane into the nucleus, thus activating gene transcription" [8, 9].

Types of STATs

In the human genome, up till now, seven kinds of STAT genes have been discovered, and they are as follows; "STAT1 chromosomal location 2q32.2, STAT2 12q13.3, STAT3 17q21.2, STAT4 2q32.), STAT5a 17q21.), STAT5b 17q21.2, STAT612q13.3" [8, 9].

Their signal transduction is included in numerous usual physiological cell procedures, counting propagation, variation, angiogenesis apoptosis and immune ruling. Irregularities may occur in its pathways, leading to abnormal STAT rules, which in turn lead to various pathological events, such as malicious alteration and "metastasis" of cells [10].

Features of the STAT Group of Proteins

All of the "STAT proteins" are made up of a quantity of functionally and as well as structurally preserved areas [11].

1. The "Src-homology 2 SH2" field, along with the "N-terminal domain ND" intercedes homo- and "heterodimerization" of STAT monomers throughout stimulation.

2. The "coiled-coil domain CCD" works as a signal of the nuclear locale by incriminating interactions between protein-protein.

3. The C-terminal "transcriptional activation domain TAD", endures "serine phosphorylation" and thus employs extra activators that are transcriptional, improving the actions of STAT pertaining to transcriptions.

4. The "DNA-binding domain DBD" is responsible for the determination of DNA association [12, 13].

Some of the STAT proteins institute isoforms by alternate mRNA interweaving or processing of "post-translational proteolytic". The isoforms that are of complete length are labelled "α isoforms", while their corresponding items that are full-length are termed "β, γ or δ" [13].

Biochemical Cascade

The STAT protein is inactivated in a latent form, and is inactivated in a monomeric form or a phosphorylated dimer form and is located in the unstimulated target cells' cytoplasm. They are quickly triggered by a variety of cytokines counting interferon (IFN) and interleukin (IL), and also growth aspects and hormones that are fixed to receptors of the membrane [14, 15].

"STAT1", "STAT3", "STAT5a", and "STAT5b" are triggered by numerous discrete and occasionally overlying ligands, while "STAT2", "STAT4" and "STAT6" are triggered by a limited cytokine.

Modes of STAT Activation

"STAT proteins" do not possess tyrosine kinase activity, so they depend on other molecules that interrelate with them to deliver this effect. Numerous methods of activations of STAT have been defined.

The Standard Janus Kinase (JAK)-STAT Path

In this cascade reaction, extracellular peptides send signals across membrane receptors, leading to a way to control transcriptase without the use of other receptors. Then, JAK phosphorylates and transphosphorylases the linked tyrosine residues, thereby providing a docking point for the SH2 domain of potential STAT molecules. Once this connection is established, JAK will "phosphorylate specific Tyr" residues (pYs) on the receptor-related STAT molecule, instigating this important pY to be bound by a receptor linked to pSTAT to the SH2 domain pSTAT. The other receptor eventually binds, leading to homodimerization or heterodimerization of STAT. Then the PSTAT-pSTAT light modulator is unrestricted from the receptor and is quickly introduced in the nucleus [16].

Receptors with Inherent Kinase Actions

Receptors like FGF, PDGF and EGF are responsible for the activation of STAT, and this happens in a direct as well as indirect method with JAK. This is also reported in the EGF gesticulating that occurs in breast cancer cell lines in humans.

G-Protein Joined Receptors

For instance, chemokine receptors for "MIP-1" and "RANTES" in T-cells trigger "STAT1" and "STAT3" upon binding of chemokine.

Non-Receptor Tyrosine Kinases

Receptors like “v-Src”, “v-Fps”, “v-Sis”, “polyoma virus middle T antigen,” and “v-Abl” and assorted kinases of protein (counting numerous MAPKs) encourage activation of STAT that is constitutive.

Stimulation of STATs Arbitrated by Additional Proteins

This assists connectors to take JAKs in near propinquity to the “STATs”, such as stimulation of “STAT3” through over-expression of “MEKK1-C” and “islet-1”.

Transcriptional Engagement

STAT participates in the surrounding DRE, leading to initiation, suppression or objective binding of transcription. They also participate in binding locations farther away from genes encoding proteins by regulating the activity of promoters and the epigenetic position of related genes, or openly directing noncoding positions (*e.g.,* “miRNAs”) [17]. The epigenetic changes induced by Stat occur in the area accountable for STAT binding and dependent on STAT formulation directive. This delivers a self-regulating effect with inhibitory or tonic activity. This means that due to cellular mutations that allow or allow access to genes, the target registry of a particular STAT may differ from one cell kind. The transcriptional activity produced by STAT is affected by other variables (such as gene selection, communication with other TFs, genomic struggle, and different STATs indicating that the same STAT molecule has different results and the length and/or intensity of the STAT signal) complex [17].

Activation and Functions of STAT Proteins

1. STAT1 participates in virus-related and bacteriological reactions, growth inhibition, stimulating cell apoptosis and inhibiting tumor growth.

2. STAT2 is important for the antiviral, immunogenic, anti-apoptotic and anti-proliferative belongings of “IFN-I”, and encourages the instigation and binding of the “STAT2”, “STAT1” heterodimer, which forms the transcription complex “ISGF3” with the DNA clinging protein “IRF9”, thereby activating the expression of “IFN-I” targets [11, 18, 19].

3. STAT3 is started by:

- A huge quantity of cytokines that make use of signing subunits of receptor comparable to "gp130" as "IL-6" (the IL-6/JAK/STAT3 signalling pathway).
- Numerous hormones like leptin, prolactin and development hormones.
- Growth features that make use of "tyrosine kinase receptors".
- Receptors that are related to kinases like JAK.
- Numerous oncogenic "non-receptor tyrosine kinases" like ABL and Src.
- By way of receptors that are toll-like.
- In reply to "oncogenic heterotrimeric G protein subunits" by way of instigation of a non-receptor "cellular tyrosine kinase, c-Src" [20].

Temporary activation of STAT3 is a key factor in restoring tissue veracity, wound curing and eventually solving the response of immune [21 - 24]. Sustained activation STAT involves synthesis, carcinogenesis, survival, metastasis, and anti-apoptosis [14].

4. STAT4, generally, its expression is limited to testis, thymus and myeloid cells [25]. STAT4 precisely intercedes "IL-12," indicating, distressing a broad array of immune cells. It is obligatory for the growth of Th1 and for the creation of "IFN-γ" [26]. Subsequent to the instigation, "STAT4" binds to many sites of the target in the genome, with the sponsor sections of genes programming for "cytokines (IFN-γ, TNF)", receptors, and features gesturing (MYD88) [27].

5. STAT5a and STAT5b are triggered in reply to the "ligand-receptor" connection of many hormones and cytokines, like prolactin (PRL), erythropoietin (EPO) and growth hormone (GH) and numerous interleukins [28]. STAT5 proteins have remained linked with a variation of cells [29 - 31], mobilization lipid [32] and development of lymphocytes [33]. "STAT5a" is included in PRL, and "STAT5b" is in GH gesticulating [13].

6. STAT6:

- Causes a response in immune cells by gesticulating IL-4 and IL-13 [34]. This causes the proliferation of B and T cells, a distinction of alternately triggered macrophages [35].
- Reregulation of IgE class substituting in B cells (in collaboration with (NF-κB) instigation) [36].
- Cell exterior molecules induction (like main "histocompatibility complex type II MHC-II") in "B cells" and in alternate triggered macrophages [37].
- Deterrence of apoptosis by way of genes that are anti-apoptotic induction, for instance, Bcl-XL.

- STAT6 is a significant contributor to the development of Th2 cells, and it reduces the creation of IL-10 [38, 39].

Inactivation of STAT Proteins

Inactivation of molecules of STAT can be achieved by common pathways, like endocytosis of internal receptors on vesicles, and subsequent degradation of the receptors *via* the "ubiquitin-proteasome" pathway [40]. Particularly inhibitory signals originate as of "protein tyrosine phosphatase (PTP)", which can act in the membrane-linked receptor kinase complex stage [41 - 43], or at the core through the phosphorylation of active STAT dimers and the reprocessing of potential STATs to play a role in the cytoplasm [44, 45]. The JAKs' devise their individual inhibitors, named "suppressor of cytokine signalling (SOCS)" proteins, that unswervingly bind to and incapacitate the kinases [46]. The manifestation of SOCS genes might be inspired by increasing the similar cellular changes activated by STAT. Therefore, the SOCS protein can play a role in the classical feedback inhibition loop, and the absenteeism of SOCS members in the cell can convert the transcriptional characteristics motivated by STAT from one STAT to another. The activated STAT protein inhibitor (PIAS) binds to the phosphorylated STAT dimer, thereby preventing DNA recognition [47]. The form of STAT ice may also have negative rules for STAT power generation, which is mainly reflected in the STAT1 and STAT3 tags [48 - 50].

Mutations Affecting STAT Signaling

Signalling that has malfunctioned because of transmutations in members of the JAK family, such as;

- JAK3 causes extreme immunodeficiency.
- "STAT1" to continuing "mucocutaneous candidiasis" and recurring contaminations of mycobacteria.
- "STAT2" amplified vulnerability to virus-related contaminations.
- "STAT3" to the "hyperglobulin E syndrome".
- "STAT5" to insensitivity pertaining to development hormones and complicated syndromes that are categorized by immunodeficiency, dwarfism and auto-immune illnesses [51, 52].

Alterations in genes of JAK-STAT are frequently found in myeloproliferative disorders, such as polycythemia vera, that has transformations in "JAK2 V617F" but are rare in solid tumors [53].

Cytokine signalling dependency is also one of the reasons for hematologic malignancies mutations. It is reported as follows that:

- "STAT5b" in hepatosplenic "γδ T-cell lymphoma".
- "STAT3" in T-cell big "granular lymphocytic leukemia" and "natural killer cell (NK)" lymphoproliferative syndromes.
- JAK3 in NK/T "cell lymphomas" [54, 55].
- Growth of tumour in hematological malignancies can be caused by abnormalities in STAT3 [56]. Large quantities of "tyrosine phosphorylated STAT5" are linked with an adverse projection in numerous "myeloid neoplasms" [57].

Cancer & STAT Family Protein

Triggered STATs, especially "STAT1", "STAT3" and "STAT5", have originated in various tumors (including vascular malignancies and solid tumors) in humans and cancer cell lines. STAT3 and STAT5 may have the greatest important role in the expansion of cancer, especially STAT3 is very captivating [58].

1. STAT1 has two appearances in cancer related to humans. It can either be an oncoprotein or a suppressor of tumour. It is a significant constituent of signalling of IFN; triggered STAT1 generally plays the role of suppressor of tumors in cells of cancer [59].

Active STAT1 mutants increase the record and countenance of some pre-apoptotic genes and cycle of the cell (such as "caspase", "Bcl-2", "Bcl-XL", "p27" and "p21WAF") [60]. Abnormal activation of STAT1 has been reported in numerous kinds of human cancers, such as breast cancer, pneumonia, lung cancer and head cancer, as well as lymphoma [61]. STAT1 has two isoforms: the longer STAT1α isoform, which is the physically dynamic type of STAT1, and also the shorter STAT1β isoform, which is the physical inhibitor of STAT1.

2. STAT2: Its anti-tumor effect and its role in immune tumors *in vivo* are still controversial. STAT2 is essential for IFNI's antiviral, immunomodulatory, anti-apoptotic and proliferative properties, leading to the belief that STAT2 has tumor-inhibiting properties [62].

3. STAT3: It is closely related to the advancement of tumor growth and immunodeficiency, and is the only STAT family member that destroys the genetic effects of embryos [63].

Active STAT3 protein prevents p53-mediated development monitoring and apoptosis [64]. STAT3 binds to the IL-6 supporter area, resulting in augmented IL-6 expression, thus forming an optimistic reaction loop on the "IL-6/JAK/STAT3" path. A comparable optimistic reaction may occur for NF-κB, because NF-κB is often over-activated in humanoid cancers and leads to the discharge of cellular changes, counting IL-6 [65]. STAT3 initiation encourages proteins that determine the proliferation tumour and endurance. It turns to convert immune cells inside the TME, thus inspiring the making of extra "proinflammatory cytokines", like "IL-1β", "IL-8", "CCL2", "CCL3", "CCL5" and "GMCSF" [66]. STAT3 upregulates factors that are immunosuppressive, counting TGF-β and IL-10; these two can also trigger STAT3 and make an additional loop that feed-forward amid STAT3 cells of cancer. STAT3 regulates negatively "NK cells", "effector T cells", "dendritic cells" and neutrophils, whereas it regulate positively regulatory T cells and MDSCs [67]. STAT3 encourages the creation of "miR-21" and "miR-181b-1", which overwhelm the tumor suppressors' countenance of the ubiquitin "carboxyl-terminal hydrolase", "PTEN" and "CYLD", correspondingly [68, 69].

4. STAT4: The degradation of STAT4 leads to the inhibition of cell transport, incursion and metastasis, which is an important part of gastric cancer metastasis [70]. The increase in STAT4 expression is confidently connected with the gravity of incursion in CRC patients. Though, the precise role of STAT4 with regard to cancer is still uncertain, because the levels of expression are high [71].

5. STAT5: Denotes two proteins, "STAT5a" and "STAT5b", which have 94% construction capacity, but are transliterated from distinct genes. Methods to promote STAT5 instigation and play important carcinogenic effects include proteins in human cancers, counting changes of epigenetic, hormone-regulated and miRNA protease pathway changes, gene amplification, and atypical growth factor markers [72]. STAT5 delivers its oncogenic commotion as follows:

- Causes anti-apoptotic messenger, abnormal response to DNA harm and invasion, and changes in the transcription or interaction of proteins and proteins [63]. The "TGF-β", "PI3K/PTEN" and "HIF1α-signaling" pathways. Antiapoptotic paths. The G1/S evolution path. The DNA impairment control path [73].

STAT5 is included in cell transport and epithelial cell incursion [74]. In continuing "myelogenous leukemia (CML)", the mediating action of BCR-ABL, as well as multiple myeloma and lymphoma, are all related to the TEL/JAK2 of cancer, which is essential for its carcinogenic effects [75]. However, STAT5 protein can similarly regulate genes that have suppressor activity of tumour. The activated STAT5 predicts a good prognosis for breast cancer patients and rhinoplasty patients. STAT5b has a hepatoprotective effect to prevent continuing liver injury [76].

6. STAT6 can organize many processes besides the immune response, including the proliferation of cancer cells, resistance to apoptosis, metastasis, epithelial cell activity, chromosome closure, and DNA damage and repair [34]. The continuous activation of STAT6 in different cancers can lead to proliferation, survival and metastasis, as well as reduced tumor resistance [34]. STAT6 signal is usually triggered in malicious cells and adjusts several genes that are essential for immune reply, irritation and propagation [77].

STAT Proteins as Targets for Treatment

STAT gesticulating can be targeted in either direct ways or indirect ways [11].

- Agents directing upstream features, for example, the "JAK1/2 inhibitor ruxolitinib" for the cure of multicellular organisms and main myelofibrosis, the "pan-JAK inhibitor tofacitinib" for the handling of arthritis, and the IL-6 antibodies siltuximab [78].
- Drugs that directly target STAT can inhibit STAT protein dimerization or disrupt "STAT DNA" bind or constrain "STAT mRNA". So far, the chief focus of drug improvement pertaining to this arena is the expansion of inhibitors of STAT3, which are essential for fetal development, but not for normal or unchanged tissues and cells [79].

STAT3 inhibitors can reduce the effect of known cancerous tumors, thereby increasing the appearance of IL-6, thus circuitously activating the JAKSTAT3 pathway that inhibits STAT3, thereby inducing p53-mediated tumor cell infection and promoting tumors Reticence of growth of the cell. Opening. On the other hand, under certain circumstances, active STAT3 may have a tumor suppressor effect. Therefore, the clinical use of STAT3 inhibitors is ultimately needed to examine the part of STAT3 in each precise kind of tumor and, perchance, in each subject [80].

STAT Engagement in Immunotherapy

As mentioned above, each STAT protein regulates its optimal immunomodulatory effect, which is mediated by the main activated cytokines. However, a single cytokine knows how to regulate the triggering of numerous STAT members. This leads to a procedure in which the consistency of the subtle and multifaceted communications of dissimilar molecules of STAT will guide the control of the immune system [81].

Suppressing the immune system (ICI) is a promising new therapy that can be used to treat many types of tumors with a response rate of less than 30%. To solve this problem, the fusion method that combines ICI and other immunosuppressive drugs is considered an important step forward [82]. The expression of "PD-1" and "PD-L1" is mostly controlled by IFN-γ-linked JAK/STAT motioning [83].

Whereas, compared with these antibodies, the degradation of "PD-1" and/or "PD-L1" by inhibitors of JAK/STAT may end in PD-1 blockers (such as pembrolizumab and nivolumab) due to condensed protein countenance. The efficacy is reduced [11]. It is proved that the degradation of JAK2 and treatment with Ruxolitinib can inhibit the countenance of "PD-L1" and regulate the infiltration and activation of cytotoxic T cells [84].

"STAT1" and "STAT3" are possible biomarkers that can be used to identify those patients that have the tendency to be more responsive with regards to immunotherapy [85 - 87].

Therapeutic Techniques of Targeting STATS

STAT3/5-Targeting RNAi

Several small molecules that inhibit cytokines and factors of growth, inhibit "STAT3 dimerization", inhibit STAT3 / STAT3 nuclear transformation, or inhibit the activity of DNA have studied the inhibitory effects of STAT3. Because of cytotoxicity and limitations of specificity, the progress of STAT3 inhibitors that are pharmacological is limited [88]. Targeting low molecular weight inhibitors with STAT3 or numerous methods that are not specific may cause many unwanted side effects. Therefore, it is necessary to deliver these inhibitors by linking these inhibitors with drugs to specificity upsurge and evade causing undesirable results [89, 90].

Afterward the introduction of siRNA, they would be assimilated into the "RNA-induced silencing complex (RISC)", one element of the complex will be detached, and the RISC will be directed by the other strand of antisense RNA to stop the conversion of other arrangements of mRNA [91]. Genetic degradation can last for 1 week in decomposing cells and several weeks in decomposing cells [92]. In general, siRNA-directed STAT3 / 5 has been shown to suppress apoptosis, cell cycle termination, and invasion of cancer cells in a variety of carcinoma cell models, including esophageal, breast, hepatocellular, prostate, colon cancers and bronchial [88, 93 - 98].

The main difficulty in developing SIRNA as a therapist is overcoming the poor distribution of SIRNA, as naked SIRNA can be broken down by extracellular RNAs in the bloodstream and, due to its molecular weight and net negative charge, cannot pass through cell membranes. To solve the problem, nanoparticles are often used to deliver naked siRNA as they protect the siRNA and help with endocytosis [92, 99].

Additional Approaches in Directing STAT3/5

- **Viral Vector**

Genetic information is naturally carried by viruses. "STAT3-directed siRNA" to subdue the propagation of cells of B16 melanoma with 95% efficacy of transduction [100]. Lentivirus vector system coordination with the LacZ correspondent synthesis system, the transmission efficiency of STAT3 mRNA is high and averages 85% in three lymphoma cells [101]. "LV-STAT3siRNA" showed a significant reduction in VEGF and MMP-2, decreased growth of cells, and a decreased invasive capacity of cancer cells. Because of their limited transgenic ability, virus-related vectors are used less frequently than non-viral vectors in the delivery of STAT3-RNAi [102].

- **Nanoparticles**

Non-viral vectors are less toxic, and easier to synthesize, and the immune response introduces siRNA than viral vectors [103]. High molecular weight polyethyleneimine can arouse the outline of siRNA in the cytoplasm by binding cationic lipids to the intracellular membrane layers, but also generating responsive species of oxygen and discharge of Ca^{2+} [104].

- **Polyethyleneimine (PEI)**

PEI has high toxicity; PEI was adapted with stearic acid (StA) to overcome high toxicity and improve the sedative effect of STAT3. IL-6 secretion increased cellular caspase3 expression and decreased VEGF creation [105].

- **Inorganic Compounds**

To improve constancy and cell absorption, nanoparticles coated with chitosan gold were used to treat miRNAomes cells to co-deliver "STAT3 siRNA" and statin siRNA and imatinib (IM). Gold nanoparticles are biocompatible, chemically inert, nanosynthetic, adaptable and have a longer blood flow. Stat3 siRNA based on plasmids presented by "$CaCl_2$-modified hydroxyapatite (HAP)" nanoparticles were able to regulate the countenance of Stat3-related downstream genes by reducing the expression of Stat3, and p-Stat3 proteins in mice with prostate cancer have been [106].

• Solid Lipid Nanoparticles

Solid lipid particles have a diameter of 10 to 1000 nanometers, including a hot round. Solid lipid particles include a hot solid lipid core matrix that can dissolve lipophilic molecules. The lipid core is steadied by surfactants. The use of an emulsifier is located on the route of administration and parenteral administration limited to. A lipid term is used here in the broad sense and comprises triglycerides, diglycerides, monoglycerides, fatty acids, steroids and wax. All types of emulsifiers (amount charged molecular weight) were used to stabilize the lipid. No association found that emulsions effectively inhibit the grouping of particles [107].

• PAMAM Dendrimer

"Polyamide dendrimers" The dendrites are the most common. In one study, "EGFR gene oligonucleotides," as if it were the cell lines PAMA dendrimers as targeted colon cancer. EGFR expression levels were significantly reduced, resulting in the genes downstream of EGFR expression and the way MAPK1 STAT5. A hot particle delivery system to deliver FLT3 ligand, and amidoamine PAMA limited to MRR1 cells AML cells. Directly from the hot particles by way of signalling inhibits FLT3 inhibition of ERK activity *in vivo* AKT and STAT5 [108].

• Exosomes

The extracellular membrane vesicles Exosoma 30-120 m in diameter and endogenous genetic material such as proteins, lipids and DNA. Infection subpopulations two, EX-L and EX-S, contains secretory proteins involved in the regulation of turns, including the "2-2 / STAT5 'means the route, which means that these nanoparticles from potential participants in the" STAT5 "targeted lorem [109].

Summary

Just ascertaining the activity of a single STAT member is not enough to correlate with the nature of the disease, but instead, it should be remembered when trying to apply a balanced (neutral) STAT-related diagnostic or therapeutic tool between family members [11].

Nuclear Factor-Kb (Nf-Kb) Tumor Transcription Factor

Definition of NF-κB

One of the essential transcription factors for human health is Nuclear factor-κB (NF-κB), which are encompassed in possession of a large number of biological and normal cellular procedures, including developmental procedures, cellular development, apoptosis, and inflammatory responses [110, 111].

Different inflammatory stimuli activate NF-κB, including infectious microbes and development factors. A number of genes are expressed through NF-κB controls for regulating immune responses to different stimuli, elevation, apoptosis, stress responses, cell development, survival, growth of a variety of stimuli, and embryogenesis [103, 112].

NF-κB Subunits

A total of five associated transcription factors are comprised within the NF-B family, specifically in mammals, which include RelA (p65), RelB, c-Rel, NF-κB1 p50, and NF-κB2 p52, which form different dimeric developments that transactivate numerous target genes through binding to the κB enhancer [113].

1. The inactive NF-B complexes reside in the cytoplasm in a complicated form with any of the inhibitory protein family members in most cells, including IκBα and other ankyrin repeat-containing proteins. When the platform is activated, the repressive protein is tarnished, and the NF-B complex enters the nucleus to moderate target gene expression [114, 115].

2. Proteasome processing is experienced within p105 and p100 for producing the mature NF-κB1 and NF-κB2 proteins (p50 and p52), resulting in IκB-like function interruption of these predecessor proteins [116].

An N-terminal DNA-binding/dimerization domain is associated with the NF-κB family, which allows the formation of homodimers and heterodimers as well as binding with a number of associated targeted DNA sequences for modulating gene expression. C-terminal transcription activation domains are comprised within Rel/Nf-Kb RelA, c-Rel and RelB, allowing them to activate targeted gene expression [117, 118]. The mature NF-B subunits are produced, including p50 and p52, after pretreatment of p105 and p100 *via* a proteasome or ubiquitin platform encompassing selective degradation of their C terminal region.

C-terminal trans-activation domains are absent in p50 and p52; hence, they do not possess an inherent competence for activating transcription and acting as transcriptional inhibitors when binding B elements as homologous markers regardless of forming dimers with other class members [119].

NF-κB Signalling Pathway

A family of inhibitors sequesters the NF-κB dimers in the cytoplasm, such as IκBs, comprising several alternatives of a sequence in less-triggered cells [120, 121]. The nuclear localization signals are masked through the IκB proteins and retain them sequestered in the cytoplasm in a sedentary state by the quality of their ankyrin repeat areas [118, 122]. It has been noted that p100 and p105 react as IκB proteins due to the occurrence of ankyrin repeats in their C-terminal halves. NF-κB dimer activation is potentiated through IκBδ degradation in a NIK-reliant non-canonical pathway with respect to developmental stimuli (Fig. **7.1**) [123].

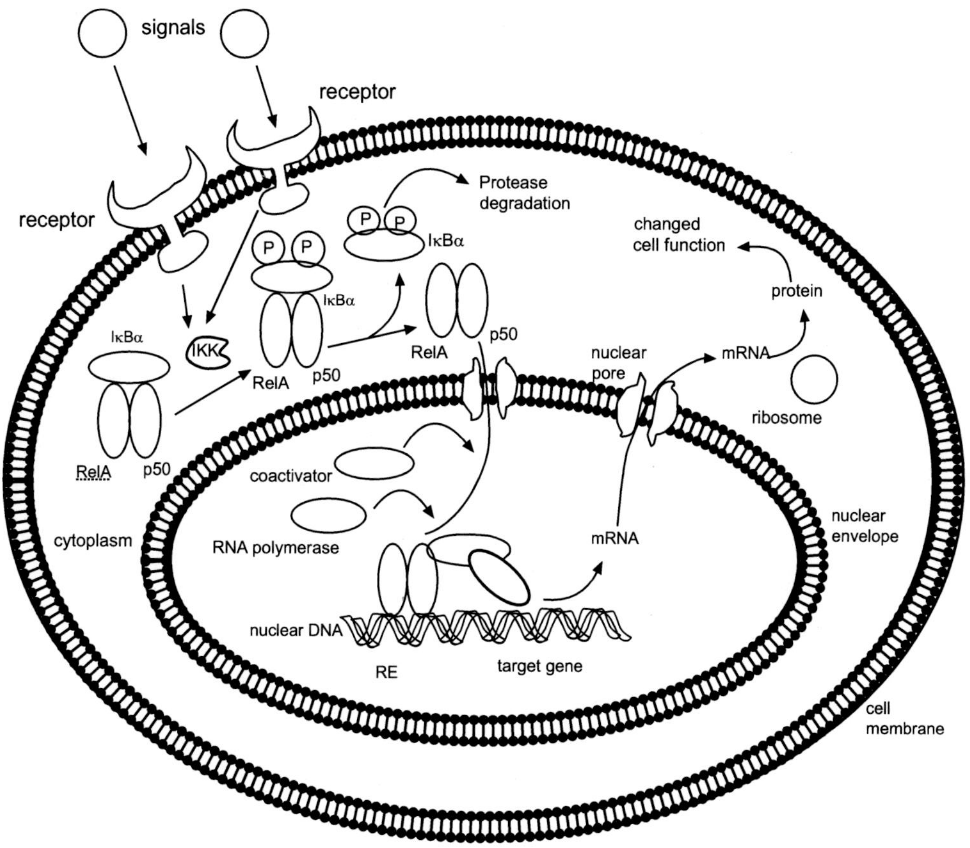

Fig. (7.1). NF-kB signalling pathway.

Canonical Pathway

Destructing IκBα allows the formation of canonical NF-κB pathway, which lead to nuclear translocation of complexes, majorly the p50/p65 dimer [124]. This destruction is done through phosphorylation using the IκB kinase (IKK) for establishing trimeric catalytic subunits [125]. Two serine remains positioned in an IκB regulatory domain are phosphorylated through the IκB kinase, leading to its proteasome degradation (Fig. **7.2**) [126, 127].

The NF-κB complex arrives in the nucleus, where it can switch the appearance of different genes, possessing DNA-binding regions with the degradation of IκB [126, 127]. Different biological procedures were provided through the activation of such genes since inflammatory circumstances or immune response [128]. Its repressor is then expressed through NF-κB, inhibiting afterward and establishing an auto-feedback platform to derive oscillating levels of NF-κB activity [126, 127]. A number of essential biological functions are thus controlled through this NF-κB pathway, including dendritic cell (DC) activation, bone metabolism regulation, lymphoid organogenesis, B-cell survival and development, and the immune system.

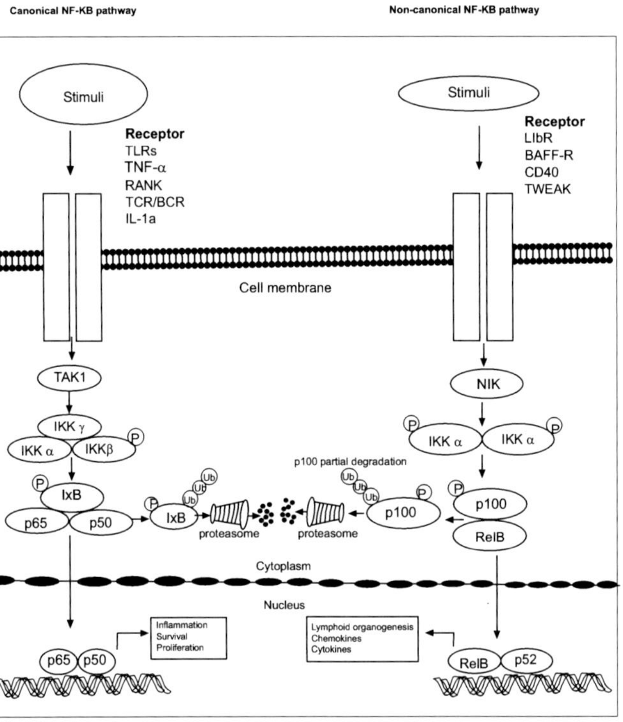

Fig. (7.2). The conical NF-kB pathway.

Non-Canonical Pathway

The RelB/p52 NF-κB complex is activated by the non-canonical NF-κB platform in the presence of the inducible dispensation of p100 as compared to the degradation of IκBα. P52 is generated after processing p100, while it further induces the nuclear translocation of the RelB/p52 heterodimer [129]. P100 is the most essential element of NF-κB2 in a majority of the cell types [130, 131]. In mammalian cells, p52 is converted through overexpressing p100 as compared to the constitutive generation of p50 from p105 [132]. An IKK complex is utilized within this platform to activate NIK for phosphorylating an IKK alpha complex that switches the IκB domain of p100 to the deliverance of p52/RelB [133]. The translocation of this heterodimer is subsequent with respect to the nucleus activating targeted genes [133, 134].

Both RelA and RelB are activated through an integrated NF-B system network, comprising of a dimer. The disrupted canonical platform will induce an abnormal cellular reaction using the non-canonical platform (Fig. **7.3**) [133, 135]. Lymphoid malignancies are related to deregulated non-canonical NF-κB signaling [136, 137]. This platform is activated through cell-differentiating or developmental spurs, including receptor activators of nuclear factor kappa-B ligand, lymphotoxin-α, and B-cell activation factor [138].

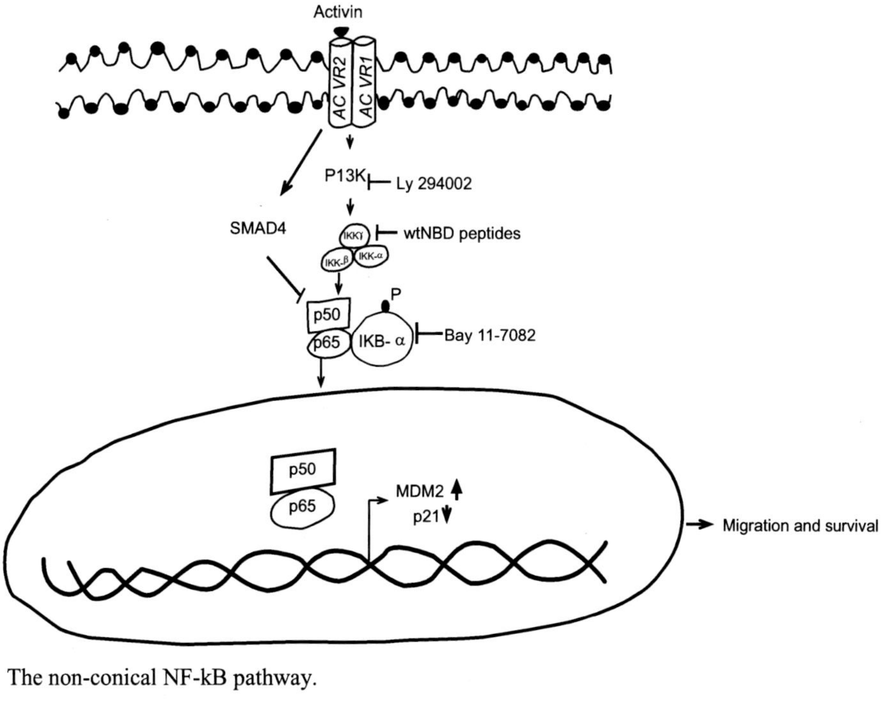

Fig. (7.3). The non-conical NF-kB pathway.

Role of NF-κB in Cancer

Cancer triggered by gene deletions, mutations, and chromosomal translocations disrupt genes for encoding NF-κB as well as IκB proteins in order to separate NF-κB aspects from their inhibitors and regulators to activate NF-κB [139]. In addition, NF-κB is regulated, in tumor cells, because of mutations in genes that encode the NF-κB transcription aspects or in genes. Moreover, factors are secreted through some tumor cells, activating NF-κB [140, 141].

Mechanisms Implicated in Tumor Generation

1. The transcription of genes is stimulated through NF-κB to encode G1 cyclins. Consequently, the cyclin D1 promotor shows the presence of a κB [110, 140, 142, 143].

2. The transcription of several targeted genes is activated through NF-κB that restrict the initiation of apoptosis by TNF-α and other pro-apoptotic elements of this family [127, 144, 145]. Cellular inhibitors of apoptosis are encompassed within the anti-apoptotic factors [127].

3. Production of chemokines is deregulated through cells with raised NF-κB, elevating migratory activity [110]. Angiogenesis is increased with the regulation of NF-κB [146].

4. Additionally, the promoters of genes identify κB sites for encoding different matrix metalloproteinases that assist in invading tumors of surrounding tissues [147]. Cancer cells destroy NF-κB into one of the enablers of the extracellular matrix [148, 149].

5. Continuous NF-κB activity is increased by reactive oxygen species in inflammation, therefore, destructing DNA of subsequent epithelial cells [150]; for instance, gastrointestinal cancer [151].

6. NF-κB acts as a Fas transcription enabler in the canonical pathway, whereas transcription repressor is the alternative to NF-κB [152].

NF-κB (Transcription Factor in Tumors)

NF-κB as a Transcription Factor

One of the main enablers of cellular stress, immune responses, and inflammation is the transcription factor NF-κB. In addition, its engagement has been widely observed in the regulation of cancer cell survival, invasion and neoplastic angiogenesis, chemical resistance, and elevation. The IκB inhibitor adversely regulates NF-κB, insulating NF-κB to the cytoplasm. The occurrence of NFκB activation is seen through the activity of IKKs, phosphorylating IKKs and enabling the degradation of IκB arbitrated by the protozoa. Afterward, the nucleus transmits NF-κB and establishes a functional heterozygote with retinal oncogene A. Direct genetic drift of NF-κB coding genes causes aberrant NFκB activity. The transactional likelihood of NF-κB is activated through AKT using different mechanisms.

The first mechanism can phosphorylate the IKK α subunit to improve IKK activity [153, 154]. IKK activity is indirectly stimulated in the second phase by targeting the phosphorylation of organic molecules in the MAPK platform, which includes p38 and the Osaka thyroid adenocarcinoma [155, 156]. The third and final platform directs the transactional domain of REL-A and elevates NF-κB activity [155, 157].

NF-κB in Brain Tumors

Due to precancerous stress signals, cytokine stimulation activates or regulates glioblastoma. Constitutive activation of the ultimate signalling networks is led by epidermal growth factor receptor amplification or demonstration of the oncogenic EGFR mutation, which includes the PI3K pathway. The binding between binder 1, tyrosine phosphatase, Grb-2 bound anchoring protein, and the src-2 domain homologation region is catalyzed through GBM cells.

Different other growth factor receptor signals activate abnormally NF-κB in GBM, activating PI3K in GBM. Platelet-derived growth factor, regardless of EGF, activates NF-κB in GBM cells as well as both of PDGF and EGF-reliant pathways [153, 158, 159]. In GBM replication, the role of NF-κB is constant with its planned contribution in GBM precursor cell biology and propagation, which is assumed to be because of the NFκB reliant parameter of cancer stem cell genes, such as cyclin D1 and CD44.

NF-κB Inhibition using Chemical Compounds

A number of different types of cancer cells rely on NF-κB signalling for development and survival after hindering NF-κB *via* chemical compounds, such as small molecule inhibitors.

- Multiple sclerosis can be treated *via* dimethyl fumarate that overwhelms NF-κB signalling effectively as well as stimulates the development of human breast cancer cells effectively [160]. On the contrary, apoptosis is caused by chronic lymphocytic leukemia cells.

- There is appealing experimental information that stimulation of NF-κB signalling changes the maximum carcinogenic attributes of both GBM cells and glioma-like cells in terms of brain cancer. Differentiation of human GSCs and reduced invasive potential is stimulated through a cytolytic peptide enabler of NF-κB.
- Clearly, SN50 caused mitigated neoplasia and elevated sensitivity to standard cytotoxic treatments utilized in TMZ, GBM, and radiation exposure in mouse xenograft models [161].

GBM cell death is induced through other NF-κB enablers such as curcumin, arsenic trioxide, parthenolide, and BAY117082 [162]. The entire surgical removal of tumors is prevented through the invasion of GBM cells into a healthy brain parenchyma [163].

Activating Mutations of NF-κB Pathway

In Eukaryotes, the NF-κB platform is a relatively conserved signalling platform where its constituents are engaged in the diagnosed chromosomal reclassifications in gene fusion and cancer cells [144, 145, 164, 165]. High expression of NF-κB family members recommend the contribution of the NF-κB platform in HL [166]. High HL is correlated with mutations of the NF-κB enabler alpha and alpha-induced tumor necrosis factor 3 [167, 168]. Inhibitors regulating NF-κB activity are restricted to NF-κB and merely release NF-κB after glycolysis [169]. NF-κB expression is encouraged and activated with the use of cytokines or cytotoxic drugs in some tumors [169 - 171].

Such induced activation can be inhibited by 1st curcumin and other derivatives. For instance, curcumin derivatives have reflected a reduction in TFR-induced expression, specifically in neuroblastoma and melanoma cells [169].

Curcumin indicates the NF-κB -inhibitory activity with other stimulating phytochemicals include capsaicin [172]. The NF-κB platform is possibly activated through 2nd Vitamin D, in the majority of the cases, inhibiting the NF-κB activation [173 - 176]. There was no evidence in reserve of NF-κB by vitamin D [177], specifically in Jurkat cells. This shows that some of the cancer cells have disturbed this platform, surprisingly, NF-κB can restrict VDR signals, and this cross-inhibition may demonstrate the corresponding high constitutive VDR expression and activated NF-κB in lymphoma cells [178].

NF-kB and Activin-Induced Colorectal Cancer Migration

Migration and cell viability are affected through NF-kBactivation after inducing genes encompassed in matrix degradation and genes in their survival [179, 180].

Cell viability is reduced by activin in colon cancer [181, 182]. The importance of NF-κB has been demonstrated for activating inflammatory cytokine with a SMAD4-based pathway [183]. Others have indicated that epithelial activation of NF-κB is essential for the growth of colitis-related colorectal cancer. The core aspect in the context of the dual pro and anti-tumor actions is based on correlation between NF-κB and activin signalling pathways [184].

NF-κB Hyperactivation and Esophageal Squamous Cell Carcinoma

NF-κB activation has been induced through the conditional loss of p120ctn in the esophagus, specifically in esophageal adenomas [185]. In recent times, human ESCC tissue upregulates NF-κB p65 expression more than cancer tissue and is, thus, related to progressive clinical-stage lymph node metastasis [186]. The occurrence of NF-κB activation is frequently observed in CRC related to colitis and focuses on the development of cancer [187]. NF-κB activation was reserved and the modifications in migration monitored include the HCT116 colon cancer cell line model system due to the important role played in activin-induced migration. HCT116 is the parent strain that lacks expression of the activin receptor, whereas its alternative is complemented by human chromosome 2, which reestablishes the expression as well as activity of the activin receptor [188].

Summary

The activity of NF-κB signalling is important for the survival of normal lymphocytes as well as the majority of the B cell tumor types, which include multiple myeloma. MM tumors are facilitated through NF-κB activation mutations to become less reliant on the bone marrow signals for activating NF-κB. The most prevalent among the types of NF-kB mutations are NFkB inducing kinase. It is also considered the core activator kinase of the subsequent NF-κB platform, even though the classical platform is further activated *via* NIK's overexpression.

WNT (Β)-CATENIN SIGNALING

Introduction

Wnt (β)-Catenin signalling pathway is required for a variety of biological activities during embryogenesis including cell development into a final cell type that involves several processes, such as cell proliferation migration and apoptosis or autophagy [189]. Oncogenic processes of the mouse mammary tumor virus were studied by Nusse and his colleague in 1982. During that period, the mouse *wnt1* gene was identified as the first element of the Wnt-signalling pathway [190]. *INT1* was the first name for Wnt1, which represented the integration site in breast tumors caused by a virus. Human *INT1* was later found to be quite analogous to mouse *INT1*, proposing that this pathway is exceptionally rationed across living beings [191]. Many other genes were discovered in mouse mammary tumor virus and linked to other genetic pathways during further analysis for proviral inclusion locales in tumors, including *INT2, INT3*, and *INT4* [192 - 194]. Wnt signalling includes Wnt proteins, receptors for Wnt proteins, and signalling modulators.

Wnt (β)-Catenin Signalingprotein

A minimum of nineteenth human proto-oncogenes has been found according to genome sequencing, which encodes a family of cysteine-rich Wnt proteins (350-400 a.a. long). These WNT glycoproteins can be further classified into twelve conserved Wntsubtypes. The proteins of WNTs are strongly conserved across a wide variety of animals, including invertebrates and mammals [195]. Cells release Wnt proteins into the non-cellular component present in the extracellular matrix, which stimulates receptor-mediated signalling pathways in neighboring cells [196, 197].

Wnt is expressed abundantly in every mammal cell. Wnt protein are globular structures with a molecular weight of about 40 kDa. The C terminal domain consists primarily of two β-sheets with six disulfide bridges, while the N terminal domain is dominated by α-helices with five disulfide bridges, while the carboxy-terminal domain consists of two β-sheets with six disulfide bridges. Wnt is extremely difficult to dissolve due to the post-translational modification in the protein structure prior to their release into the extracellular cytoplasmic milieu. The post-translational modifications involve glycosylation and palmitoylation and are required for Wnt activity [198, 199]. Porcupin (Porc), an endoplasmic reticulum protein, glycosylates and palmitoylates Wnt protein, then Wntlessproteins (Wls) transport it to the plasma membrane [200]. Porc or Wls deficiency inhibits Wnt proteins function, which causes birth defects [201, 202]. Wnt proteins appear to function in direct communication through cell-cell or cell-matrix contact and also function in distant tissue through indirect communication. The stimulation of the Wnt receptor initiates three signalling pathways:

1. Wnt/β-catenin signalling pathway (Canonical).

2. β-catenin-independent signalling pathway (Non-canonical), also referred to as the noncanonical planar cell polarity (PCP) pathway [203].

3. Wnt/Ca^{2+} signalling pathway.

Wnt/β-catenin signalling is the most considered pathway, and it is the focus of this section.

Wnt/β-Catenin Signalling Receptor: Frizzled and LRP5/6

The Frizzled receptor proteins (Fz or Fzd) and the lipopolysaccharide receptor proteins 5 and 6 (LRP5 and LRP6) are both two fundamental receptor families for Wnt/-catenin signaling. Fz and LRP5/6 receptor complex binds to Wnt lipoprotein *via* its large N-terminal extra-cellular cysteine-rich domain. Fz family is a seven-pass transmembrane protein receptor and functions as Wnt signaling's primary receptor [204, 205]. Fz protein belongs to the G-protein-coupled (GPCRs) membrane receptor superfamily. Wnt and Fz proteins interact in a not restricted manner; one Wnt protein interacts with number of Fz proteins. The lipid hanging out of the Wnt protein integrates into a hydrophobic cavity in Fz, demonstrated by the Wnt-Frizzled binding configuration [206]. In contrast to the Fz protein, LRP6 has diverse restricting locales for various Wnt proteins [207].

Wnt/β-Catenin Signaling Modulators

Aside from the notable receptors Frizzled and LRP, the table below lists a variety of other extracellular ligands that modulate Wnt/-catenin signalling (Table **7.1**). Wnt signalling modulators may either act as an antagonist or an agonist. An antagonist binds to the Wnt receptor but not triggers a reaction and instead blocks it. Opposite to that is the agonist modulators which bind to the receptor and generate a reaction within the cell. R-spondins are an example of an activator modulator [208]. To stimulate the Fz/LRP complex and promote Wnt signaling, R-spondins bind to other cell surface members of the Leucine-rich repeat-containing G-protein coupled receptor 5 (LGR5) family [209 - 211]. ZNRF3 and RNF3 are transmembrane proteins and function as a down regulator for the Wnt signalling pathway *via* their E3 ubiquitin ligases' effect on Frizzled proteins, allowing these receptors to turn over which lead to inhibition of the Wnt signalling [212, 213].

Wnt Signalling Functions in Cancer Progression

Cell proliferation, metastasis and apoptosis are controlled by the Wnt/β-catenin signalling pathway [224]. Genes involved in Wnt pathway are often mutated in tumors, demonstrating that they play key role in carcinogenesis. Colorectal cancer is identified with a significant increase in β-catenin and TC4 expression levels and with a significant decrease in APC and AXIN2 in expression level [225 - 227]. Furthermore, deletion in the LRP5 receptor leads to down-regulation in the Wnt pathway in hyper-parathyroid tumors [228]. Moreover, a mutation in LEF1 and AXIN1 has been connected to the downregulation of the Wnt signalling pathway in sebaceous skin tumors and hepatocellular carcinoma [229, 230].

Table 7.1. Wnt antagonists and agonists.

Modulator	Annotation	Effect	Function
sFRPs	Secreted Frizzled-related proteins	Wnt antagonists	Inhibit β-catenin and noncanonical signalling through binding to Wnt and Fz [214].
WIF	Wnt inhibitory protein	Wnt antagonists	Inhibit β-catenin and noncanonical signalling through binding to Wnt [214].
DKK	Dickkopffamily	Wnt antagonists	Inhibit Wnt/ β-catenin signalling as they are LRP5/6 antagonists ligands which cause interruption of Wnt- Fz-LRP6 complex production or cause degradation of LRP6 through Kremen transmembrane protein (Krm) [215, 216].
SOST	Sclerostin	Wnt antagonists	Inhibit Wnt/ β-catenin signalling as they are LRP5/6 antagonists ligands. *In vitro*,it can interrupt Wnt-induced Fz-LRP6 complex [217 - 219].
SHISA	Shisafamily member	Wnt antagonists	Inhibit Wnt/ β-catenin signalling as they bound Fz proteins in the endoplasmic reticulum and blocking them from reaching the cell surface [220].
Cer	Xenopus Cerberus	Wnt antagonists	Inhibit Wnt/ β-catenin signalling through binding to Wnt protein [221].
BMP	bone morphogenetic protein	Wnt antagonists	Inhibit Wnt/ β-catenin signalling through binding to Wnt protein [221].
IGFBP-4	Insulin-like growth-factor bindingprotein-4	Wnt antagonists	Besides to role in modulating IGF signaling, it inhibits Wnt/ β-catenin signalling through binding to both Fz and LRP6 [222].
Norrin	Norrie disease protein	Wnt agonists	It is the FZD4 ligand that works through FZD4 and LRP5/6 to activate the Fz/LRP complex, which therefore activates Wnt signalling during retinal vascularization [223].

NOTCH AND HEDGEHOG SIGNALLING PATHWAYS

Introduction

WNT, NOTCH, and HH signalling pathways are fundamental regulators that influence cell differentiation and proliferation. Embryonic lethality frequently occurs when a single gene of the three pathways is depleted [231]. Adult gene mutations in these pathways, which likely result in signalling activation, have been linked to the cancer progression [232 - 234]. Hedgehog and Notch pathways' function in cancer progression has been widely investigated [235, 236]. They are major signalling pathways that are commonly triggered in a variety of tumors. In addition to their role in tumor initiation, they are usually enhanced in many tumors processes, such as tumor progression and metastasis. Furthermore, they play a key role in the regulation of the cancer stem cell [237]. The NOTCH and HH signalling pathways have significant cellular signals integration, highlighting how complicated the tumor micro-environmental signals can be.

Notch Signalling Pathway

The Notch signalling pathway was initially introduced in 1917 during a study of Drosophila melanogaster that revealed notches development in the wings as a result of a genetic disorder [238]. The Notch signalling is fundamental for different platforms and critical for the growth of various organs such as the hematopoietic system [239, 240]. Furthermore, this pathway is essential during embryonic development because it greatly influences patterns for the cell to cell interactions that define each cell's fate and facilitate various cell differentiation [241]. In addition to that, several studies have demonstrated that the notch signalling pathway has a significant effect as an oncogene as well as tumor suppression [237, 242]. Dysregulation of the notch pathway has been linked to tumor development. For instance, when the Notch signalling pathway is activated, CSC development and survival are promoted [243, 244]. Some neoplasms caused by Notch pathway dysregulation include diffuse large B-cell lymphoma (DLBCL) and T-cell acute lymphoblastic leukaemia (T-ALL) [245, 246]. Furthermore, dysregulation of this pathway also has some negative impacts. Some of the impacts can cause human birth defects, such as cerebral autosomal dominant arteriopathy with subcortical infarcts and leukoencephalopathy (CADASIL), Allagile syndrome (ALGS), and spondylocostaldysostosis (SCDO), and Hajdu-Cheney syndrome (HCS) [247 - 250].

The Components and Process of Notch Signalling Pathways

The Notch signalling pathways in vertebrate consists of 4 NOTCH receptors and 5 Notch ligands: the receptors are Notch1, Notch2, Notch3 and Notch4, and the ligands are Jagged-1 (JAG1), Jagged-2 (JAG2), Delta-like-1 (Dll-1), Delta-like-3 (Dll-3) and Delta-like-4 (Dll-4) [251]. The mediation between the receptor and the ligand is done by the fringe family of glycosyltransferases, constituting lunatic, maniac, and radical fringe which offer extra specificity for receptor-ligand interactions [240]. The ligands-receptors interaction initiates the pathway's activation, which prompts the Notch receptors to undergo a series of consecutive proteolytic cleavages as a result of this. The receptor's proteolytic cleavage is necessary for signaling.

1. While transportation through the Golgi apparatus, the first cleavage incident occurs which is controlled by Furin-like convertases, leading to the development of heterodimeric transmembrane Notch protein [239, 240, 252, 253].

2. A second Notch cleavage incident occurs extracellularly when the Notch ligands are recognized on the surface of other nearby cells catalyzed by ADAM10, a member of the ADAM metalloproteases.

3. The third cleavage occurs intracellularly by γ-secretase, which is known to release a notch intracellular domain (NICD) [239, 240].

Construction of a transcriptional activation complex appears when the NICD release and translocate to the nucleus, then, it joins bind the transcription factor CSL/RBP-Jk. At this phase, a member of Mastermind-like (MAML) family member is recruited in the process so that transcription of target genes can be enabled to stimulate the expression of a number of genes such as Myc, and CyclinD [239, 240, 254, 255].

The Hedgehog Signalling Pathway

The hedgehog pathway (HH) was identified for the first time in 1980 [256]. It has important involvement throughout embryonic development and the regeneration of various tissues and organs. The main function of this pathway is to improve embryonic structure and composition, in addition to its key role in adult tissue homeostasis [257]. Consequently, abnormal embryonic development as well as adult tumor progression, and cell proliferation likely arise as a result of HH pathway dysregulation, such as overexertion or mutations in this pathway's genes [258 - 261]. It is also reported that HH pathways are associated with *in vitro* and *in vivo* cancer metastasis [237]. Furthermore, this pathway has a recognized function in other diseases, for instance, it has been implicated in holoprosencephaly, basal cell carcinomas, Gorlin syndrome, and medulloblastomas [262]. Other functions of the pathway also include the survival of progenitor cells and multiple stem cell differentiation while continuing the undifferentiated state [263]. However, the conclusions are inconsistent, with reports from many experiments contradicting each other [264, 265].

The Components and Process of Hedgehog Signalling Pathway

Hedgehog signalling pathway involves three ligand proteins in a mammal, which are sonic (Shh), Indian (Ihh), and desert (Dhh). The two stages hedgehog signalling mechanism have described are as follows:

1- At the signal-secreting cells: HH is usually adjusted by adding cholesterol post-translationally, which triggers a self-cleavage process. After that, they go through a palmitoylation event which is catalyzed by acyltransferase Skinny HH. HH protein is released from the cells with the help of dispatched protein (disp), a 12-pass transmembrane protein [257, 266].

2- At the signal-receiving cells: HH proteins bind to the HH receptor, which is comprised of Patched 12-pass transmembrane protein receptors with the support of the CDON coreceptors, and bioregional CDON-restricting protein. This interaction removes the repression of the 7-pass transmembrane protein smoothened (Smo). Smoprotein remains inactive by the patched receptors if the HH protein-receptor interaction is missing [257, 266].

The activation of the Smo protein will be followed by the initiation of a downstream signalling transduction process that induces or downregulates the expression of the target genes. For example, the glioma-associated oncogene homologue isoforms (Gli-1,-2,-3) are activated in the cytoplasm and translocate to the nucleus as a result of Smo's downstream signalling activation. Gli-1,-2,-3 are transcription factors that regulate the expression of target genes, most genes of the cell cycle and proapoptotic signals genes [267].

Since the HH pathway plays a pivotal role from embryogenesis to adulthood, mutations or changes in its gene expression and their downstream components may result in development of a wide range of genetic disorders at various pathway stages. Noriaki *et al.* summarized a number of abnormalities in hedgehog-related genes that cause genetic disorders (Table **7.2**). Abnormalities in hedgehog-related genes rarely occur as full gene deletion in humans. Instead, HH genomic mutations commonly encode proteins with insufficient or suboptimal activity [268].

Table 7.2. Genetic disorders associated with mutations in hedgehog-related genes.

Gene Name	Annotation	Gene Product	-
Shh	Sonic Hedgehog	Signal secreted factor	Holoprosencephaly (HPE)
Dhh	Desert Hedgehog	Signal secreted factor	Gonadal dysgenesis
Ihh	Indian Hedgehog	Signal secreted factor	Brachydactyly, acrocapitofemoral dysplasia
HHAT	Hedgehog acyltransferase	Transmembrane acyltransferase at ER	Holoprosencephaly (HPE)
Disp	Dispatched	Membrane receptor	Holoprosencephaly (HPE)
Scube2	Signal Peptide, CUB Domain and EGF Like Domain Containing 2	Secreted and membrane-tethered	Colorectal Cancer
Chmp1a	Charged Multivesicular body Protein 1a	Endosomal protein (ESCRT-III)	Pontocerebellar hypoplasia
Ext1	ExostosinGlycosyltransferase 1	Glycosyltransferase	Hereditary multiple exostoses

(Table 7.2) cont.....

Gene Name	Annotation	Gene Product	-
NPC1	Niemann Pick type C1	Cholesterol transporter with transmembrane domains	Ataxia, dysphagia
DHCR7	7-dehydrocholesterol reductase	Enzyme	Smith-Lemli-Opitz syndrome (SLOS)
EHD1	EPS15-Homology Domain-containing protein 1	Membrane-binding protein	Not linked to disease
GPC3	Glypican-3	Heparan sulfate proteoglycan	Simpson-Golabi-Behmel overgrowth syndrome (SGBS)
Ptch1	Patched1	12-span transmembrane protein	Gorlin's syndrome, basal cell carcinoma, basal cell nevus syndrome
Ptch2	Patched2	12-span transmembrane protein	Medulloblastoma, basal cell carcinoma, basal cell nevus syndrome
Smo	Smoothened	G-protein coupled receptor	Curry-Jones Syndrome
Hhip	Hedgehoginteracting protein 1	Membrane protein	Chronic obstructive pulmonary disease (COPD)
Gas1	Growth-arrestspecific 1	GPI-anchored cell surface protein	Holoprosencephaly (HPE)
Cdo/Cdon	Cell-adhesion molecule-related, downregulated by oncogenes	Membrane protein of Immunoglobulin superfamily	Holoprosencephaly (HPE)
Boc	Brother of Cdo	Membrane protein of Immunoglobulin superfamily	Holoprosencephaly
LRP2	Low density lipoprotein related protein 2	Single-span receptor	Donnai-Barrow syndrome
CK1α	Casein kinase 1a	Serine/threonine kinase	Colorectal cancer
GRK2	G protein-coupled receptor kinase 2	Serine/threonine kinase	Granulosa cell tumors, thyroid carcinoma
β-Arr2	β-Arrestin2	GPCR modulator	Hepatocellular carcinoma
Kif3a	Kinesin Family Member 3A	Kinesin-like protein	Usher's syndrome
Kif7	Kinesin family member 7	Signal mediators-Kinesin 4 family	Acrocallosal syndromes, Joubert syndrome, Meckel syndrome
SuFu	Suppressor of Fused	Signal mediators-scaffold protein	Joubert syndrome, medulloblastoma, basal cell carcinoma, basal cell nevus syndrome

(Table 7.2) cont.....

Gene Name	Annotation	Gene Product	-
Spop	Speckle-type POZ protein	Signal mediators- E3 ubiquitin ligase adaptor	Prostate cancer
Gli1	GLI family zinc finger 1	Transcription factor	Ellis–van Creveld syndrome
Gli2	GLI family zinc finger 2	Transcription factor	Holoprosencephaly (HPE)
Gli3	GLI family zinc finger 3	Transcription factor	Greigcephalopolysyndactyly syndrome (GCPS)

CONCLUSION

Transcription factors are frequently deregulated in the pathogeneses of human cancer and involve in several carcinogenesis activities such as Proliferation, survival, metabolism, invasion, and metastasis. As a result, targeting transcription factors can be extremely effective in treating different types of cancers.

CONSENT FOR PUBLICATION

Not applicable.

CONFLICT OF INTEREST

The author declares no conflict of interest, financial or otherwise.

ACKNOWLEDGEMENTS

We thank King Abdullah International Medical Research Center (KAIMRC) and Um Al Qura University for their technical support.

REFERENCES

[1] Tilley WD, Clarke CL, Birrell SN, Bruchovsky N. Hormones and cancer: new insights, new challenges. Trends Endocrinol Metab 2001; 12(5): 186-8. [http://dx.doi.org/10.1016/S1043-2760(01)00393-9] [PMID: 11592245]

[2] Brivanlou AH, Darnell JE Jr. Signal transduction and the control of gene expression. Science 2002; 295(5556): 813-8. [http://dx.doi.org/10.1126/science.1066355] [PMID: 11823631]

[3] Thakur JK, Yadav A, Yadav G. Molecular recognition by the KIX domain and its role in gene regulation. Nucleic Acids Res 2014; 42(4): 2112-25. [http://dx.doi.org/10.1093/nar/gkt1147] [PMID: 24253305]

[4] Grandori C, Cowley SM, James LP, Eisenman RN. The Myc/Max/Mad network and the transcriptional control of cell behavior. Annu Rev Cell Dev Biol 2000; 16(1): 653-99. [http://dx.doi.org/10.1146/annurev.cellbio.16.1.653] [PMID: 11031250]

[5] Eisenman RN. Deconstructing Myc: Figure 1. Genes Dev 2001; 15(16): 2023-30. [http://dx.doi.org/10.1101/gad928101] [PMID: 11511533]

[6] Wu L, Timmers C, Maiti B, *et al.* The E2F1–3 transcription factors are essential for cellular proliferation. Nature 2001; 414(6862): 457-62. [http://dx.doi.org/10.1038/35106593] [PMID: 11719808]

[7] Eymin B, Karayan L, Séité P, *et al.* Human ARF binds E2F1 and inhibits its transcriptional activity. Oncogene 2001; 20(9): 1033-41. [http://dx.doi.org/10.1038/sj.onc.1204220] [PMID: 11314038]

[8] Darnell JE Jr. STATs and gene regulation. Science 1997; 277(5332): 1630-5. [http://dx.doi.org/10.1126/science.277.5332.1630] [PMID: 9287210]

[9] Teiten M-H, Blasius R, Morceau F, Diederich M, Dicato M. Signaling Chains 2007. [http://dx.doi.org/10.1016/B0-08-045044-X/00083-3]

[10] Bowman T, Garcia R, Turkson J, Jove R. STATs in oncogenesis. Oncogene 2000; 19(21): 2474-88. [http://dx.doi.org/10.1038/sj.onc.1203527] [PMID: 10851046]

[11] Darnell JE Jr, Kerr M, Stark GR. Jak-STAT pathways and transcriptional activation in response to IFNs and other extracellular signaling proteins. Science 1994; 264(5164): 1415-21. [http://dx.doi.org/10.1126/science.8197455] [PMID: 8197455]

[12] Abroun S, Saki N, Ahmadvand M, Asghari F, Salari F, Rahim F. STATs: An Old Story, Yet Mesmerizing. Cell J 2015; 17(3): 395-411. [http://dx.doi.org/10.22074/cellj.2015.1] [PMID: 26464811]

[13] Lim CP, Cao X. Structure, function, and regulation of STAT proteins. Mol Biosyst 2006; 2(11): 536-50. [http://dx.doi.org/10.1039/b606246f] [PMID: 17216035]

[14] Bromberg JF. Activation of STAT proteins and growth control. BioEssays 2001; 23(2): 161-9. [http://dx.doi.org/10.1002/1521-1878(200102)23:2<161::AID-BIES1023>3.0.CO;2-0] [PMID: 11169589]

[15] Schindler CW. Series Introduction: JAK-STAT signaling in human disease. J Clin Invest 2002; 109(9): 1133-7. [http://dx.doi.org/10.1172/JCI0215644] [PMID: 11994400]

[16] Reich NC. STATs get their move on. JAKSTAT. 2013; 2(4): e27080. [http://dx.doi.org/10.4161/jkst.27080]

[17] Villarino AV, Kanno Y, O'Shea JJ. Mechanisms and consequences of Jak–STAT signaling in the immune system. Nat Immunol 2017; 18(4): 374-84. [http://dx.doi.org/10.1038/ni.3691] [PMID: 28323260]

[18] Levy DE, Darnell JE Jr. STATs: transcriptional control and biological impact. Nat Rev Mol Cell Biol 2002; 3(9): 651-62. [http://dx.doi.org/10.1038/nrm909] [PMID: 12209125]

[19] Stark GR, Kerr IM, Williams BRG, Silverman RH, Schreiber RD. How cells respond to interferons. Annu Rev Biochem 1998; 67(1): 227-64. [http://dx.doi.org/10.1146/annurev.biochem.67.1.227] [PMID: 9759489]

[20] Ram PT, Iyengar R. G protein coupled receptor signaling through the Src and Stat3 pathway: role in proliferation and transformation. Oncogene 2001; 20(13): 1601-6. [http://dx.doi.org/10.1038/sj.onc.1204186] [PMID: 11313907]

[21] Fielding CA, McLoughlin RM, McLeod L, *et al.* IL-6 regulates neutrophil trafficking during acute inflammation *via* STAT3. J Immunol 2008; 181(3): 2189-95. [http://dx.doi.org/10.4049/jimmunol.181.3.2189] [PMID: 18641358]

[22] Chang HY, Sneddon JB, Alizadeh AA, *et al.* Gene expression signature of fibroblast serum response predicts human cancer progression: similarities between tumors and wounds. PLoS Biol 2004; 2(2): e7.

[http://dx.doi.org/10.1371/journal.pbio.0020007] [PMID: 14737219]

[23] Sano S, Itami S, Takeda K, *et al.* Keratinocyte-specific ablation of Stat3 exhibits impaired skin remodeling, but does not affect skin morphogenesis. EMBO J 1999; 18(17): 4657-68. [http://dx.doi.org/10.1093/emboj/18.17.4657] [PMID: 10469645]

[24] Huynh J, Chand A, Gough D, Ernst M. Therapeutically exploiting STAT3 activity in cancer — using tissue repair as a road map. Nat Rev Cancer 2019; 19(2): 82-96. [http://dx.doi.org/10.1038/s41568-018-0090-8] [PMID: 30578415]

[25] Bacon CM, Petricoin EF III, Ortaldo JR, *et al.* Interleukin 12 induces tyrosine phosphorylation and activation of STAT4 in human lymphocytes. Proc Natl Acad Sci USA 1995; 92(16): 7307-11. [http://dx.doi.org/10.1073/pnas.92.16.7307] [PMID: 7638186]

[26] Yamamoto K, Quelle FW, Thierfelder WE, *et al.* Stat4, a novel gamma interferon activation site-binding protein expressed in early myeloid differentiation. Mol Cell Biol 1994; 14(7): 4342-9. [http://dx.doi.org/10.1128/MCB.14.7.4342] [PMID: 8007943]

[27] Good SR, Thieu VT, Mathur AN, *et al.* Temporal induction pattern of STAT4 target genes defines potential for Th1 lineage-specific programming. J Immunol 2009; 183(6): 3839-47. [http://dx.doi.org/10.4049/jimmunol.0901411] [PMID: 19710469]

[28] Hennighausen L, Robinson GW. Interpretation of cytokine signaling through the transcription factors STAT5A and STAT5B. Genes Dev 2008; 22(6): 711-21. [http://dx.doi.org/10.1101/gad.1643908] [PMID: 18347089]

[29] Floyd ZE, Stephens JM. STAT5A promotes adipogenesis in nonprecursor cells and associates with the glucocorticoid receptor during adipocyte differentiation. Diabetes 2003; 52(2): 308-14. [http://dx.doi.org/10.2337/diabetes.52.2.308] [PMID: 12540601]

[30] Lee J, Seong S, Kim JH, *et al.* STAT5 is a key transcription factor for IL-3-mediated inhibition of RANKL-induced osteoclastogenesis. Sci Rep 2016; 6(1): 30977. [http://dx.doi.org/10.1038/srep30977] [PMID: 27485735]

[31] Richard AJ, Stephens JM. The role of JAK–STAT signaling in adipose tissue function. Biochim Biophys Acta Mol Basis Dis 2014; 1842(3): 431-9. [http://dx.doi.org/10.1016/j.bbadis.2013.05.030] [PMID: 23735217]

[32] Kaltenecker D, Mueller KM, Benedikt P, *et al.* Adipocyte STAT5 deficiency promotes adiposity and impairs lipid mobilisation in mice. Diabetologia 2017; 60(2): 296-305. [http://dx.doi.org/10.1007/s00125-016-4152-8] [PMID: 27858140]

[33] Heltemes-Harris LM, Farrar MA. The role of STAT5 in lymphocyte development and transformation. Curr Opin Immunol 2012; 24(2): 146-52. [http://dx.doi.org/10.1016/j.coi.2012.01.015] [PMID: 22342169]

[34] Hebenstreit D, Wirnsberger G, Horejshoeck J, Duschl A. Signaling mechanisms, interaction partners, and target genes of STAT6. Cytokine Growth Factor Rev 2006; 17(3): 173-88. [http://dx.doi.org/10.1016/j.cytogfr.2006.01.004] [PMID: 16540365]

[35] Martinez FO, Helming L, Gordon S. Alternative activation of macrophages: an immunologic functional perspective. Annu Rev Immunol 2009; 27(1): 451-83. [http://dx.doi.org/10.1146/annurev.immunol.021908.132532] [PMID: 19105661]

[36] Iciek LA, Delphin SA, Stavnezer J. CD40 cross-linking induces Ig epsilon germline transcripts in B cells *via* activation of NF-kappaB: synergy with IL-4 induction. J Immunol 1997; 158(10): 4769-79. [PMID: 9144491]

[37] Takeda K, Tanaka T, Shi W, *et al.* Essential role of Stat6 in IL-4 signalling. Nature 1996; 380(6575): 627-30. [http://dx.doi.org/10.1038/380627a0] [PMID: 8602263]

[38] Yao Y, Li W, Kaplan MH, Chang CH. Interleukin (IL)-4 inhibits IL-10 to promote IL-12 production

by dendritic cells. J Exp Med 2005; 201(12): 1899-903.
[http://dx.doi.org/10.1084/jem.20050324] [PMID: 15967820]

[39] Ansel KM, Djuretic I, Tanasa B, Rao A. Regulation of th2 differentiation and *Il4* locus accessibility. Annu Rev Immunol 2006; 24(1): 607-56.
[http://dx.doi.org/10.1146/annurev.immunol.23.021704.115821] [PMID: 16551261]

[40] Kim TK, Maniatis T. Regulation of interferon-gamma-activated STAT1 by the ubiquitin-proteasome pathway. Science 1996; 273(5282): 1717-9.
[http://dx.doi.org/10.1126/science.273.5282.1717] [PMID: 8781235]

[41] Meyer J, Jücker M, Ostertag W, Stocking C. Carboxyl-truncated STAT5beta is generated by a nucleus-associated serine protease in early hematopoietic progenitors. Blood 1998; 91(6): 1901-8.
[http://dx.doi.org/10.1182/blood.V91.6.1901] [PMID: 9490672]

[42] Irie-Sasaki J, Sasaki T, Matsumoto W, *et al.* CD45 is a JAK phosphatase and negatively regulates cytokine receptor signalling. Nature 2001; 409(6818): 349-54.
[http://dx.doi.org/10.1038/35053086] [PMID: 11201744]

[43] David M, Chen HE, Goelz S, Larner AC, Neel BG. Differential regulation of the alpha/beta interferon-stimulated Jak/Stat pathway by the SH2 domain-containing tyrosine phosphatase SHPTP1. Mol Cell Biol 1995; 15(12): 7050-8.
[http://dx.doi.org/10.1128/MCB.15.12.7050] [PMID: 8524272]

[44] Haspel RL, Salditt-Georgieff M, Darnell JE Jr. The rapid inactivation of nuclear tyrosine phosphorylated Stat1 depends upon a protein tyrosine phosphatase. EMBO J 1996; 15(22): 6262-8.
[http://dx.doi.org/10.1002/j.1460-2075.1996.tb01016.x] [PMID: 8947049]

[45] David M, Grimley PM, Finbloom DS, Larner AC. A nuclear tyrosine phosphatase downregulates interferon-induced gene expression. Mol Cell Biol 1993; 13(12): 7515-21.
[http://dx.doi.org/10.1128/MCB.13.12.7515] [PMID: 8246969]

[46] Krebs DL, Hilton DJ. SOCS proteins: negative regulators of cytokine signaling. Stem Cells 2001; 19(5): 378-87.
[http://dx.doi.org/10.1634/stemcells.19-5-378] [PMID: 11553846]

[47] Shuai K. Modulation of STAT signaling by STAT-interacting proteins. Oncogene 2000; 19(21): 2638-44.
[http://dx.doi.org/10.1038/sj.onc.1203522] [PMID: 10851063]

[48] Wakahara R, Kunimoto H, Tanino K, *et al.* Phospho-Ser727 of STAT3 regulates STAT3 activity by enhancing dephosphorylation of phospho-Tyr705 largely through TC45. Genes Cells 2012; 17(2): 132-45.
[http://dx.doi.org/10.1111/j.1365-2443.2011.01575.x] [PMID: 22233524]

[49] Ng IHW, Ng DCH, Jans DA, Bogoyevitch MA. Selective STAT3-α or -β expression reveals spliceform-specific phosphorylation kinetics, nuclear retention and distinct gene expression outcomes. Biochem J 2012; 447(1): 125-36.
[http://dx.doi.org/10.1042/BJ20120941] [PMID: 22799634]

[50] Baran-Marszak F, Feuillard J, Najjar I, *et al.* Differential roles of STAT1 and STAT1 in fludarabine-induced cell cycle arrest and apoptosis in human B cells. Blood 2004; 104(8): 2475-83.
[http://dx.doi.org/10.1182/blood-2003-10-3508] [PMID: 15217838]

[51] O'Shea JJ, Schwartz DM, Villarino AV, Gadina M, McInnes IB, Laurence A. The JAK-STAT pathway: impact on human disease and therapeutic intervention. Annu Rev Med 2015; 66(1): 311-28.
[http://dx.doi.org/10.1146/annurev-med-051113-024537] [PMID: 25587654]

[52] Klammt J, Neumann D, Gevers EF, *et al.* Dominant-negative STAT5B mutations cause growth hormone insensitivity with short stature and mild immune dysregulation. Nat Commun 2018; 9(1): 2105.
[http://dx.doi.org/10.1038/s41467-018-04521-0] [PMID: 29844444]

[53] Nicolae A, Xi L, Pham TH, *et al.* Mutations in the JAK/STAT and RAS signaling pathways are common in intestinal T-cell lymphomas. Leukemia 2016; 30(11): 2245-7. [http://dx.doi.org/10.1038/leu.2016.178] [PMID: 27389054]

[54] Shahmarvand N, Nagy A, Shahryari J, Ohgami RS. Mutations in the signal transducer and activator of transcription family of genes in cancer. Cancer Sci 2018; 109(4): 926-33. [http://dx.doi.org/10.1111/cas.13525] [PMID: 29417693]

[55] Teramo A, Gattazzo C, Passeri F, *et al.* Intrinsic and extrinsic mechanisms contribute to maintain the JAK/STAT pathway aberrantly activated in T-type large granular lymphocyte leukemia. Blood 2013; 121(19): 3843-54. [http://dx.doi.org/10.1182/blood-2012-07-441378]

[56] Maurer B, Nivarthi H, Wingelhofer B, *et al.* High activation of STAT5A drives peripheral T-cell lymphoma and leukemia. Haematologica 2020; 105(2): 435-47. [http://dx.doi.org/10.3324/haematol.2019.216986] [PMID: 31123029]

[57] Moriggl R, Sexl V, Kenner L, *et al.* Stat5 tetramer formation is associated with leukemogenesis. Cancer Cell 2005; 7(1): 87-99. [http://dx.doi.org/10.1016/j.ccr.2004.12.010] [PMID: 15652752]

[58] Benekli M, Baumann H, Wetzler M. Targeting signal transducer and activator of transcription signaling pathway in leukemias. J Clin Oncol 2009; 27(26): 4422-32. [http://dx.doi.org/10.1200/JCO.2008.21.3264] [PMID: 19667270]

[59] Koromilas AE, Sexl V. The tumor suppressor function of STAT1 in breast cancer. JAK-STAT 2013; 2(2): e23353. [http://dx.doi.org/10.4161/jkst.23353] [PMID: 24058806]

[60] Zhang Y, Molavi O, Su M, Lai R. The clinical and biological significance of STAT1 in esophageal squamous cell carcinoma. BMC Cancer 2014; 14(1): 791. [http://dx.doi.org/10.1186/1471-2407-14-791] [PMID: 25355139]

[61] Arzt L, Kothmaier H, Halbwedl I, Quehenberger F, Popper HH. Signal transducer and activator of transcription 1 (STAT1) acts like an oncogene in malignant pleural mesothelioma. Virchows Arch 2014; 465(1): 79-88. [http://dx.doi.org/10.1007/s00428-014-1584-8] [PMID: 24838635]

[62] Gamero AM, Young MR, Mentor-Marcel R, *et al.* STAT2 contributes to promotion of colorectal and skin carcinogenesis. Cancer Prev Res (Phila) 2010; 3(4): 495-504. [http://dx.doi.org/10.1158/1940-6207.CAPR-09-0105] [PMID: 20233899]

[63] Dorritie KA, McCubrey JA, Johnson DE. STAT transcription factors in hematopoiesis and leukemogenesis: opportunities for therapeutic intervention. Leukemia 2014; 28(2): 248-57. [http://dx.doi.org/10.1038/leu.2013.192] [PMID: 23797472]

[64] Yu H, Jove R. The STATs of cancer — new molecular targets come of age. Nat Rev Cancer 2004; 4(2): 97-105. [http://dx.doi.org/10.1038/nrc1275] [PMID: 14964307]

[65] Tilborghs S, Corthouts J, Verhoeven Y, *et al.* The role of Nuclear Factor-kappa B signaling in human cervical cancer. Crit Rev Oncol Hematol 2017; 120: 141-50. [http://dx.doi.org/10.1016/j.critrevonc.2017.11.001] [PMID: 29198328]

[66] Lederle W, Depner S, Schnur S, *et al.* IL-6 promotes malignant growth of skin SCCs by regulating a network of autocrine and paracrine cytokines. Int J Cancer 2011; 128(12): 2803-14. [http://dx.doi.org/10.1002/ijc.25621] [PMID: 20726000]

[67] Kortylewski M, Kujawski M, Wang T, *et al.* Inhibiting Stat3 signaling in the hematopoietic system elicits multicomponent antitumor immunity. Nat Med 2005; 11(12): 1314-21. [http://dx.doi.org/10.1038/nm1325] [PMID: 16288283]

[68] Basu R, Whitley SK, Bhaumik S, *et al.* IL-1 signaling modulates activation of STAT transcription factors to antagonize retinoic acid signaling and control the TH17 cell–iTreg cell balance. Nat Immunol 2015; 16(3): 286-95.
[http://dx.doi.org/10.1038/ni.3099] [PMID: 25642823]

[69] Iliopoulos D, Jaeger SA, Hirsch HA, Bulyk ML, Struhl K. STAT3 activation of miR-21 and miR-181b-1 *via* PTEN and CYLD are part of the epigenetic switch linking inflammation to cancer. Mol Cell 2010; 39(4): 493-506.
[http://dx.doi.org/10.1016/j.molcel.2010.07.023] [PMID: 20797623]

[70] Zhou X, Xia Y, Su J, Zhang G. Down-regulation of miR-141 induced by *Helicobacter pylori* promotes the invasion of gastric cancer by targeting STAT4. Cell Physiol Biochem 2014; 33(4): 1003-12.
[http://dx.doi.org/10.1159/000358671] [PMID: 24732377]

[71] Li S, Sheng B, Zhao M, Shen Q, Zhu H, Zhu X. The prognostic values of signal transducers activators of transcription family in ovarian cancer. Biosci Rep 2017; 37(4): BSR20170650.
[http://dx.doi.org/10.1042/BSR20170650] [PMID: 28536310]

[72] Wang Y, Cai D, Brendel C, *et al.* Adaptive secretion of granulocyte-macrophage colony-stimulating factor (GM-CSF) mediates imatinib and nilotinib resistance in BCR/ABL+ progenitors *via* JAK-2/STAT-5 pathway activation. Blood 2007; 109(5): 2147-55.
[http://dx.doi.org/10.1182/blood-2006-08-040022] [PMID: 17090651]

[73] Koppikar P, Lui VWY, Man D, *et al.* Constitutive activation of signal transducer and activator of transcription 5 contributes to tumor growth, epithelial-mesenchymal transition, and resistance to epidermal growth factor receptor targeting. Clin Cancer Res 2008; 14(23): 7682-90.
[http://dx.doi.org/10.1158/1078-0432.CCR-08-1328] [PMID: 19047094]

[74] Carlesso N, Frank DA, Griffin JD. Tyrosyl phosphorylation and DNA binding activity of signal transducers and activators of transcription (STAT) proteins in hematopoietic cell lines transformed by Bcr/Abl. J Exp Med 1996; 183(3): 811-20.
[http://dx.doi.org/10.1084/jem.183.3.811] [PMID: 8642285]

[75] Schwaller J, Parganas E, Wang D, *et al.* Stat5 is essential for the myelo- and lymphoproliferative disease induced by TEL/JAK2. Mol Cell 2000; 6(3): 693-704.
[http://dx.doi.org/10.1016/S1097-2765(00)00067-8] [PMID: 11030348]

[76] Metón I, Boot EPJ, Sussenbach JS, Steenbergh PH. Growth hormone induces insulin-like growth factor-I gene transcription by a synergistic action of STAT5 and HNF-1α. FEBS Lett 1999; 444(2-3): 155-9.
[http://dx.doi.org/10.1016/S0014-5793(99)00064-2] [PMID: 10050749]

[77] Chen J, Gong C, Mao H, *et al.* E2F1/SP3/STAT6 axis is required for IL-4-induced epithelial-mesenchymal transition of colorectal cancer cells. Int J Oncol 2018; 53(2): 567-78.
[http://dx.doi.org/10.3892/ijo.2018.4429] [PMID: 29901191]

[78] Sarzi-Puttini P, Ceribelli A, Marotto D, Batticciotto A, Atzeni F. Systemic rheumatic diseases: From biological agents to small molecules. Autoimmun Rev 2019; 18(6): 583-92.
[http://dx.doi.org/10.1016/j.autrev.2018.12.009] [PMID: 30959214]

[79] Leeman RJ, Lui VWY, Grandis JR. STAT3 as a therapeutic target in head and neck cancer. Expert Opin Biol Ther 2006; 6(3): 231-41.
[http://dx.doi.org/10.1517/14712598.6.3.231] [PMID: 16503733]

[80] Lee HJ, Zhuang G, Cao Y, Du P, Kim HJ, Settleman J. Drug resistance *via* feedback activation of Stat3 in oncogene-addicted cancer cells. Cancer Cell 2014; 26(2): 207-21.
[http://dx.doi.org/10.1016/j.ccr.2014.05.019] [PMID: 25065853]

[81] Kang YH, Biswas A, Field M, Snapper SB. STAT1 signaling shields T cells from NK cell-mediated cytotoxicity. Nat Commun 2019; 10(1): 912.
[http://dx.doi.org/10.1038/s41467-019-08743-8] [PMID: 30796216]

[82] van Dam PA, Verhoeven Y, Trinh XB, *et al.* RANK/RANKL signaling inhibition may improve the effectiveness of checkpoint blockade in cancer treatment. Crit Rev Oncol Hematol 2019; 133: 85-91. [http://dx.doi.org/10.1016/j.critrevonc.2018.10.011] [PMID: 30661662]

[83] Weinstein S, Toker IA, Emmanuel R, *et al.* Harnessing RNAi-based nanomedicines for therapeutic gene silencing in B-cell malignancies. Proc Natl Acad Sci USA 2016; 113(1): E16-22. [http://dx.doi.org/10.1073/pnas.1519273113] [PMID: 26699502]

[84] Chen M, Pockaj B, Andreozzi M, *et al.* JAK2 and PD-L1 Amplification Enhance the Dynamic Expression of PD-L1 in Triple-negative Breast Cancer. Clin Breast Cancer 2018; 18(5): e1205-15. [http://dx.doi.org/10.1016/j.clbc.2018.05.006] [PMID: 29933930]

[85] Zemek RM, De Jong E, Chin WL, *et al.* Sensitization to immune checkpoint blockade through activation of a STAT1/NK axis in the tumor microenvironment. Sci Transl Med 2019; 11(501): eaav7816.
[http://dx.doi.org/10.1126/scitranslmed.aav7816] [PMID: 31316010]

[86] Attili I, Karachaliou N, Bonanno L, *et al.* TAT3 as a potential immunotherapy biomarker in oncogene-addicted non-small cell lung cancer. Ther Adv Med Oncol 2018; 10: 1758835918763744. [http://dx.doi.org/10.1177/1758835918763744]

[87] Nakayama Y, Mimura K, Tamaki T, *et al.* Phospho-STAT1 expression as a potential biomarker for anti-PD-1/anti-PD-L1 immunotherapy for breast cancer. Int J Oncol 2019; 54(6): 2030-8. [http://dx.doi.org/10.3892/ijo.2019.4779] [PMID: 31081058]

[88] Xiong H, Hong J, Du W, *et al.* Roles of STAT3 and ZEB1 proteins in E-cadherin down-regulation and human colorectal cancer epithelial-mesenchymal transition. J Biol Chem 2012; 287(8): 5819-32. [http://dx.doi.org/10.1074/jbc.M111.295964] [PMID: 22205702]

[89] Turkson J. STAT proteins as novel targets for cancer drug discovery. Expert Opin Ther Targets 2004; 8(5): 409-22.
[http://dx.doi.org/10.1517/14728222.8.5.409] [PMID: 15469392]

[90] Turkson J, Jove R. STAT proteins: novel molecular targets for cancer drug discovery. Oncogene 2000; 19(56): 6613-26.
[http://dx.doi.org/10.1038/sj.onc.1204086] [PMID: 11426647]

[91] de Fougerolles A, Vornlocher HP, Maraganore J, Lieberman J. Interfering with disease: a progress report on siRNA-based therapeutics. Nat Rev Drug Discov 2007; 6(6): 443-53. [http://dx.doi.org/10.1038/nrd2310] [PMID: 17541417]

[92] Peer D, Lieberman J. Special delivery: targeted therapy with small RNAs. Gene Ther 2011; 18(12): 1127-33.
[http://dx.doi.org/10.1038/gt.2011.56] [PMID: 21490679]

[93] Zhang W, Sun H, Shi X, *et al.* SENP1 regulates hepatocyte growth factor-induced migration and epithelial-mesenchymal transition of hepatocellular carcinoma. Tumour Biol 2016; 37(6): 7741-8. [http://dx.doi.org/10.1007/s13277-015-4406-y] [PMID: 26695141]

[94] Xu X, Dong Z, Li Y, *et al.* The upregulation of signal transducer and activator of transcription 5-dependent microRNA-182 and microRNA-96 promotes ovarian cancer cell proliferation by targeting forkhead box O3 upon leptin stimulation. Int J Biochem Cell Biol 2013; 45(3): 536-45. [http://dx.doi.org/10.1016/j.biocel.2012.12.010] [PMID: 23262295]

[95] Kunigal S, Lakka SS, Sodadasu PK, Estes N, Rao JS. Stat3-siRNA induces Fas-mediated apoptosis in vitro and in vivo in breast cancer. Int J Oncol 2009; 34(5): 1209-20.
[PMID: 19360334]

[96] Yang Q, Li M, Wang T, Xu H, Zang W, Zhao G. Effect of STAT5 silenced by siRNA on proliferation apoptosis and invasion of esophageal carcinoma cell line Eca-109. Diagn Pathol 2013; 8(1): 132. [http://dx.doi.org/10.1186/1746-1596-8-132] [PMID: 23915238]

[97] Choi JK, Kim KH, Park H, Park SR, Choi BH. Granulocyte macrophage-colony stimulating factor shows anti-apoptotic activity in neural progenitor cells *via* JAK/STAT5-Bcl-2 pathway. Apoptosis : an international journal on programmed cell death 2011; 16(2): 127-34. [http://dx.doi.org/10.1007/s10495-010-0552-2]

[98] Gu L, Vogiatzi P, Puhr M, *et al.* Stat5 promotes metastatic behavior of human prostate cancer cells in vitro and in vivo. Endocr Relat Cancer 2010; 17(2): 481-93. [http://dx.doi.org/10.1677/ERC-09-0328] [PMID: 20233708]

[99] Tatiparti K, Sau S, Kashaw S, Iyer A. siRNA Delivery Strategies: A Comprehensive Review of Recent Developments. Nanomaterials (Basel) 2017; 7(4): 77. [http://dx.doi.org/10.3390/nano7040077] [PMID: 28379201]

[100] Wang X, Liu P, Liu H, *et al.* Delivery of interferons and siRNA targeting STAT3 using lentiviral vectors suppresses the growth of murine melanoma. Cancer Gene Ther 2012; 19(12): 822-7. [http://dx.doi.org/10.1038/cgt.2012.65] [PMID: 23018621]

[101] Anastasov N, Klier M, Koch I, *et al.* Efficient shRNA delivery into B and T lymphoma cells using lentiviral vector-mediated transfer. J Hematop 2009; 2(1): 9-19. [http://dx.doi.org/10.1007/s12308-008-0020-x] [PMID: 19669218]

[102] Yang G, Huang C, Cao J, Huang KJ, Jiang T, Qiu ZJ. Lentivirus-mediated shRNA interference targeting STAT3 inhibits human pancreatic cancer cell invasion. World J Gastroenterol 2009; 15(30): 3757-66. [http://dx.doi.org/10.3748/wjg.15.3757] [PMID: 19673016]

[103] Baeuerle PA, Henkel T. Function and activation of NF-kappa B in the immune system. Annu Rev Immunol 1994; 12(1): 141-79. [http://dx.doi.org/10.1146/annurev.iy.12.040194.001041] [PMID: 8011280]

[104] Zhao Y, Zheng C, Zhang L, Chen Y, Ye Y, Zhao M. Knockdown of STAT3 expression in SKOV3 cells by biodegradable siRNA–PLGA/CSO conjugate micelles. Colloids Surf B Biointerfaces 2015; 127: 155-63. [http://dx.doi.org/10.1016/j.colsurfb.2015.01.034] [PMID: 25677339]

[105] Alshamsan A, Hamdy S, Samuel J, El-Kadi AOS, Lavasanifar A, Uludağ H. The induction of tumor apoptosis in B16 melanoma following STAT3 siRNA delivery with a lipid-substituted polyethylenimine. Biomaterials 2010; 31(6): 1420-8. [http://dx.doi.org/10.1016/j.biomaterials.2009.11.003] [PMID: 19913908]

[106] Liang ZW, Guo BF, Li Y, *et al.* Plasmid-based Stat3 siRNA delivered by hydroxyapatite nanoparticles suppresses mouse prostate tumour growth in vivo. Asian J Androl 2011; 13(3): 481-6. [http://dx.doi.org/10.1038/aja.2010.167] [PMID: 21297658]

[107] Ma Y, Zhang X, Xu X, *et al.* STAT3 Decoy Oligodeoxynucleotides-Loaded Solid Lipid Nanoparticles Induce Cell Death and Inhibit Invasion in Ovarian Cancer Cells. PLoS One 2015; 10(4): e0124924. [http://dx.doi.org/10.1371/journal.pone.0124924] [PMID: 25923701]

[108] Najar AG, Pashaei-Asl R, Omidi Y, Farajnia S, Nourazarian AR. EGFR antisense oligonucleotides encapsulated with nanoparticles decrease EGFR, MAPK1 and STAT5 expression in a human colon cancer cell line. Asian Pac J Cancer Prev 2013; 14(1): 495-8. [http://dx.doi.org/10.7314/APJCP.2013.14.1.495] [PMID: 23534780]

[109] Zhang H, Freitas D, Kim HS, *et al.* Identification of distinct nanoparticles and subsets of extracellular vesicles by asymmetric flow field-flow fractionation. Nat Cell Biol 2018; 20(3): 332-43. [http://dx.doi.org/10.1038/s41556-018-0040-4] [PMID: 29459780]

[110] Karin M, Cao Y, Greten FR, Li ZW. NF-κB in cancer: from innocent bystander to major culprit. Nat Rev Cancer 2002; 2(4): 301-10. [http://dx.doi.org/10.1038/nrc780] [PMID: 12001991]

[111] Nakajima S, Kitamura M. Bidirectional regulation of NF-κB by reactive oxygen species: A role of

unfolded protein response. Free Radic Biol Med 2013; 65: 162-74.
[http://dx.doi.org/10.1016/j.freeradbiomed.2013.06.020] [PMID: 23792277]

[112] Tak PP, Firestein GS. NF-κB: a key role in inflammatory diseases. J Clin Invest 2001; 107(1): 7-11.
[http://dx.doi.org/10.1172/JCI11830] [PMID: 11134171]

[113] Sun SC. Non-canonical NF-κB signaling pathway. Cell Res 2011; 21(1): 71-85.
[http://dx.doi.org/10.1038/cr.2010.177] [PMID: 21173796]

[114] Vallabhapurapu S, Karin M. Regulation and function of NF-kappaB transcription factors in the immune system. Annu Rev Immunol 2009; 27(1): 693-733.
[http://dx.doi.org/10.1146/annurev.immunol.021908.132641] [PMID: 19302050]

[115] Hayden MS, Ghosh S. Shared principles in NF-kappaB signaling. Cell 2008; 132(3): 344-62.
[http://dx.doi.org/10.1016/j.cell.2008.01.020] [PMID: 18267068]

[116] Sun SC, Ley SC. New insights into NF-κB regulation and function. Trends Immunol 2008; 29(10): 469-78.
[http://dx.doi.org/10.1016/j.it.2008.07.003] [PMID: 18775672]

[117] Senftleben U, Cao Y, Xiao G, *et al.* Activation by IKKalpha of a second, evolutionary conserved, NF-κ B signaling pathway. Science 2001; 293(5534): 1495-9.
[http://dx.doi.org/10.1126/science.1062677] [PMID: 11520989]

[118] Karin M, Ben-Neriah Y. Phosphorylation meets ubiquitination: the control of NF-[κ]B activity. Annu Rev Immunol 2000; 18(1): 621-63.
[http://dx.doi.org/10.1146/annurev.immunol.18.1.621] [PMID: 10837071]

[119] Guan H, Hou S, Ricciardi RP. DNA binding of repressor nuclear factor-kappaB p50/p50 depends on phosphorylation of Ser337 by the protein kinase A catalytic subunit. J Biol Chem 2005; 280(11): 9957-62.
[http://dx.doi.org/10.1074/jbc.M412180200] [PMID: 15642694]

[120] Perkins ND. Integrating cell-signalling pathways with NF-κB and IKK function. Nat Rev Mol Cell Biol 2007; 8(1): 49-62.
[http://dx.doi.org/10.1038/nrm2083] [PMID: 17183360]

[121] Oeckinghaus A, Ghosh S. The NF-kappaB family of transcription factors and its regulation. Cold Spring Harb Perspect Biol 2009; 1(4): a000034.
[http://dx.doi.org/10.1101/cshperspect.a000034] [PMID: 20066092]

[122] Tilstra JS, Clauson CL, Niedernhofer LJ, Robbins PD. NF-κB in aging and disease. Aging Dis 2011; 2(6): 449-65.
[PMID: 22396894]

[123] Lo JC, Basak S, James ES, *et al.* Coordination between NF-κB family members p50 and p52 is essential for mediating LTβR signals in the development and organization of secondary lymphoid tissues. Blood 2006; 107(3): 1048-55.
[http://dx.doi.org/10.1182/blood-2005-06-2452] [PMID: 16195333]

[124] Hoffmann A, Levchenko A, Scott ML, Baltimore D. The IkappaB-NF-kappaB signaling module: temporal control and selective gene activation. Science 2002; 298(5596): 1241-5.
[http://dx.doi.org/10.1126/science.1071914] [PMID: 12424381]

[125] May MJ, D'Acquisto F, Madge LA, Glöckner J, Pober JS, Ghosh S. Selective inhibition of NF-kappaB activation by a peptide that blocks the interaction of NEMO with the IkappaB kinase complex. Science 2000; 289(5484): 1550-4.
[http://dx.doi.org/10.1126/science.289.5484.1550] [PMID: 10968790]

[126] Karin M, Delhase M. The IκB kinase (IKK) and NF-κB: key elements of proinflammatory signalling Seminars in immunology. Elsevier 2000; pp. 85-98.

[127] Karin M, Lin A. NF-κB at the crossroads of life and death. Nat Immunol 2002; 3(3): 221-7.

[http://dx.doi.org/10.1038/ni0302-221] [PMID: 11875461]

[128] Hayden MS, West AP, Ghosh S. NF-κB and the immune response. Oncogene 2006; 25(51): 6758-80. [http://dx.doi.org/10.1038/sj.onc.1209943] [PMID: 17072327]

[129] Solan NJ, Miyoshi H, Carmona EM, Bren GD, Paya CV. RelB cellular regulation and transcriptional activity are regulated by p100. J Biol Chem 2002; 277(2): 1405-18. [http://dx.doi.org/10.1074/jbc.M109619200] [PMID: 11687592]

[130] Derudder E, Dejardin E, Pritchard LL, Green DR, Körner M, Baud V. RelB/p50 dimers are differentially regulated by tumor necrosis factor-α and lymphotoxin-β receptor activation: critical roles for p100. J Biol Chem 2003; 278(26): 23278-84. [http://dx.doi.org/10.1074/jbc.M300106200] [PMID: 12709443]

[131] Coope HJ, Atkinson PG, Huhse B, *et al.* CD40 regulates the processing of NF-kappaB2 p100 to p52. EMBO J 2002; 21(20): 5375-85. [http://dx.doi.org/10.1093/emboj/cdf542] [PMID: 12374738]

[132] Xiao G, Harhaj EW, Sun SC. NF-kappaB-inducing kinase regulates the processing of NF-kappaB2 p100. Mol Cell 2001; 7(2): 401-9. [http://dx.doi.org/10.1016/S1097-2765(01)00187-3] [PMID: 11239468]

[133] Bonizzi G, Bebien M, Otero DC, *et al.* Activation of IKKα target genes depends on recognition of specific κB binding sites by RelB:p52 dimers. EMBO J 2004; 23(21): 4202-10. [http://dx.doi.org/10.1038/sj.emboj.7600391] [PMID: 15470505]

[134] Basak S, Shih VFS, Hoffmann A. Generation and activation of multiple dimeric transcription factors within the NF-kappaB signaling system. Mol Cell Biol 2008; 28(10): 3139-50. [http://dx.doi.org/10.1128/MCB.01469-07] [PMID: 18299388]

[135] Novack DV, Yin L, Hagen-Stapleton A, *et al.* The IkappaB function of NF-kappaB2 p100 controls stimulated osteoclastogenesis. J Exp Med 2003; 198(5): 771-81. [http://dx.doi.org/10.1084/jem.20030116] [PMID: 12939342]

[136] Jost PJ, Ruland J. Aberrant NF-κB signaling in lymphoma: mechanisms, consequences, and therapeutic implications. Blood 2007; 109(7): 2700-7. [http://dx.doi.org/10.1182/blood-2006-07-025809] [PMID: 17119127]

[137] Rong ZT, Gong XJ, Sun HB, Li YM, Ji H. Protective effects of oleanolic acid on cerebral ischemic damage *in vivo* and H_2O_2-induced injury *in vitro*. Pharm Biol 2011; 49(1): 78-85. [http://dx.doi.org/10.3109/13880209.2010.499130] [PMID: 20684747]

[138] Hayden MS, Ghosh S. NF-κB in immunobiology. Cell Res 2011; 21(2): 223-44. [http://dx.doi.org/10.1038/cr.2011.13] [PMID: 21243012]

[139] Prasad S, Ravindran J, Aggarwal BB. NF-κB and cancer: how intimate is this relationship. Mol Cell Biochem 2010; 336(1-2): 25-37. [http://dx.doi.org/10.1007/s11010-009-0267-2] [PMID: 19823771]

[140] Guttridge DC, Albanese C, Reuther JY, Pestell RG, Baldwin AS Jr. NF-kappaB controls cell growth and differentiation through transcriptional regulation of cyclin D1. Mol Cell Biol 1999; 19(8): 5785-99. [http://dx.doi.org/10.1128/MCB.19.8.5785] [PMID: 10409765]

[141] Ben-Neriah Y, Karin M. Inflammation meets cancer, with NF-κB as the matchmaker. Nat Immunol 2011; 12(8): 715-23. [http://dx.doi.org/10.1038/ni.2060] [PMID: 21772280]

[142] Hinz M, Krappmann D, Eichten A, Heder A, Scheidereit C, Strauss M. NF-kappaB function in growth control: regulation of cyclin D1 expression and G0/G1-to-S-phase transition. Mol Cell Biol 1999; 19(4): 2690-8. [http://dx.doi.org/10.1128/MCB.19.4.2690] [PMID: 10082535]

[143] Cao Y, Bonizzi G, Seagroves TN, *et al.* IKKalpha provides an essential link between RANK signaling and cyclin D1 expression during mammary gland development. Cell 2001; 107(6): 763-75. [http://dx.doi.org/10.1016/S0092-8674(01)00599-2] [PMID: 11747812]

[144] Van Antwerp DJ, Martin SJ, Kafri T, Green DR, Verma IM. Suppression of TNF-α-Induced Apoptosis by NF-κB. Science 1996; 274(5288): 787-9. [http://dx.doi.org/10.1126/science.274.5288.787] [PMID: 8864120]

[145] Beg AA, Baltimore D. An essential role for NF-kappaB in preventing TNF-alpha-induced cell death. Science 1996; 274(5288): 782-4. [http://dx.doi.org/10.1126/science.274.5288.782] [PMID: 8864118]

[146] Lane BR, Liu J, Bock PJ, *et al.* Interleukin-8 and growth-regulated oncogene alpha mediate angiogenesis in Kaposi's sarcoma. J Virol 2002; 76(22): 11570-83. [http://dx.doi.org/10.1128/JVI.76.22.11570-11583.2002] [PMID: 12388718]

[147] Overall CM, López-Otín C. Strategies for MMP inhibition in cancer: innovations for the post-trial era. Nat Rev Cancer 2002; 2(9): 657-72. [http://dx.doi.org/10.1038/nrc884] [PMID: 12209155]

[148] Pickup MW, Mouw JK, Weaver VM. The extracellular matrix modulates the hallmarks of cancer. EMBO Rep 2014; 15(12): 1243-53. [http://dx.doi.org/10.15252/embr.201439246] [PMID: 25381661]

[149] Bartok B, Firestein GS. Fibroblast-like synoviocytes: key effector cells in rheumatoid arthritis. Immunol Rev 2010; 233(1): 233-55. [http://dx.doi.org/10.1111/j.0105-2896.2009.00859.x] [PMID: 20193003]

[150] Grivennikov SI, Greten FR, Karin M. Immunity, inflammation, and cancer. Cell 2010; 140(6): 883-99. [http://dx.doi.org/10.1016/j.cell.2010.01.025] [PMID: 20303878]

[151] Gambhir S, Vyas D, Hollis M, Aekka A, Vyas A. Nuclear factor kappa B role in inflammation associated gastrointestinal malignancies. World J Gastroenterol 2015; 21(11): 3174-83. [http://dx.doi.org/10.3748/wjg.v21.i11.3174] [PMID: 25805923]

[152] Liu F, Bardhan K, Yang D, *et al.* NF-κB directly regulates Fas transcription to modulate Fas-mediated apoptosis and tumor suppression. J Biol Chem 2012; 287(30): 25530-40. [http://dx.doi.org/10.1074/jbc.M112.356279] [PMID: 22669972]

[153] Romashkova JA, Makarov SS. NF-κB is a target of AKT in anti-apoptotic PDGF signalling. Nature 1999; 401(6748): 86-90. [http://dx.doi.org/10.1038/43474] [PMID: 10485711]

[154] Nidai Ozes O, Mayo LD, Gustin JA, Pfeffer SR, Pfeffer LM, Donner DB. NF-κB activation by tumour necrosis factor requires the Akt serine–threonine kinase. Nature 1999; 401(6748): 82-5. [http://dx.doi.org/10.1038/43466] [PMID: 10485710]

[155] Madrid LV, Mayo MW, Reuther JY, Baldwin AS Jr. Akt stimulates the transactivation potential of the RelA/p65 Subunit of NF-kappa B through utilization of the Ikappa B kinase and activation of the mitogen-activated protein kinase p38. J Biol Chem 2001; 276(22): 18934-40. [http://dx.doi.org/10.1074/jbc.M101103200] [PMID: 11259436]

[156] Kane LP, Mollenauer MN, Xu Z, Turck CW, Weiss A. Akt-dependent phosphorylation specifically regulates Cot induction of NF-kappa B-dependent transcription. Mol Cell Biol 2002; 22(16): 5962-74. [http://dx.doi.org/10.1128/MCB.22.16.5962-5974.2002] [PMID: 12138205]

[157] Sizemore N, Leung S, Stark GR. Activation of phosphatidylinositol 3-kinase in response to interleukin-1 leads to phosphorylation and activation of the NF-kappaB p65/RelA subunit. Mol Cell Biol 1999; 19(7): 4798-805. [http://dx.doi.org/10.1128/MCB.19.7.4798] [PMID: 10373529]

[158] Downward J. Mechanisms and consequences of activation of protein kinase B/Akt. Curr Opin Cell

Biol 1998; 10(2): 262-7.
[http://dx.doi.org/10.1016/S0955-0674(98)80149-X] [PMID: 9561851]

[159] Smith D, Shimamura T, Barbera S, Bejcek BE. NF-κB controls growth of glioblastomas/astrocytomas. Mol Cell Biochem 2007; 307(1-2): 141-7.
[http://dx.doi.org/10.1007/s11010-007-9593-4] [PMID: 17828582]

[160] Kastrati I, Siklos MI, Calderon-Gierszal EL, *et al.* Dimethyl Fumarate Inhibits the Nuclear Factor κB Pathway in Breast Cancer Cells by Covalent Modification of p65 Protein. J Biol Chem 2016; 291(7): 3639-47.
[http://dx.doi.org/10.1074/jbc.M115.679704] [PMID: 26683377]

[161] Zhang L, Ren X, Cheng Y, *et al.* The NFκB inhibitor, SN50, induces differentiation of glioma stem cells and suppresses their oncogenic phenotype. Cancer Biol Ther 2014; 15(5): 602-11.
[http://dx.doi.org/10.4161/cbt.28158] [PMID: 24557012]

[162] Zanotto-Filho A, Braganhol E, Schröder R, *et al.* NFκB inhibitors induce cell death in glioblastomas. Biochem Pharmacol 2011; 81(3): 412-24.
[http://dx.doi.org/10.1016/j.bcp.2010.10.014] [PMID: 21040711]

[163] Chandrika G, Natesh K, Ranade D, Chugh A, Shastry P. Suppression of the invasive potential of Glioblastoma cells by mTOR inhibitors involves modulation of NFκB and PKC-α signaling. Sci Rep 2016; 6(1): 22455.
[http://dx.doi.org/10.1038/srep22455] [PMID: 26940200]

[164] Fracchiolla NS, Lombardi L, Salina M, *et al.* Structural alterations of the NF-kappa B transcription factor lyt-10 in lymphoid malignancies. Oncogene 1993; 8(10): 2839-45.
[PMID: 8378093]

[165] Neri A, Chang CC, Lombardi L, *et al.* B cell lymphoma-associated chromosomal translocation involves candidate oncogene lyt-10, homologous to NF-κB p50. Cell 1991; 67(6): 1075-87.
[http://dx.doi.org/10.1016/0092-8674(91)90285-7] [PMID: 1760839]

[166] Barth TFE, Martin-Subero JI, Joos S, *et al.* Gains of 2p involving the REL locus correlate with nuclear c-Rel protein accumulation in neoplastic cells of classical Hodgkin lymphoma. Blood 2003; 101(9): 3681-6.
[http://dx.doi.org/10.1182/blood-2002-08-2577] [PMID: 12511414]

[167] Lake A, Shield LA, Cordano P, *et al.* Mutations of *NFKBIA*, encoding IκBα, are a recurrent finding in classical Hodgkin lymphoma but are not a unifying feature of non-EBV-associated cases. Int J Cancer 2009; 125(6): 1334-42.
[http://dx.doi.org/10.1002/ijc.24502] [PMID: 19507254]

[168] Schmitz R, Hansmann ML, Bohle V, *et al.* TNFAIP3 (A20) is a tumor suppressor gene in Hodgkin lymphoma and primary mediastinal B cell lymphoma. J Exp Med 2009; 206(5): 981-9.
[http://dx.doi.org/10.1084/jem.20090528] [PMID: 19380639]

[169] Vinod BS, Antony J, Nair HH, *et al.* Mechanistic evaluation of the signaling events regulating curcumin-mediated chemosensitization of breast cancer cells to 5-fluorouracil. Cell Death Dis 2013; 4(2): e505.
[http://dx.doi.org/10.1038/cddis.2013.26] [PMID: 23429291]

[170] Surh YJ, Han SS, Keum YS, Seo HJ, Lee SS. Inhibitory effects of curcumin and capsaicin on phorbol ester-induced activation of eukaryotic transcription factors, NF-κB and AP-1. Biofactors 2000; 12(1-4): 107-12.
[http://dx.doi.org/10.1002/biof.5520120117] [PMID: 11216470]

[171] Sandur SK, Deorukhkar A, Pandey MK, *et al.* Curcumin modulates the radiosensitivity of colorectal cancer cells by suppressing constitutive and inducible NF-kappaB activity. Int J Radiat Oncol Biol Phys 2009; 75(2): 534-42.
[http://dx.doi.org/10.1016/j.ijrobp.2009.06.034] [PMID: 19735878]

[172] Yeon KY, Kim SA, Kim YH, *et al.* Curcumin produces an antihyperalgesic effect *via* antagonism of TRPV1. J Dent Res 2010; 89(2): 170-4.
[http://dx.doi.org/10.1177/0022034509356169] [PMID: 20040737]

[173] Geldmeyer-Hilt K, Heine G, Hartmann B, Baumgrass R, Radbruch A, Worm M. 1,25-dihydroxyvitamin D3 impairs NF-κB activation in human naïve B cells. Biochem Biophys Res Commun 2011; 407(4): 699-702.
[http://dx.doi.org/10.1016/j.bbrc.2011.03.078] [PMID: 21420936]

[174] Yu XP, Bellido T, Manolagas SC. Down-regulation of NF-kappa B protein levels in activated human lymphocytes by 1,25-dihydroxyvitamin D3. Proc Natl Acad Sci USA 1995; 92(24): 10990-4.
[http://dx.doi.org/10.1073/pnas.92.24.10990] [PMID: 7479923]

[175] Harant H, Wolff B, Lindley IJD. 1α,25-Dihydroxyvitamin D_3 decreases DNA binding of nuclear factor-κB in human fibroblasts. FEBS Lett 1998; 436(3): 329-34.
[http://dx.doi.org/10.1016/S0014-5793(98)01153-3] [PMID: 9801142]

[176] Chen Y, Kong J, Sun T, *et al.* 1,25-Dihydroxyvitamin D3 suppresses inflammation-induced expression of plasminogen activator inhibitor-1 by blocking nuclear factor-κB activation. Arch Biochem Biophys 2011; 507(2): 241-7.
[http://dx.doi.org/10.1016/j.abb.2010.12.020] [PMID: 21176770]

[177] Shifera AS, Leong D, Hardin JA. Vitamin D does not modulate NF-κB activity in Jurkat T cells. Immunol Lett 2010; 131(2): 151-8.
[http://dx.doi.org/10.1016/j.imlet.2010.04.001] [PMID: 20385167]

[178] Farmer PK, He X, Schmitz ML, Rubin J, Nanes MS. Inhibitory effect of NF-κB on 1,25-dihydroxyvitamin D_3 and retinoid X receptor function. Am J Physiol Endocrinol Metab 2000; 279(1): E213-20.
[http://dx.doi.org/10.1152/ajpendo.2000.279.1.E213] [PMID: 10893342]

[179] Ghosh-Choudhury N, Mandal CC, Ghosh-Choudhury N, Ghosh Choudhury G. Simvastatin induces derepression of PTEN expression *via* NFκB to inhibit breast cancer cell growth. Cell Signal 2010; 22(5): 749-58.
[http://dx.doi.org/10.1016/j.cellsig.2009.12.010] [PMID: 20060890]

[180] Han SS, Yun H, Son DJ, *et al.* NF-κB/STAT3/PI3K signaling crosstalk in iMycEμ B lymphoma. Mol Cancer 2010; 9(1): 97.
[http://dx.doi.org/10.1186/1476-4598-9-97] [PMID: 20433747]

[181] Jung BH, Beck SE, Cabral J, *et al.* Activin type 2 receptor restoration in MSI-H colon cancer suppresses growth and enhances migration with activin. Gastroenterology 2007; 132(2): 633-44.
[http://dx.doi.org/10.1053/j.gastro.2006.11.018] [PMID: 17258738]

[182] Bauer J, Sporn JC, Cabral J, Gomez J, Jung B. Effects of activin and TGFβ on p21 in colon cancer. PLoS One 2012; 7(6): e39381.
[http://dx.doi.org/10.1371/journal.pone.0039381] [PMID: 22761777]

[183] Wamsley JJ, Kumar M, Allison DF, *et al.* Activin upregulation by NF-κB is required to maintain mesenchymal features of cancer stem-like cells in non-small cell lung cancer. Cancer Res 2015; 75(2): 426-35.
[http://dx.doi.org/10.1158/0008-5472.CAN-13-2702] [PMID: 25432175]

[184] Greten FR, Eckmann L, Greten TF, *et al.* IKKbeta links inflammation and tumorigenesis in a mouse model of colitis-associated cancer. Cell 2004; 118(3): 285-96.
[http://dx.doi.org/10.1016/j.cell.2004.07.013] [PMID: 15294155]

[185] Stairs DB, Bayne LJ, Rhoades B, *et al.* Deletion of p120-catenin results in a tumor microenvironment with inflammation and cancer that establishes it as a tumor suppressor gene. Cancer Cell 2011; 19(4): 470-83.
[http://dx.doi.org/10.1016/j.ccr.2011.02.007] [PMID: 21481789]

[186] Ping FM, Liu GJ, Liu ZJ, *et al.* Expression of RKIP, E-cadherin and NF-kB p65 in esophageal squamous cell carcinoma and their correlations. Int J Clin Exp Pathol 2015; 8(9): 10164-70. [PMID: 26617724]

[187] Puliyappadamba VT, Hatanpaa KJ, Chakraborty S, Habib AA. The role of NF-κB in the pathogenesis of glioma. Mol Cell Oncol 2014; 1(3): e963478. [http://dx.doi.org/10.4161/23723548.2014.963478] [PMID: 27308348]

[188] Shin HM, Kim MH, Kim BH, *et al.* Inhibitory action of novel aromatic diamine compound on lipopolysaccharide-induced nuclear translocation of NF-κB without affecting IκB degradation. FEBS Lett 2004; 571(1-3): 50-4. [http://dx.doi.org/10.1016/j.febslet.2004.06.056] [PMID: 15280016]

[189] Valenta T, Hausmann G, Basler K. The many faces and functions of β-catenin. EMBO J 2012; 31(12): 2714-36. [http://dx.doi.org/10.1038/emboj.2012.150] [PMID: 22617422]

[190] Nusse R, Varmus HE. Many tumors induced by the mouse mammary tumor virus contain a provirus integrated in the same region of the host genome. Cell 1982; 31(1): 99-109. [http://dx.doi.org/10.1016/0092-8674(82)90409-3] [PMID: 6297757]

[191] van Ooyen A, Kwee V, Nusse R. The nucleotide sequence of the human int-1 mammary oncogene; evolutionary conservation of coding and non-coding sequences. EMBO J 1985; 4(11): 2905-9. [http://dx.doi.org/10.1002/j.1460-2075.1985.tb04021.x] [PMID: 2998762]

[192] Dickson C, Smith R, Brookes S, Peters G. Tumorigenesis by mouse mammary tumor virus: Proviral activation of a cellular gene in the common integration region int-2. Cell 1984; 37(2): 529-36. [http://dx.doi.org/10.1016/0092-8674(84)90383-0] [PMID: 6327073]

[193] Gallahan D, Callahan R. Mammary tumorigenesis in feral mice: identification of a new int locus in mouse mammary tumor virus (Czech II)-induced mammary tumors. J Virol 1987; 61(1): 66-74. [http://dx.doi.org/10.1128/jvi.61.1.66-74.1987] [PMID: 3023708]

[194] Roelink H, Wagenaar E, Lopes da Silva S, Nusse R. Wnt-3, a gene activated by proviral insertion in mouse mammary tumors, is homologous to int-1/Wnt-1 and is normally expressed in mouse embryos and adult brain. Proc Natl Acad Sci USA 1990; 87(12): 4519-23. [http://dx.doi.org/10.1073/pnas.87.12.4519] [PMID: 2162045]

[195] Cadigan KM, Nusse R. Wnt signaling: a common theme in animal development. Genes Dev 1997; 11(24): 3286-305. [http://dx.doi.org/10.1101/gad.11.24.3286] [PMID: 9407023]

[196] Pai SG, Carneiro BA, Mota JM, *et al.* Wnt/beta-catenin pathway: modulating anticancer immune response. J Hematol Oncol 2017; 10(1): 101. [http://dx.doi.org/10.1186/s13045-017-0471-6] [PMID: 28476164]

[197] Niehrs C. The complex world of WNT receptor signalling. Nat Rev Mol Cell Biol 2012; 13(12): 767-79. [http://dx.doi.org/10.1038/nrm3470] [PMID: 23151663]

[198] Willert K, Brown JD, Danenberg E, *et al.* Wnt proteins are lipid-modified and can act as stem cell growth factors. Nature 2003; 423(6938): 448-52. [http://dx.doi.org/10.1038/nature01611] [PMID: 12717451]

[199] Hofmann K. A superfamily of membrane-bound O -acyltransferases with implications for Wnt signaling. Trends Biochem Sci 2000; 25(3): 111-2. [http://dx.doi.org/10.1016/S0968-0004(99)01539-X] [PMID: 10694878]

[200] Takada R, Satomi Y, Kurata T, *et al.* Monounsaturated fatty acid modification of Wnt protein: its role in Wnt secretion. Dev Cell 2006; 11(6): 791-801. [http://dx.doi.org/10.1016/j.devcel.2006.10.003] [PMID: 17141155]

[201] Grzeschik KH, Bornholdt D, Oeffner F, *et al.* Deficiency of PORCN, a regulator of Wnt signaling, is associated with focal dermal hypoplasia. Nat Genet 2007; 39(7): 833-5. [http://dx.doi.org/10.1038/ng2052] [PMID: 17546031]

[202] Port F, Kuster M, Herr P, *et al.* Wingless secretion promotes and requires retromer-dependent cycling of Wntless. Nat Cell Biol 2008; 10(2): 178-85. [http://dx.doi.org/10.1038/ncb1687] [PMID: 18193032]

[203] Clevers H, Nusse R. Wnt/β-catenin signaling and disease. Cell 2012; 149(6): 1192-205. [http://dx.doi.org/10.1016/j.cell.2012.05.012] [PMID: 22682243]

[204] Logan CY, Nusse R. The Wnt signaling pathway in development and disease. Annu Rev Cell Dev Biol 2004; 20(1): 781-810. [http://dx.doi.org/10.1146/annurev.cellbio.20.010403.113126] [PMID: 15473860]

[205] He X, Semenov M, Tamai K, Zeng X. LDL receptor-related proteins 5 and 6 in Wnt/β-catenin signaling:Arrows point the way. Development 2004; 131(8): 1663-77. [http://dx.doi.org/10.1242/dev.01117] [PMID: 15084453]

[206] Janda CY, Waghray D, Levin AM, Thomas C, Garcia KC. Structural basis of Wnt recognition by Frizzled. Science 2012; 337(6090): 59-64. [http://dx.doi.org/10.1126/science.1222879] [PMID: 22653731]

[207] Gong Y, Bourhis E, Chiu C, *et al.* Wnt isoform-specific interactions with coreceptor specify inhibition or potentiation of signaling by LRP6 antibodies. PLoS One 2010; 5(9): e12682. [http://dx.doi.org/10.1371/journal.pone.0012682] [PMID: 20856934]

[208] de Lau W, Barker N, Low TY, *et al.* Lgr5 homologues associate with Wnt receptors and mediate R-spondin signalling. Nature 2011; 476(7360): 293-7. [http://dx.doi.org/10.1038/nature10337] [PMID: 21727895]

[209] Glinka A, Dolde C, Kirsch N, *et al.* LGR4 and LGR5 are R-spondin receptors mediating Wnt/β-catenin and Wnt/PCP signalling. EMBO Rep 2011; 12(10): 1055-61. [http://dx.doi.org/10.1038/embor.2011.175] [PMID: 21909076]

[210] Carmon KS, Gong X, Lin Q, Thomas A, Liu Q. R-spondins function as ligands of the orphan receptors LGR4 and LGR5 to regulate Wnt/β-catenin signaling. Proc Natl Acad Sci USA 2011; 108(28): 11452-7. [http://dx.doi.org/10.1073/pnas.1106083108] [PMID: 21693646]

[211] Kwon MS, Park B, Kim HM, Kim S. Leucine-rich repeat-containing G-protein coupled receptor 5/GPR49 activates G12/13-Rho GTPase pathway. Mol Cells 2013; 36(3): 267-72. [http://dx.doi.org/10.1007/s10059-013-0173-z] [PMID: 23912594]

[212] Koo BK, Spit M, Jordens I, *et al.* Tumour suppressor RNF43 is a stem-cell E3 ligase that induces endocytosis of Wnt receptors. Nature 2012; 488(7413): 665-9. [http://dx.doi.org/10.1038/nature11308] [PMID: 22895187]

[213] Hao HX, Xie Y, Zhang Y, *et al.* ZNRF3 promotes Wnt receptor turnover in an R-spondin-sensitive manner. Nature 2012; 485(7397): 195-200. [http://dx.doi.org/10.1038/nature11019] [PMID: 22575959]

[214] Bovolenta P, Esteve P, Ruiz JM, Cisneros E, Lopez-Rios J. Beyond Wnt inhibition: new functions of secreted Frizzled-related proteins in development and disease. J Cell Sci 2008; 121(6): 737-46. [http://dx.doi.org/10.1242/jcs.026096] [PMID: 18322270]

[215] Mao B, Wu W, Davidson G, *et al.* Kremen proteins are Dickkopf receptors that regulate Wnt/β-catenin signalling. Nature 2002; 417(6889): 664-7. [http://dx.doi.org/10.1038/nature756] [PMID: 12050670]

[216] Semënov MV, Tamai K, Brott BK, Kühl M, Sokol S, He X. Head inducer Dickkopf-1 is a ligand for Wnt coreceptor LRP6. Curr Biol 2001; 11(12): 951-61.

[http://dx.doi.org/10.1016/S0960-9822(01)00290-1] [PMID: 11448771]

[217] Itasaki N, Jones CM, Mercurio S, *et al.* Wise, a context-dependent activator and inhibitor of Wnt signalling. Development 2003; 130(18): 4295-305. [http://dx.doi.org/10.1242/dev.00674] [PMID: 12900447]

[218] Semënov M, Tamai K, He X. SOST is a ligand for LRP5/LRP6 and a Wnt signaling inhibitor. J Biol Chem 2005; 280(29): 26770-5. [http://dx.doi.org/10.1074/jbc.M504308200] [PMID: 15908424]

[219] Li X, Zhang Y, Kang H, *et al.* Sclerostin binds to LRP5/6 and antagonizes canonical Wnt signaling. J Biol Chem 2005; 280(20): 19883-7. [http://dx.doi.org/10.1074/jbc.M413274200] [PMID: 15778503]

[220] Yamamoto A, Nagano T, Takehara S, Hibi M, Aizawa S. Shisa promotes head formation through the inhibition of receptor protein maturation for the caudalizing factors, Wnt and FGF. Cell 2005; 120(2): 223-35. [http://dx.doi.org/10.1016/j.cell.2004.11.051] [PMID: 15680328]

[221] Piccolo S, Agius E, Leyns L, *et al.* The head inducer Cerberus is a multifunctional antagonist of Nodal, BMP and Wnt signals. Nature 1999; 397(6721): 707-10. [http://dx.doi.org/10.1038/17820] [PMID: 10067895]

[222] Zhu W, Shiojima I, Ito Y, *et al.* IGFBP-4 is an inhibitor of canonical Wnt signalling required for cardiogenesis. Nature 2008; 454(7202): 345-9. [http://dx.doi.org/10.1038/nature07027] [PMID: 18528331]

[223] Xu Q, Wang Y, Dabdoub A, *et al.* Vascular development in the retina and inner ear: control by Norrin and Frizzled-4, a high-affinity ligand-receptor pair. Cell 2004; 116(6): 883-95. [http://dx.doi.org/10.1016/S0092-8674(04)00216-8] [PMID: 15035989]

[224] Yang K, Wang X, Zhang H, *et al.* The evolving roles of canonical WNT signaling in stem cells and tumorigenesis: implications in targeted cancer therapies. Lab Invest 2016; 96(2): 116-36. [http://dx.doi.org/10.1038/labinvest.2015.144] [PMID: 26618721]

[225] Morin PJ, Sparks AB, Korinek V, *et al.* Activation of beta-catenin-Tcf signaling in colon cancer by mutations in beta-catenin or APC. Science 1997; 275(5307): 1787-90. [http://dx.doi.org/10.1126/science.275.5307.1787] [PMID: 9065402]

[226] Bass AJ, Lawrence MS, Brace LE, *et al.* Genomic sequencing of colorectal adenocarcinomas identifies a recurrent VTI1A-TCF7L2 fusion. Nat Genet 2011; 43(10): 964-8. [http://dx.doi.org/10.1038/ng.936] [PMID: 21892161]

[227] Liu W, Dong X, Mai M, *et al.* Mutations in AXIN2 cause colorectal cancer with defective mismatch repair by activating β-catenin/TCF signalling. Nat Genet 2000; 26(2): 146-7. [http://dx.doi.org/10.1038/79859] [PMID: 11017067]

[228] Björklund P, Åkerström G, Westin G. An LRP5 receptor with internal deletion in hyperparathyroid tumors with implications for deregulated WNT/beta-catenin signaling. PLoS Med 2007; 4(11): e328. [http://dx.doi.org/10.1371/journal.pmed.0040328] [PMID: 18044981]

[229] Takeda H, Lyle S, Lazar AJF, Zouboulis CC, Smyth I, Watt FM. Human sebaceous tumors harbor inactivating mutations in LEF1. Nat Med 2006; 12(4): 395-7. [http://dx.doi.org/10.1038/nm1386] [PMID: 16565724]

[230] Satoh S, Daigo Y, Furukawa Y, *et al.* AXIN1 mutations in hepatocellular carcinomas, and growth suppression in cancer cells by virus-mediated transfer of AXIN1. Nat Genet 2000; 24(3): 245-50. [http://dx.doi.org/10.1038/73448] [PMID: 10700176]

[231] Vanamerongen R, Berns A. Knockout mouse models to study Wnt signal transduction. Trends Genet 2006; 22(12): 678-89. [http://dx.doi.org/10.1016/j.tig.2006.10.001] [PMID: 17045694]

[232] Amakye D, Jagani Z, Dorsch M. Unraveling the therapeutic potential of the Hedgehog pathway in cancer. Nat Med 2013; 19(11): 1410-22.
[http://dx.doi.org/10.1038/nm.3389] [PMID: 24202394]

[233] Lobry C, Oh P, Aifantis I. Oncogenic and tumor suppressor functions of Notch in cancer: it's NOTCH what you think. J Exp Med 2011; 208(10): 1931-5.
[http://dx.doi.org/10.1084/jem.20111855] [PMID: 21948802]

[234] Polakis P. Wnt signaling in cancer. Cold Spring Harb Perspect Biol 2012; 4(5): a008052.
[http://dx.doi.org/10.1101/cshperspect.a008052] [PMID: 22438566]

[235] Vinson KE, George DC, Fender AW, Bertrand FE, Sigounas G. The Notch pathway in colorectal cancer. Int J Cancer 2016; 138(8): 1835-42.
[http://dx.doi.org/10.1002/ijc.29800] [PMID: 26264352]

[236] Papadopoulos V, Tsapakidis K, Riobo Del Galdo NA, *et al.* The prognostic significance of the hedgehog signaling pathway in colorectal cancer. Clin Colorectal Cancer 2016; 15(2): 116-27.
[http://dx.doi.org/10.1016/j.clcc.2016.02.010] [PMID: 27032873]

[237] Nwabo KAH, Takam KP, Tagne SR, *et al.* Developmental pathways associated with cancer metastasis: Notch, Wnt, and Hedgehog. Cancer Biol Med 2017; 14(2): 109-20.
[http://dx.doi.org/10.20892/j.issn.2095-3941.2016.0032] [PMID: 28607802]

[238] Morgan TH. The theory of the gene. Am Nat 1917; 51(609): 513-44.
[http://dx.doi.org/10.1086/279629]

[239] Sandy AR, Jones M, Maillard I. Notch Signaling and Development of the Hematopoietic System.Notch Signaling in Embryology and Cancer. New York, NY: Springer US 2012; pp. 71-88.
[http://dx.doi.org/10.1007/978-1-4614-0899-4_6]

[240] Andersson ER, Sandberg R, Lendahl U. Notch signaling: simplicity in design, versatility in function. Development 2011; 138(17): 3593-612.
[http://dx.doi.org/10.1242/dev.063610] [PMID: 21828089]

[241] Lai EC. Notch signaling: control of cell communication and cell fate. Development 2004; 131(5): 965-73.
[http://dx.doi.org/10.1242/dev.01074] [PMID: 14973298]

[242] Rallis G, Koletsa T, Saridaki Z, *et al.* Association of Notch and Hedgehog Pathway Activation With Prognosis in Early-stage Colorectal Cancer. Anticancer Res 2019; 39(4): 2129-38.
[http://dx.doi.org/10.21873/anticanres.13326] [PMID: 30952759]

[243] Sikandar SS, Pate KT, Anderson S, *et al.* NOTCH signaling is required for formation and self-renewal of tumor-initiating cells and for repression of secretory cell differentiation in colon cancer. Cancer Res 2010; 70(4): 1469-78.
[http://dx.doi.org/10.1158/0008-5472.CAN-09-2557] [PMID: 20145124]

[244] Leow CC, Romero MS, Ross S, Polakis P, Gao WQ. Hath1, down-regulated in colon adenocarcinomas, inhibits proliferation and tumorigenesis of colon cancer cells. Cancer Res 2004; 64(17): 6050-7.
[http://dx.doi.org/10.1158/0008-5472.CAN-04-0290] [PMID: 15342386]

[245] Lee S, Kumano K, Nakazaki K, *et al.* Gain-of-function mutations and copy number increases of Notch2 in diffuse large B-cell lymphoma. Cancer Sci 2009; 100(5): 920-6.
[http://dx.doi.org/10.1111/j.1349-7006.2009.01130.x] [PMID: 19445024]

[246] Weng AP, Ferrando AA, Lee W, *et al.* Activating mutations of NOTCH1 in human T cell acute lymphoblastic leukemia. Science 2004; 306(5694): 269-71.
[http://dx.doi.org/10.1126/science.1102160] [PMID: 15472075]

[247] Bulman MP, Kusumi K, Frayling TM, *et al.* Mutations in the human Delta homologue, DLL3, cause axial skeletal defects in spondylocostal dysostosis. Nat Genet 2000; 24(4): 438-41.

[http://dx.doi.org/10.1038/74307] [PMID: 10742114]

[248] Simpson MA, Irving MD, Asilmaz E, *et al.* Mutations in NOTCH2 cause Hajdu-Cheney syndrome, a disorder of severe and progressive bone loss. Nat Genet 2011; 43(4): 303-5. [http://dx.doi.org/10.1038/ng.779] [PMID: 21378985]

[249] Joutel A, Corpechot C, Ducros A, *et al.* Notch3 mutations in CADASIL, a hereditary adult-onset condition causing stroke and dementia. Nature 1996; 383(6602): 707-10. [http://dx.doi.org/10.1038/383707a0] [PMID: 8878478]

[250] Li L, Krantz ID, Deng Y, *et al.* Alagille syndrome is caused by mutations in human Jagged1, which encodes a ligand for Notch1. Nat Genet 1997; 16(3): 243-51. [http://dx.doi.org/10.1038/ng0797-243] [PMID: 9207788]

[251] Artavanis-Tsakonas S, Rand MD, Lake RJ. Notch signaling: cell fate control and signal integration in development. Science 1999; 284(5415): 770-6. [http://dx.doi.org/10.1126/science.284.5415.770] [PMID: 10221902]

[252] Baron M. An overview of the Notch signalling pathway. Semin Cell Dev Biol 2003; 14(2): 113-9. [http://dx.doi.org/10.1016/S1084-9521(02)00179-9] [PMID: 12651094]

[253] Logeat F, Bessia C, Brou C, *et al.* The Notch1 receptor is cleaved constitutively by a furin-like convertase. Proc Natl Acad Sci USA 1998; 95(14): 8108-12. [http://dx.doi.org/10.1073/pnas.95.14.8108] [PMID: 9653148]

[254] Fehon RG, Kooh PJ, Rebay I, *et al.* Molecular interactions between the protein products of the neurogenic loci Notch and Delta, two EGF-homologous genes in Drosophila. Cell 1990; 61(3): 523-34. [http://dx.doi.org/10.1016/0092-8674(90)90534-L] [PMID: 2185893]

[255] Nichols JT, Miyamoto A, Olsen SL, D'Souza B, Yao C, Weinmaster G. DSL ligand endocytosis physically dissociates Notch1 heterodimers before activating proteolysis can occur. J Cell Biol 2007; 176(4): 445-58. [http://dx.doi.org/10.1083/jcb.200609014] [PMID: 17296795]

[256] Nusslein-Volhard C, Wieschaus E. Mutations affecting segment number and polarity in Drosophila. A Cen Nat: Twenty-One Discover Changed. Sci World 2003; 267.

[257] Varjosalo M, Taipale J. Hedgehog: functions and mechanisms. Genes Dev 2008; 22(18): 2454-72. [http://dx.doi.org/10.1101/gad.1693608] [PMID: 18794343]

[258] McMahon AP, Ingham PW, Tabin CJ. Developmental roles and clinical significance of Hedgehog signaling. 2003.

[259] Johnson RL, Rothman AL, Xie J, *et al.* Human homolog of patched, a candidate gene for the basal cell nevus syndrome. Science 1996; 272(5268): 1668-71. [http://dx.doi.org/10.1126/science.272.5268.1668] [PMID: 8658145]

[260] Dahmane N, Lee J, Robins P, Heller P, Altaba AR. Activation of the transcription factor Gli1 and the Sonic hedgehog signalling pathway in skin tumours. Nature 1997; 389(6653): 876-81. [http://dx.doi.org/10.1038/39918] [PMID: 9349822]

[261] Taylor MD, Liu L, Raffel C, *et al.* Mutations in SUFU predispose to medulloblastoma. Nat Genet 2002; 31(3): 306-10. [http://dx.doi.org/10.1038/ng916] [PMID: 12068298]

[262] Mullor JL, Sánchez P, Altaba AR. Pathways and consequences: Hedgehog signaling in human disease. Trends Cell Biol 2002; 12(12): 562-9. [http://dx.doi.org/10.1016/S0962-8924(02)02405-4] [PMID: 12495844]

[263] Varnat F, Duquet A, Malerba M, *et al.* Human colon cancer epithelial cells harbour active HEDGEHOG-GLI signalling that is essential for tumour growth, recurrence, metastasis and stem cell survival and expansion. EMBO Mol Med 2009; 1(6-7): 338-51.

[http://dx.doi.org/10.1002/emmm.200900039] [PMID: 20049737]

[264] Alinger B, Kiesslich T, Datz C, *et al.* Hedgehog signaling is involved in differentiation of normal colonic tissue rather than in tumor proliferation. Virchows Arch 2009; 454(4): 369-79. [http://dx.doi.org/10.1007/s00428-009-0753-7] [PMID: 19280222]

[265] Chatel G, Ganeff C, Boussif N, *et al.* Hedgehog signaling pathway is inactive in colorectal cancer cell lines. Int J Cancer 2007; 121(12): 2622-7. [http://dx.doi.org/10.1002/ijc.22998] [PMID: 17683069]

[266] Melichar H, Kang J. Integrated morphogen signal inputs in γδ *versus* αβ T-cell differentiation. Immunol Rev 2007; 215(1): 32-45. [http://dx.doi.org/10.1111/j.1600-065X.2006.00469.x] [PMID: 17291277]

[267] Lauth M, Bergstrom Å, Shimokawa T, Toftgard R. Inhibition of GLI-mediated transcription and tumor cell growth by small-molecule antagonists. Proc Natl Acad Sci USA 2007; 104(20): 8455-60. [http://dx.doi.org/10.1073/pnas.0609699104] [PMID: 17494766]

[268] Sasai N, Toriyama M, Kondo T. Hedgehog Signal and Genetic Disorders. Front Genet 2019; 10(1103): 1103. [http://dx.doi.org/10.3389/fgene.2019.01103] [PMID: 31781166]

CHAPTER 8

Epigenetic and Genetics Factors

Abeer A. Alsofyani[1,*] and **Yazan Samih Said**[2]

[1] *King Abdullah International Medical Research Center, King Saud Bin Abdulaziz University for Health Sciences, Jeddah, Saudi Arabia*

[2] *King Fahad Specialist Hospital, Dammam, Saudi Arabia*

Abstract: Despite variations in the morphology and behaviors of human body cells, every single cell in our body is composed of identical DNA material. The variation in cell phenotypes is a result of a specific regulatory mechanism known as epigenetics, by which gene expression undergoes some modifications without the actual nucleotide sequence being affected [1]. This phenomenon is accomplished through several mechanisms, such as cytosine residue methylation, modifications of histone units, and RNA interference. Therefore, epigenetics performs a key function in embryonic growth and development, cellular RNA expression, gene imprinting, and silencing of females' X chromosomes [2]. Any impairment in these mechanisms may cause various human disorders, including cancer [3]. In carcinogenesis, defective epigenetic machinery at several distinct levels results in abnormal cellular functions [4].

This chapter highlights epigenetics' importance in cancer development and its potential applications for cancer treatment.

Keywords: Cancer, Epigenetics, Histone, Methylation, miRNA.

MOLECULAR MACHINERY FOR METHYLATING DNA

DNA methylation is a central epigenetic process occurring in DNA, as it regulates gene expression and cell differentiation without altering nucleotide sequences [5, 6]. DNA methylation changes dynamically as cells develop, but the process becomes static as they begin to differentiate. This distinctive regulatory modification is indispensable for proper development, managing the expression of particular genes in specific tissues, allowing a cell to terminate DNA transcription, silencing one of the X chromosomes, and facilitating genomic imprinting.

* **Corresponding author Abeer A. Alsofyani:** King Abdullah International Medical Research Center, King Saud Bin Abdulaziz University for Health Sciences, Jeddah, Saudi Arabia; E-mail: alsofyaniab@gmail.com

Faris Q.B. Alenzi (Ed.)

Normally, methylation occurs primarily in regions where cytosine-guanine dinucleotide repeats are highly condensed, also known as CpG islands [7]. Throughout our genome, CpG sites are not randomly distributed, and most cytosine residues are methylated. Around 70% of promoters contain these clusters, which are unmethylated to keep euchromatic conformation and allow transcription factors to bind in order to initiate gene expression [5, 8]. The methylation machinery is propelled by the DNA methyltransferase (DNMT) family [2]. This enzyme family used SAM as a group donor to add the CH3 group to cytosine [9]. DNMTs are classified into three major types: DNMT1, DNMT2, and DNMT3. The latter has three sub-members: DNMT3A, DNMT3B, and DNMT3L [2]. DNMT1 is a maintenance enzyme that has a high affinity toward the hemimethylated region in the DNA helix. During cell division, the methylating activity of DNMT1 mimics the methylation process that takes place prior to DNA replication by binding to anew synthesized DNA. Further, The DNMT1 protein also helps to restore DNA methylation [10].

In contrast to other members, DNMT2 shows no enzyme activity, and its role in DNA methylation is still largely unknown; however, it appears to be involved in methylating the amino acid tRNA cytosine. A DNMT3 enzyme family is usually involved in *de novo* methylation. *De novo* methylation occurs during gametogenesis through both DNMT3A and DNMT3B. In the case of DNMT3L, it is involved in the *de novo* methylating regulatory factor in extraembryonic tissue [11].

These covalent modifications can be removed at distinct development levels from the DNA helix through a mechanism called DNA demethylation. TET enzymes catalyze the conversion of 5-methylcytosine to 5-hydroxymethylcytosine using oxygen atoms to demethylate DNA [12, 13]. There are two types of demethylations: active and passive. Active DNA demethylation is an enzyme-driven process that demethylates methylated cytosine residues by removing the methyl group from these residues. Passive DNA demethylation takes place during successive stages of replication, leading to the loss of 5-methylcytosine [12].

MOLECULAR MACHINERY FOR HISTONE MODIFICATION

Acetylation of Lysine

Histone lysine (K) undergoes acetylation\ deacetylation through the involvement of two antagonistic enzymes; acetyltransferases (HATs) and deacetylases (HDACs) [14]. HATs allocate acetyl groups to the side chains of lysine by using acetyl CoA as a cofactor. In turn, it promotes DNA liberation by diminishing positive charges on lysine residues, consequently enhancing its approachability to transcription factors and RNA polymerase complexes [15, 16]. There are three main groups of HATs: p300/CBP, MYST (which includes MOZ, MOF, TIP60, HBO1), and GNAT (which includes GCN5, PCAF) [17]. There are many cytoplasmic acetyltransferases, including MCM3AP, ARD1 and TFIIB, which can also acetylate-free histones and newly synthesized histones [18]. Moreover, acetyltransferases are capable of acetylating many non-histone proteins, allowing them to regulate the DNA binding, protein stability, and enzymatic functions [19].

Conversely, HDACs stop the histone acetylation process by restoring the lysine residue's positive charge and creating a closed chromatin conformation, allowing stabilization of the chromatin structure and controlling the gene silencing [15]. Human HDACs have four major classes [16, 20]. Together, these classes promote the closure of chromatin and the repression of gene expression. Moreover, as part of epigenetic modifications, HDAC removes acetyl groups from many non-histone proteins [21]. As transcriptional corepressors, HDACs typically form various functional complexes with other class members. HDAC1 and HDAC2 are usually present together within three distinct complexes NURD, Sin3a, and Co-REST complexes. It has been shown that the purified forms of HDAC1 and HDAC2 exhibit weak deacetylation activity [22]. HDAC3 increases its activity by forming complexes with the SMRT and NCoR. Moreover, HDAC1, HDAC2, HDAC4, HDAC5, and HDAC7 deacetylases interact with NCoR without forming a complex [23 - 25]. Therefore, existing HDAC members made it difficult to distinguish which activity is responsible for a specific action. Thus, inhibitors targeting HDACs activity are now being developed as potential cancer therapy.

Methylation of Histone

During both the differentiation and development process, histone methylation occurs in a reversible and dynamic manner. As opposed to acetylation, methylation leaves the charge unchanged on lysine and arginine residues [15]. Gene activity can be induced or inhibited by methylating histones. For instance, a methyl group can inhibit gene expression at H4K20, H3K9, and H3K27, while methylating lysine at H3K79, H3K36, and H3K4 can activate gene expression [26].

Methylation of Lysine

Six major classes of histone lysine methyltransferase (HKMTs) can methylate the N-terminal lysine. Aside from KMT4, all HKMTs possess an equivalent SET motif that is necessary for enzymatic catalysis [15, 27, 28]. These enzymes catalyze methyl transfer to amino groups on the side chains of lysine using SAM molecules as a methyl donor [15, 16]. HKMTs are characterized as particular enzymes that can distinguish between different methylated forms of histone lysine and between distinct lysine. Additionally, HKMTs play an intrinsic role in controlling the degree of lysine methylation. For instance, the DIM5 methylation enzyme specifically trimethylates H3K9 21 [29].

Methylation of Arginine

In addition to lysine, histones also contain arginine residues at their N-terminal tails that become methylated by arginine methyltransferases (PRMTs). Protein PRMTs are classified into three distinct groups; group I catalyze asymmetric dimethylation, while group II catalyzes arginine dimethylation in a symmetric way. Type III contains only PRMT7 [30 - 32]. PRMT2 (Rme2a and Rme2s) recognized by sequence homology to other PRMT members. It is thought that PRMT2 induces arginine methylation by it co-activating with the androgen receptor [33] and hormone receptor [34]. A group of these enzymes methylates arginine within histones as well as non-histone substrates [30].

Lysine and arginine methyltransferases are distinguished from other SAM-dependent methyltransferases by a specific catalytic active site. Remarkably, the binding site of lysine/arginine methyltransferases is characterized by two faces, opposite to each other. One is a site for SAM, and the other is a site for peptidyl acceptor [35]. By understanding this unique enzyme's active site, a targeted therapy may be discovered that is capable of distinguishing among different histone methyltransferases.

Arginine/Lysine Histone Demethylation

Histone demethylases (HDMs) are categorized into two groups; lysine-specific demethylase (LSDs) and JMJC-containing demethylases [36]. Specifically, LSDs (LSD1 and LSD2) remove the methyl group from monomethylated and dimethylated lysine residues in a FAD-dependent way [37, 38]. Researchers have shown that LSD1 demethylates H3K9 and activates androgen receptor-targeted genes by forming a complex with the androgen receptor [37]. H3K4me1 and H3K4me2 are demethylated by LSD1 complexed with Co-REST [39].

JMJC-containing demethylases have the capacity to demethylate each methylated lysine form [40]. A JMJC domain containing JHDM1A demethylates lysine residues H3K36me1\2. At the same time, JMJD6 removes the methyl group from arginine residues; H3R2 and H4R3 [41]. Arginine deamination is a demethylation process where methylated arginine is converted to citrulline by arginine demethylase (PADI4), resulting in neutralizes the positive charge of the arginine residues [42].

Histone Phosphorylation

Dynamic phosphorylation of histone tails occurs primarily on tyrosine, serine, and threonine residues [43]. Two enzymes control histone phosphorylation levels by adding and removing other modifications: histone kinases and phosphatases [44]. The phosphorylation process modifies the conformation of chromatin, and the interaction between transcription factors as the amino ends get negatively charged [15, 45]. Phosphorylated H3S10 is tightly combined with H3K14 and H3K9 to induce transcriptional activation [46, 47]. Further, phosphorylating H2AX (γH2AX) contributes greatly to the healing of DNA breaks [48]. Histone phosphorylation marks can be removed by dephosphorylation enzymes, resulting in gene expression repression.

Other Modifications

Histone modifications are not limited only to methylation, acetylation, and phosphorylation. However, an excessive number of other modifications have also been described for histone modifications, including ubiquitylation and neddylation [15, 49, 50], sumoylation [51], deimination or citrullination [42], and β-N-acetylglucosamine [52], butyrylation and propionylation [53], ADP ribosylation [54], proline isomerization [55], lysine crotonylation [56], biotinylation [57], tyrosine hydroxylation [58], and N-formylation [59]. Overall, all types of histone modifications either exert their effects directly by altering the chromatin conformation or by regulating the binding of modifier molecules.

Mechanism of Histone Modifications

The modification of histones is critical for DNA duplication, repair, and gene transcription. This chapter will focus on gene transcription regulation, however. Histone modifications operate through two mechanisms. Firstly, direct structural perturbation of entire chromatin, and the second is recruiting when nonhistone proteins are recruited to the sites of modification.

Direct Structural Perturbation

Higher-order chromatin can be disrupted either by adjusting the total charge, as in acetylation and phosphorylation of histones or adding new molecules, as in ubiquitylation. When histones are modified through acetylation and phosphorylation, this can reduce the binding between histones and DNA. Thus, this causes the chromatin to unravel, allowing proteins involved in transcription to access the DNA [15].

Acetylated regions are widely distributed throughout the genome, which can effectively neutralize the charge on histone tails. This allows the structure of chromatin to unfold [60]. Enhancers and promoters are the two regions enriched with acetylated lysine facilitating the access of transcription factors [61]. However, not all the acetylation can change higher-order structures as with acetylated H4K16 [62].

Compared with histone acetylation, histone phosphorylation is a specific site modification that undoubtedly changes chromatin's overall structure. Such modification adds a negatively charged phosphate group to the histone tail that alters chromatin conformation [44]. Ubiquitylation is another mechanism that effectively induces an overall structural change of the nucleosome by adding a ubiquitin molecule, 76-amino acid polypeptide, to histone lysins. Unlike other histone modifications, ubiquitylation results in an extremely larger covalent alteration, which will perturb chromatin structure [63]. A further way to influence nucleosome interactions with DNA and/or complexes is to remove at least 21 amino acids from the H3 histone N-terminal tail by histone tail clipping [15, 64].

Regulating the Binding of Chromatin Factor

Another mechanism for histone modifications is the recruitment of chromatin-associated factors (Fig. **8.1**). Depending on the type of modification and nucleosomal features, a set of non-histone proteins can recognize specifically modified histones by their distinct domains within them. As an example, chromodomain-like proteins are highly attracted to methylated lysine sites, bromodomain-related proteins are attracted to acetylated regions, and phosphorylated sites are attracted to 14-3-3 proteins [60].

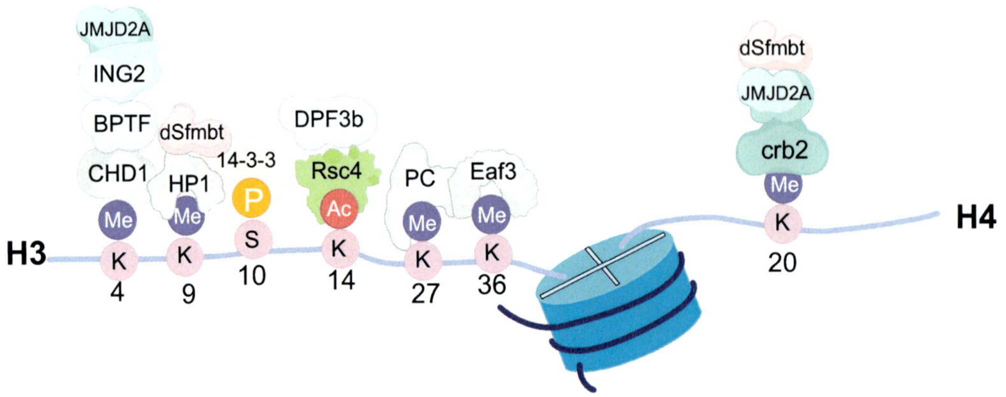

Fig. (8.1). Binding of selected proteins to modified histones through their specific domains. Created with BioRender.com.

Bromodomain PHD Finger Transcription Factor (BPTF) can recognize trimethylated H3K4 through its PHD domain. As a results, the recruited BPTF binds to the SNF2L ATPase and promotes H0XC8 gene expression [65]. Inhibitor of growth II (ING II) proteins belong to the ING family, also have a PHD domain that can read H3K4me3 tags on the histone tail and recruit histone acetyltransferase (HAT) or histone deacetylase (HDAC) to the site [66]. Additionally, ING II can tether the repressive histone deacetylases complex (mSin3a-HDAC1) to active the proliferation-particular genes after DNA damage *via* DNA-damaging agents [66, 67]. CHD1 (a histone lysine demethylase) and JMJD2A (an ATPase) are other H3K4me3 binding proteins that bind to the methylated site *via* tandem chromodomains and Tudor domains, respectively [68, 69].

A Specific methylation on the histone (H3K27me and H3K9me) is considered a marker for recruiting proteins that allow gene expression silencing. As an example, HP1-protein interacts with H3K9-me3 to control gene silencing. The formed H3K9me3-HP1 complex then activates both methyltransferase activity and deacetylase enzymes [60, 70, 71].

Once acetyl groups are added to lysine residues, bromodomain-related proteins can read those marks and mediate chromatin structural change [72]. For instance, the chromatin-remodeling complex Swi2/Snf2 comprises a bromodomain that recognizes acetylated lysine and binds to it, resulting in open the chromatin for transcription factors [73]. Tandem Ph.D. fingers of DPF3b can recognize the acetylated sites on the H3 and form a complex with an H3K14ac, which in turn attracts the BAF complex to acetylated histones [74].

Histone Modification Communications

The diversity of possible modifications on the histone's tail creates a cross-talk among modifications, leading to an additional complexity level to control the overall chromatin structure (Fig. **8.2**) [15]. Systematically, such cross-take may occur by several different mechanisms. Firstly, different modifications are competing on the same site(s) of the histone, creating a form of antagonism between them. Particularly, histone lysine is a targeted residue for methylation, acetylation, and/or ubiquitylation. Secondly, modifying the site where an enzyme recognizes its substrate could affect its activity [55]. Thirdly, in some cases, an adjoining modification, for example, can interfere with the binding of a protein. HP1's ability to bind to methylated H3K9 might be disrupted by phosphorylation [75]. In *S. pombe*, binding of spChp1 to H3K9me is inhibited due to the acetylation of H3K4 83 [76]. Fourthly, the recognition of substrate by its enzyme may depend on another modification. For example, phosphorylation at H3S10 allows GCN5 acetyltransferase to recognize H3 effectively [77]. Several histone modifications can communicate with each other. For tri-methylated H3K4, for example, H2B ubiquitination is necessary [60].

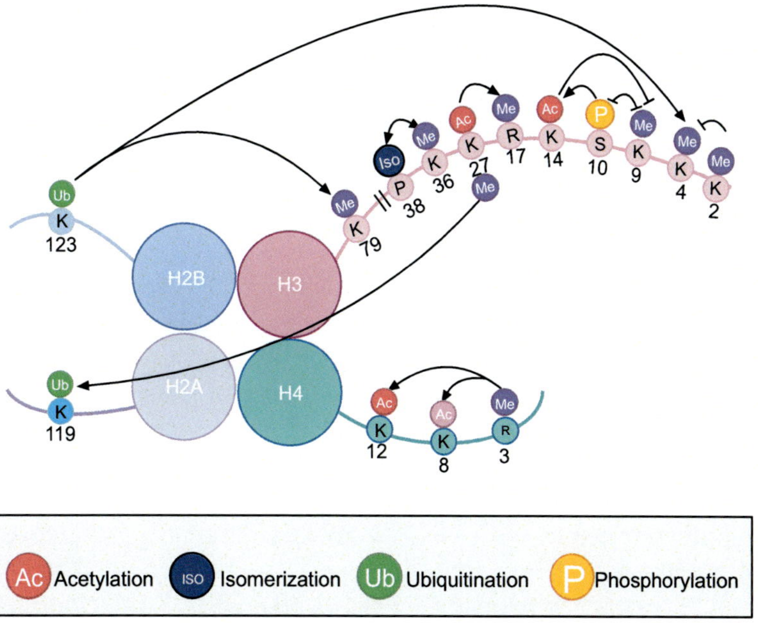

Fig. (8.2). Communication between histone modifications. In the illustration, an arrow depicts the positive impact, while a flat head shows the destructive effect. Adapted from reference [15] and created with BioRender.com.

CHROMATIN REMODELING COMPLEXES

DNA packaging and unpackaging are dynamically balanced through collaboration between a set of specialized proteins [78]. A nucleosome is a repeating unit of chromatin structure that can be moving or ejecting *via* chromatin remodeling complexes (remodelers), altering chromatin's packaging state. The precise mechanism of how the remodeler complexes target specific sites and alter the whole nucleosome and chromatin structure remains elusive. However, similarities and differences between these complexes give us an idea of how chromatin remodelers act. Remodeling complexes must first recognize their binding sides on the nucleosome or DNA and bind to it, controlling chromatin's packaging/unpackaging state and various biological processes [79, 80].

Extensive studies have attempted to demonstrate the pattern of how the complexes bind to their substrate. SWI/SNF complex, for example, recognizes specific structural sites on the DNA and nucleosome and binds to them with high affinity. In contrast, the ISWI complex interacts with DNA with low affinity and forms an unstable complex [80, 81].

Remodeler Families

Remodeling complexes perform multiple functions that ensure the proper conformation of chromatin structure and functions for either gene transcription activation or repression. Functionally, chromatin remodelers can be grouped into three sets. Set of remodelers named assembly remodelers assist in the assembly and spacing of nucleosomes following DNA replication [82], where assembly-related complexes such as ISWI and CHD are recruited to the site. At which, remodeling complexes form tightly nucleosome arrays *via* the establishment of canonical octameric nucleosomes and positioning of nucleosomes in a fixed distance. These functional properties for ISWI and CHD complexes result in gene silencing (Fig. **8.3A**) [83 - 86]. Another set of chromatin remodelers is called access remodelers (such as SWI/SNF family) that enhance accessibility for transcription factors (activators or repressors) to bind DNA at promoters or enhancers regions. Mechanistically, a nucleosome-access remodeler slides nucleosomes together with DNA, removes a part of a nucleosome or evicts the whole nucleosome. Thus, remodeling complexes activate the chromatin opening process for gene expression (Fig. **8.3B**) [87, 88]. Another further set of remodelers is editing remodelers, who exchange the first canonical histone with a histone variant to restructure the nucleosome. Good examples of editing remodelers are the INO80 subfamily (INO80, p400, and SRCAP) which have unique editing functions (Fig. **8.3C**) [89, 90].

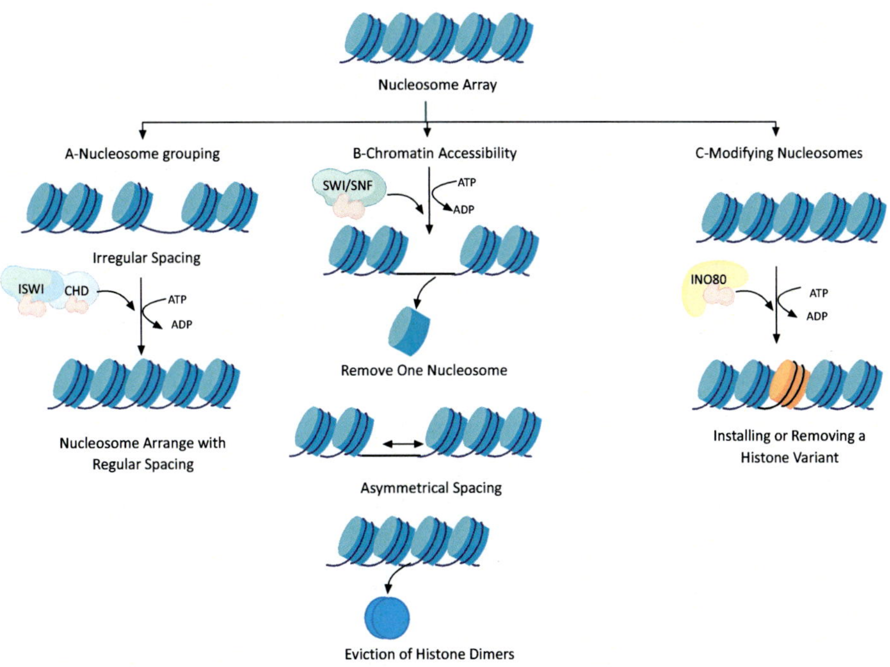

Fig. (8.3). Functional classification of chromatin remodelers. All four use ATP hydrolysis to do their related function. **A** - Nucleosome assembly: ISWI and CHD subfamily remodelers can collect the chromatins of the random deposited histones and form a nucleosome array with comparatively fixed distance. **B**- Chromatin access: mainly, SWI/SNF subfamily remodelers can act on a nucleosome array to facilitate chromatin access by irregular repositioning nucleosomes (nucleosomal sliding), evicting histone's octamer or ejecting histone dimers. This function not restricted to SWI/SNF subfamily, certain CHD and NO80C remodelers have a role chromatin access. **C**-Nucleosome editing: primarily INO80 subfamily remodelers can replace H2A-H2B dimer with H2A.Z variants (selected histone). Adapted from reference [90] and created with BioRender.com.

Although several ATPase remodelers have distinct biological functions during normal development, they are not required for cell viability, as seen with other subfamilies [91 - 93]. In so doing, any structural abnormality within a subunit of such a remodeler would result in an abnormal cell with aberrant pathways leading to cell transformation. Recent technological advances have provided a unique opportunity for discovering new links between cancer development and chromatin remodeling complexes.

MICRORNAS

Endogenous microRNA (miRNA) is a small, noncoding RNA, which controls gene activities. The miRNAs act by interacting with messenger RNA (mRNA) in order to repress gene translation [94].

Profiling of miRNAs and profound sequencing studies confirm that miRNA levels are changed in many malignancies. This information would be utilized to diagnose, prognosis, and classify tumors [95]. At present, thousands of genes have been annotated as human miRNA precursors that are being processed as mature miRNA sequences. However, many miRNAs are characterized by unknown functions. All levels of the biogenesis of miRNAs are highly regulated, specifically, the transcription level of miRNAs, the transport, the binding of the RISC to miRNAs, and its degradation.

Interactions between miRNA and their targets begin after miRNAs have attached to specific mRNAs, leading to translational suppression [96]. In addition to regulating gene expression by pairing with related mRNAs, miRNAs serve as ligands to stimulate signaling pathways. For example, miRNA-21/miRNA-29a produced by tumor cells adhere directly to toll-like receptor 7 or 8 on the surface of immune cells and cause a metastatic inflammatory response. Most likely, this will cause a tumor to grow and spread [97].

AN ANALYSIS OF EPIGENETIC GENE SILENCING IN CANCER

Several alterations happen to the cell during its transformation, resulting in abnormal gene expression patterns. However, the explosion of studies has enhanced our understanding of the mechanisms behind gene expression dysregulations; much more effort is required to expand our knowledge of these mechanisms. Changes in epigenetic modifications, including inappropriate DNA methylation within control regions, alteration in histone post-translation, an aberration in epigenetic modifying enzymes, mutations within chromatin remodeling subunits, and alteration regulatory microRNA, can be linked to both tumor initiation and progression (Fig. **8.4**).

Aberrant DNA Methylation in Cancer

In certain circumstances, genomes are often subjected to epigenetic changes due to extended exposure to pathogenic agents, carcinogenic substances, hormonal imbalances, abnormal mutations in mediators' genes, or any other epigenetic disturbance leading to DNA methylation instability throughout the genome. The following three general patterns can be observed in transformed cells: cancer genome hypomethylation, promoter hypermethylation, and mutations within 5-methylcytosine containing sequences. A dysfunction in the methylation remodeler's enzyme is the cause for abnormal DNA methylation (Table **8.1**). There has been considerable evidence that cancers overexpress DNMT1, and DNMT3 (a and b). A high level of DNMT1 expression was observed in ovarian

[98], gliomas [99], pancreas [100, 101], and esophageal cancer [102]. It has also been described that DNMT3a level was elevated in vulvar carcinomas [103], testicular cancer [104], and various solid cancers. Similarly, oncogenesis has also been linked with the disruption of DNA demethylation enzymes TET. By overexpressing TET1 and TET2, the global level of 5-methylated cytosine can be decreased [105]. Breast and prostate cancer are characterized by tumor penetration due to loss TET1 [106]. In the course of myeloid cancer. TET2 plays a tumor-inhibiting role, and ~15% of patients harbor a mutation in the TET2 gene [107, 108].

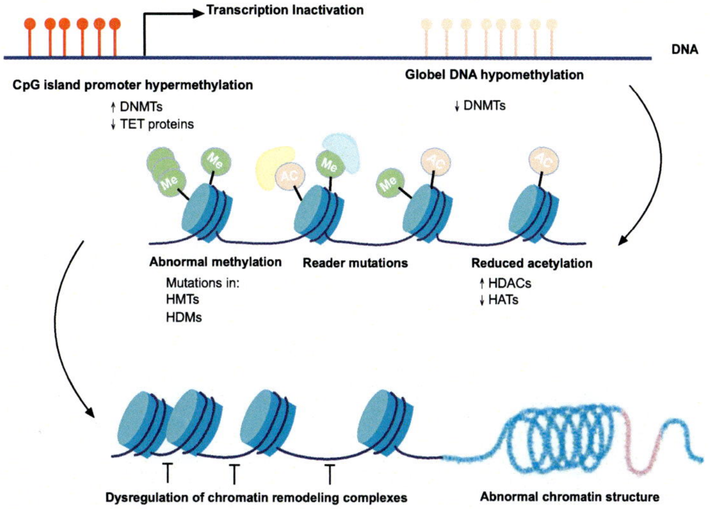

Fig. (8.4). Overview of several epigenetic alterations in cancer. Gene transcriptional inactivation is usually caused by CpG island promoter hypermethylation, global DNA hypomethylation, changes in histone modification and chromatin remodeling complexes. These main aspects of cancer epigenome resulting in the formation of abnormal chromatin structure. AC: acetylated, Me: methylated. Methylated cytosine is indicated by dark lollipop and unmethylated cytosine is indicated by light lollipop. Created with BioRender.com.

Table 8.1. Dysregulation of DNA methylation/demethylation enzymes in cancer.

Enzyme		Dysregulation	Tumor Types
DNA methyltransferases	DNMT1	Upregulated	AML, CML, breast, lung, bladder colorectal, glioma, pancreatic, esophageal, thyroid, and ovarian cancer
		Downregulated	Cervical and prostate cancer
	DNMT3a	Upregulated	Cervical, breast, gastric, prostate cancer, ovarian, and testicular cancer
		Downregulated	Lymphoma, AML, colorectal, and lung cancer
	DNMT3b	Upregulated	CML, AML, colorectal, prostate glioma, cervical, and bladder cancer

(Table 8.1) cont.....

Enzyme		Dysregulation	Tumor Types
DNA demethylases	TET1	Upregulated	AML, ovarian, breast, and renal cancer
		Downregulated	Gastric, prostate cancer, hepatocellular, and nasopharyngeal carcinoma
	TET2	Downregulated	Breast, CML, MDS, AML, colorectal prostate, and gastric cancer
	TET3	Downregulated	Ovarian cancer

DNA Hypomethylation

Feinberg and Vogelstein were the first who report the methylation loss phenomena in cancer genomes that were recently defined as hallmarks of cancers. They found that colon adenomas display hypomethylation in some of the genes compared with normal epithelium cells [103, 104]. Several subsequent studies have confirmed recurrent overall genomic hypomethylation in tumors relative to normal tissues [105 - 107]. In this regard, hypomethylation is predicted to cause metastasis and progression of cancer more commonly than hypomethylation [108]. In many instances, deficiency of DNA methylation is linked with transcription reactivation, permitting transcription of oncogenes, repeats, and transposable elements that lead to genomic instability [109, 110]. Oncogene activation is predicted to be correlated with the reduction of methylation levels [111, 112].

In global hypomethylation, 5-methylcytosine content throughout the genome is decreased. There is a significant reduction in methylated 5-methylcytosine in tumor cells, specifically in repetitive sequences [113]. Hypomethylated repetitive DNA sequences are observed frequently in constitutive centromeric satellite alpha, juxtacentromeric satellite 2, and interspersed repeats (LINEs and SINEs) [114 - 116]. Indeed, multiple copies of hypomethylated repeats destabilized all the chromosomal rearrangement in the cell, as seen in Wilms' tumor [117].

Hypomethylation of specific loci of a gene frequently occurs in cancer cells. For example, c-Myc is acts as a regulator of chromatin structure throughout histone acetylation [118 - 120]. Hypomethylated protooncogene c-Myc was observed in hepatocellular carcinoma [121], gastric cancer [122], and acute leukemia. In addition, DNA hypomethylation at alleles of the imprinted gene IGF2 may result in abnormal IGF2 expression, a characteristic often found in tumor cells. It is also possible that IGF2 may act as a predictor for cancer susceptibility as it is detected in normal colon tissues and peripheral blood [123]. Hypomethylation of IGF2 could be a potential biomarker for colorectal cancer [124], and colon neoplasia [125], and esophageal squamous cell carcinoma [126]. As seen in several cancers, hypermethylation of DNA also contributes to the distribution of normally methylated microRNAs, such as miR-196b miRNA196b [127], and miRNA200a\200b [128].

DNA Hypermethylation

DNA methylation patterns are significantly altered during the development of tumors, indicating that these changes occur early in cellular transformation. A cancer cell exhibits increased methylation within CpG rich regions, resulting in transcriptional silencing of genes associated with cancer-suppressive functions (Table **8.2**). It is, therefore, possible to use these erroneously hypermethylated regions to predict the passage of the disease. Currently, it is unclear what causes promoter hypermethylation in cancer. It could be due to the interaction between DNMT1 and specific DNA-binding proteins [129]. Hypermethylation frequency of MGMT was found in 19.44% of HPV-negative oral and oropharyngeal tumors, and it is suggested as a potential biomarker for predict patients' responsiveness to cisplatin chemotherapy [130]. Abnormal methylation has been associated with a patient's clinical features and susceptibility to cancer, diagnosis, and prognosis. In breast cancer, hypermethylated DAPK1 was linked to poor overall survival [131, 132].

Table 8.2. An important cellular pathway is disrupted by hypermethylation of the major genes.

Pathways	Hypermethylated Genes
DNA repair	MGMT, BRCA1, hMLH1, WRN
Cell cycle	p16INK4a, p15INK4b, Rb, CCND2
Apoptosis	DAPK, TP73, WIF-1, TMS1
Metastasis	PCDH10, CDH13
Detoxification	GSTP1
Ras signaling	RASSF1, NOREIA
Wnt signaling	APC, DKK1, IGFBP-3
P53 pathway	p14ARF, HIC1, p73
Tyrosine kinase pathway	SYK, SOCS1, SOCS3
Transcription factors	ID4, GATA4, GATA5
Homeobox genes	PAX6, HOXA9
Angiogenesis	VHL

A meta-analysis study revealed that DAPK1 promoter hypermethylation was associated with aggressive cervical neoplasia and could be used as a diagnostic mark for distinguishing cervical cancer from cancer-free tissues [133].

Furthermore, downregulated DAPK1 in a patient with gastric cancer was correlated with late stage of disease [134].

DNA hypermethylation affects several genes that regulate multiple cellular pathway that seen in cancer. As an example, a tumor repressor gene RASSF1 negatively regulates cell cycle progression [135]. Abnormal methylation of RASSF1A was observed to be associated with cancer stage [136], lymph node metastasis and overall survival in nasopharyngeal carcinomas [137]. Previously, it was suggested that the promoter methylation of RASSF1A could be used as a biomarker to detect HNSCC [138]. Further, epigenetic silencing of RASSF1A was found to increase uterine cervix cancer risk [139].

The function of SFRP1 is essential for controlling cell viability and cell maturation [140]. Epigenetic silencing of SFRP1 was reported in several cancers, indicating that SFRP1 has tumor-suppressive roles [141]. Downregulation of SFRP1 by promoter hypermethylation was linked with tumor grade and stage and worse overall survival [142, 143]. In colorectal cancer patients, methylated RASGRF1 served as a putative biomarker of overall survival [144]. Taking it all together, promoter hypermethylation in certain genes could be useful to predict cancer progression, metastasis, and resistance therapies.

Despite the recent advances in anti-tumoral regimens, most cancer patients develop drug resistance, making it a major issue in cancer treatment. Several therapy resistance and predicting response to anti-tumor therapy have been linked to certain genes' promoter methylation status [145]. For instance, aberrant hypermethylation of MGMT, a DNA repair enzyme, induced tumor cell's chemoresistance. As a result, methylated MGMT can be used as a useful marker for response to temozolomide, and cyclophosphamide in cases of brain tumor and diffuse large B-cell lymphoma, respectively [146 - 148]. Inactivated TGFBI *via* promoter's hypermethylation showed an alternative mechanism to induce Trastuzumab resistance in breast cancer [149]. Additionally, resistance to 5-Fluorouracil (5-FU) was associated with hypermethylation NKX6.1 [150], CHL1, CCNEI, CCNDBP1, DDX43, and PON3 [151] in colorectal cancer and TFAP2E in gastric cancer [152]. Resistance to cisplatin was also recorded to hypermethylated MT1G, GPR56, RASSF1, and PDE3A in lung cancer [153, 154], KCNQ1, and CSF3R in hepatocellular cancer [155, 156].

On the other side, transcriptional silencing mediated by hypermethylation can be reverted for some genes. For instance, DNMT inhibitor 5-azacytidine has been proven to effectively treat hematological neoplasms and various solid tumors by inhibiting DNA methylation [145]. Restoring the expression of methylated GAS5 in adriamycin-resistant cells (SGC-7901/ADM) showed significant decreases in tumor growth and apoptosis following Adriamycin treatment [157]. In lung cancer, drug resistance is correlated with hypermethylation of the TRAIL gene [158]. Using a demethylating reagent to demethylate TRAIL methylation results in restoring sensitivity to the treatment [88]. Based on these findings, it is possible that abnormal DNA methylation might be a potential cause of cancer drug resistance.

Aberrant Histone Modification in Cancer

Histone modification is an integral part of epigenetic gene regulation that controls both chromatin arrangement and gene expression; thus, it is no surprise that abnormal alterations in histone modification are associated with cancer development (Table **8.3**). One of the examples of deviant histone modification in tumorigenesis is an aberrant activity of histone acetyltransferases (HATs). Dysregulated HAT1 was seen in lung cancer, hepatocellular carcinoma, nasopharyngeal cancer, pancreatic cancer, and esophageal carcinoma. Such dysregulation shows an effect on cell apoptosis, proliferation, differentiation and cisplatin resistance [159 - 162].

Table 8.3. Dysregulation of selected histone modifier enzymes in human cancer.

Enzyme		Dysregulation	Tumor Types
Histone acetylases	HAT1	Upregulated	Pancreatic, hepatocellular carcinoma, and esophageal carcinoma
		Downregulated	Lung cancer
	GCN5L2 (GCN5)	Upregulated	Breast, and colorectal cancer
	HTATIP (TIP60)	Upregulated	Prostate and liver cancer
		Downregulated	Bladder, breast, and colorectal cancer
	MYST1 (MOF)	Upregulated	Prostate cancer
Histone acetylases	MYST2 (HBO1)	Upregulated	Leukemia, ovarian, bladder, breast, and pancreatic cancer
	MYST3 (MOZ)	Upregulated	Leukemia, colorectal cancer, breast cancer
	MYST4 (MORF)	Upregulated	Leukemia
	CBP (CREBBP, KAT3A)	Upregulated	Leukemia, lung, gastric, ovarian, prostate, and hepatocellular carcinoma
		Downregulated	Lung, and prostate cancer
	P300 (EP300, KAT3B)	Upregulated	leukemia, lung, breast, colorectal, nasopharyngeal, gastric, prostate, and cervical cancer

(Table 8.3) cont.....

Enzyme		Dysregulation	Tumor Types
Histone deacetylase	HDAC1	Upregulated	Ovarian, colorectal, and gastric, pancreatic cancer
	HDAC2	Upregulated	Lung, colorectal, pancreatic, ovarian, breast, and prostate cancer
	HDAC3	Upregulated	Lung, colorectal, pancreatic, breast, prostate, esophageal, cervical, breast cancer
	KMT2A (KMT2A)	Upregulated	Lymphoid, myeloid leukemias, and pancreatic cancer
	EZH2 (KMT6)	Upregulated	Breast cancer
		Mutation	B cell lymphoma
	RIZ1 (KMT8)	Mutation	Liver, breast, and gastric cancer
	PFM2 (PRDM5)	Downregulated	Colorectal, gastric, and cervical cancer
	NSD1	Translocation	AML
		Mutations	Sotos syndrome
		Epigenetic Silencing	Gliomas, and neuroblastoma
	NSD2	Translocation	Multiple myeloma
	NSD3	Translocation	Leukemia
		Amplification	Breast cancer
Arginine methyltransferases	PRMT1 (HCP)	Upregulated	Breast, colon, and gastric cancer
	PRMT2	Downregulated	Breast cancer
	PRMT8	Upregulated	Ovarian and gastric cancer
Histone demethylases	KDM1A (LSD1)	Upregulated	Breast, prostate, and liver cancer
	KDM2B (FBXL10)	Mutation	Lymphoma
		Downregulated	Brain, and glioblastoma multiforme
	KMD4D (JMJD2D)	Upregulated	Colorectal cancer
	KDM7B (JHDM1F)	Upregulated	Colorectal, prostate, and gastric cancer

GCN5 and PCAF are two members of histone acetyltransferases [163]. The increase in GCN5 levels is linked with lung, colorectal, and breast cancer [163 - 165]. Additionally, overexpressed GCN5 has been shown to affect genes involved in the Smad signaling pathway and PI3K signaling pathway [165, 166]. PCAF, by contrast, is a tumor suppressor that involves in cell cycling processes [167]. Downregulated PCAF was seen in gastric, breast, and prostate cancer [167 - 169].

The reduction of PCAF is coupled with 5-fluorouracill impedance [170]. Furthermore, low PCAF expression might be a potential marker for invasive and aggressive tumors.

Lysine residue is also methylated by the DOT1L enzyme. Apparated expression of such an enzyme is correlated with mixed lineage leukemia due to chromosomal translocations rather than solid tumors [171]. Chromosomal rearrangements resulting in gene fusion are frequently seen in different kinds of leukemia. Different rearrangements of acetyltransferase MYST2 (HBO1), MYST3, and MYST4 have been observed in leukemia. MYST2 was identified as a new NUP98-MYST2 fusion in CMML, leading to increased classical monocytes, myelodysplasia, and cachexia [172]. MYST3 gene located at 8p11.2 was commonly fused to transcription regulator genes such as NCOA1 [173], NCOA2 [174], NCOA3 and CBP/CREBB [175].

Trimethylated H3K27 (H3K27me3) negatively controls gene transcription by establishing a compact chromatin structure to mediate gene silencing [176]. A significant increase in H3K27me3 level was seen in esophageal, breast, pancreatic, and ovarian cancers [177 - 179]. Histone-lysine methyltransferases - EZH2 process trimethylation for H3K27 [180]. The EZH2 gene is overexpressed in the bladder, breast, kidneys, lungs, and hematological cancers [181 - 185]. A substantial increase in tumor development, invasion, and H3K27me3 levels is associated with an upregulated expression of EZH2 [186]. Aberration in the H3K27me3 level can also result from somatic mutations in the UTX enzyme that mediate the removal of H3K27me3 marks, as seen in myeloma [187].

Loss of UTX activity was found in breast cancer invasiveness [188]. The trimethylation of H3K4 (H3K4me3) promotes transcriptional activation, and it is largely present in promoters of active genes [38]. H3K4 is hypomethylated in a variety of tumors, and its altered levels could serve as a prognostic marker [189 - 191].

KMT2A, a SET1 member of the histone methyltransferases family, catalyzes the methylation of H3K4. The pancreatic and head and neck cancerous tissues are highly expressed KMT2A, it promotes cells' self-renewal *via* the Wnt-catenin pathway, and influences transcription of PD-L1 [192, 193]. It was also observed that KMT2D overexpression is strongly linked to poor outcomes in gastric cancer [194]. A high level of SMYD3 expression can be observed in liver, breast, and colon malignancies [195, 196]. Additionally, the methylation mark on H3K4me3 can be removed by HDMs; LSD1 and JARID1 [39]. In the case of LSD1, its level is significantly elevated in multiple cancers [197 - 201]. Another family of HDMs is JARID1, which is found upregulated in colorectal, breast, and hypopharyngeal carcinoma. Overexpressed JARID1B contributes to the cell's proliferative activity and invasion [202 - 204].

ROLE OF MICRORNA IN CANCER

It has been demonstrated conclusively that human cancers display dysregulated miRNA expression *via* a variety of mechanisms, such as defects in miRNA transcription, alterations in epigenetic regulation, and malfunctions in miRNA biosynthesis.

Inactivation or Amplification of miRNA Genes

Malignant cells can express abnormal miRNAs as compared to normal cells because of changes in the miRNAs copy numbers [205]. miRNA amplification has been reported in lung cancers and B-cell lymphomas [206]. Translocation of the miRNA-17–92 gene was also detected in lymphoblastic leukemia [207]. Additional investigations revealed that many miRNA genes are found in cancer-related regions. Some of these regions may contain tumor suppressor genes, and oncogenes or may have certain breakpoints [208]. In sum, the expression of abnormal miRNAs in malignant cells may result from the depletion or amplification of genomic loci containing miRNA genes [95].

A Transcriptional Control Mechanism for miRNAs

Different transcription factors are required, including c-Myc and p5, to regulate miRNA expression. These factors work together, so that miRNA expression is carefully controlled to ensure standard transcription. Therefore, dysregulation of such factors may promote tumor growth. Many malignancies have elevated c-Myc levels that trigger the onco-activation of miRNA17–92 [209]. In accordance, c-Myc can suppress the transcriptional activity of tumor-suppressive miRNA-30 [210].

The tumor suppressor p53 is commonly mutated in cancer. The p53 gene network regulates many genes, including miRNA. miRNA-34 exhibits similar phenotypes to p53 in cancer tissues, suggesting that p53 and miRNA-34 share the same regulatory pathway [211].

Dysregulated Epigenetic Changes

Epigenetic modifications have long played a prominent role in cancer, including global hypomethylation, disruption of histone modification, and hypermethylation of tumor suppressor genes. miRNAs may be susceptible to epigenetic regulation in the same manner as protein-coding genes [212, 213]. It appears that the demethylation of DNA can promote the expression of miRNA, which may function as a tumor suppressor and defends the concept of epigenetic control of miRNA expression in cancer development.

Role of Altered miRNA Expression in Cancer

It has been demonstrated that dysregulated miRNA disrupts all six features of cancer. In view of atypical miRNA levels in the malignant cell, dysregulated miRNAs are supposed to directly affect tumor initiation and progression by dysregulating one or more cancer hallmarks [214].

Achieving resistance to growth suppressors and continuing proliferative signaling are the primary hallmarks of cancer. In certain conditions, miRNAs may function either as suppressive or oncogenic miRNAs.

miRNA regulates p53 function differently, modulating p53 levels and their activities in a feedback loop. Malignant cells that lack p53 function or its miRNA targets may display the ability to resist cell death. Multiple cancers are frequently characterized by a high level of miRNA-21. Through inhibiting Apaf-1 expression and decreasing Fas ligand levels, miRNA-21 serves as an anti-apoptotic molecule in lung tumors [215].

The role that microRNAs play in the EMT and cancer dissemination is becoming increasingly evident. It has been found that miRNA-155 overexpression causes the EMT and invasion of tumors [216].

It is also possible that miRNA is involved in inducing angiogenesis by altering its expression in cancer cells. Many miRNAs may have an important role in angiogenesis [217]. There are several miRNAs that are continuously and highly induced by hypoxia, including miRNA-210 and miRNA-424 [218].

In summary, miRNA expression is dysregulated in various types of cancer. Dysregulated miRNA expression can cause a tumor to initiate or progress in several different ways. Additionally, miRNAs may act to promote tumor occurrence by targeting specific targets even though they have multiple targets. Moreover, miRNAs have been proposed as promising tools for diagnosing, monitoring, and treating human cancers. In this context, establishing the roles of miRNAs in tumorigenesis and identifying their targets will be major challenges.

CHROMATIN REMODELING COMPLEXES AND CANCER

Much more work has been done linking chromatin remodeling complexes to cancer development. Whole-genome sequencing has shown that several remodeler genes are commonly mutated, indicating that mutations in some subunits are associated with certain cancers that may drive cell growth and differentiation, as shown in Table **8.4**. In addition to dysregulating the expression of oncogenes and tumor suppressors that is essential for cancer development, many chromatin remodeling complexes have nononcogene function that is imperative for the malignant cell to retain its characteristics and maintain its growth signals, such as NURF, RSF, and CERF remodelers' complexes [219, 220].

Table 8.4. Chromatin remodelers differentially regulated by cancerous cells.

Family	Subunit	Dysregulation	Tumor Types
ISWI family	BPTF	Upregulated	Myeloma
		Downregulated	Lymphoma
	SMARCA1	Downregulated	melanoma
	RSF1	Upregulated	Liver, oral, gallbladder, colon, bladder, rectal, prostate, ovarian, and nasopharyngeal cancer
	BAZ1A	Upregulated	Kidney caner
	SMARCA5	Upregulated	Ovarian, and breast cancer
	BAZ2A	Upregulated	Pancreatic cancer
	BAZ1B	Upregulated	Lung cancer
SWI/SNF family	PBRM1 (BAF180)	Inactivating mutation	Renal cancer
		Deletion	Pancreatic cancer
	SMARCD1	Downregulated	Ovarian, and lung cancer
		Upregulated	Gastric cancer
	SMARCA4 (BRG1)	Upregulated	melanoma and prostate cancer
		Inactivating mutation	Burkitt lymphoma, renal, and ovarian cancer
	ACTL6A (BAF53a)	Upregulated	Cervix, and Rhabdomyosarcoma
	SMARCE1 (BAF57)	Upregulated	Prostate, and bladder cancer
	SMARCC1 (BAF155)	Upregulated	Melanoma, liver, and prostate cancer
	ARID1A (BAF250A)	Inactivating mutation	Burkitt lymphoma, liver, pancreatic, renal, and endometrial cancer
	ARID1B (BAF250B)	Deletions	Pancreatic cancer
	ARID2 (BAF200)	Inactivating mutation	Lung cancer
	CAF1	Upregulated	Cervix cancer
	ACTA1	Upregulated	Lymphoma, and pancreatic cancer

(Table 8.4) cont.....

Family	Subunit	Dysregulation	Tumor Types
CHD family	MBD2	Downregulated	Esophagus cancer
	GATAD2B	Upregulated	Leukemia
	MTA1	Upregulated	Ovarian, oral and tonsil, breast, gastric, gallbladder, liver, colon, colorectal, pancreatic, lung, endometrial, prostate cancer cervical cancer
	MTA2	Upregulated	Breast and liver cancer
	CHD3	Upregulated	Colorectal cancer
	CHD7	Upregulated	Liver cancer
	CHD8	Inactivating mutation	Gastric, and breast cancer
		Downregulated	Prostate cancer
INO80 family	YY1	Upregulated	pancreatic, and melanoma cancer
	IES6	Downregulated	Esophagus
	INO80	Upregulated	Leukemia
	MRGBP	Upregulated	Bladder cancer
	RUVBL2	Upregulated	Myeloma, and bladder cancer

NURD is a chromatin remodeler that requires ATP for its activity and functions as a histone deacetylase [220]. NURD complexes are important in controlling the G1/S checkpoint, in which NURD deacetylates p53 to regulate the expression of p21, allowing cell cycle progression [221]. Therefore, a lack of the NURD complex leads to cell cycle arrest.

The MBD2-containing NURD complex is distinctive in its capability to bind methylated cytosine within promoter areas to inhibit gene activities *via* interaction with both histone methyltransferases and deacetylases [222, 223]. Thus, the NURD complex and DNA methylation function together to silence key genes [224]. Several NURD subunits have been studied in several cancers [224 - 226]. For example, overexpression of metastasis-associated proteins (MTA1, MTA2, and MTA3) is linked with cellular invasion in various cancers [227]. NURD remodeling complex comprises CHD4 and CHD5. CHD4 performs a vital role in transcription and DNA deterioration [228, 229]. It has been shown that CHD4 interacts with oxidative DNA damage sites, promoting the assembly of repressive chromatin [230]. CHD4 can also interact with transcriptional repressors NAB2 and ZIP, which are regulators of several cellular signaling pathways [229, 231]. CHD4 overexpression has been linked to tumor progression and worse patient outcomes in several cancers [230, 232]. CHD5 has several similarities with CHD4. CHD5 participates in many biological functions, including regulating gene transcription and maintaining genomic integrity [233]. It has been shown that the expression of CHD5 is essential to inhibit the G2/M checkpoint gene WEE1 [234]. CHD5 expression is commonly downregulated in diverse neoplasms and is linked with poor outcomes [235 - 238]. Downregulated CHD5 was strongly linked with a higher tumor stage [237].

Additionally, CHD5 expression is associated with suppressed EMT markers, stem cell markers, and other oncogenes in colorectal, renal, and breast cancers [237, 239, 240]. The nucleosome remodeling factor (NURF) belongs to ISWI-containing complexes primarily purified from *Drosophila melanogaster* [241]. It contains PHD finger within its BPTF subunit that interacts directly with trimethylated histone H3 at lysine four residue (H3K4me3) to regulate Hox gene expression during development [65, 242].

NURF belongs to ISWI-containing complexes primarily purified from *Drosophila melanogaster* [241]. It contains the PHD finger within its BPTF subunit, which interacts directly with trimethylated lysine residue (H3K4me3) in order to regulate Hox gene expression during development [65, 242]. Many malignancies are linked to abnormal expression of BPTF, including glioma, melanoma, colorectal cancer, and hepatocellular carcinoma [243 - 246]. As a result, it contributes to cancer progression and reduced survival rate.

Although the catalytic units of the NURF complex are similar to those of dACF and dCHRAC; it does not enhance nucleosome assembly or regulated spacing. It is more involved in the nucleosome sliding process [79]. It has been shown that NURF is essential for larval blood cell development. Mutations in NURF subunits prompt the neoplastic transformation of circulating larval hemocytes, causing melanotic tumors [247]. NURF positively regulates several biological pathways making them a potential targeted therapy [248, 249].

ARID1A (known as BAF250A) is an SWI/SNF subfamily, and it functions as an inhibiting gene. Mutations in ARID1A are commonly found in ovarian, pancreatic, and gastric cancer, and the most common mutations reported are nonsense mutations. Thus, downregulated ARID1A is associated with poor survival outcomes [250]. Mouse embryos with ARID1A mutations develop heart and neural tube defects and extraembryonic vasculature, leading to embryonic lethality [251]. Similarly, deletion in ARID1A mice has been associated with a reduced survival rate for cancer and high-grade tumors. ARID1A deficiency has also been linked to a global increase in histone markers through Myc induction, which promotes uncontrolled protein expression [252]. Functionally, ARID1A controls the expression of many proteins in p53 pathways, such as CDKN1A (p21) and SMAD3, through direct interaction with p53 target gene promoters [253].

Thus, the ability of remodeler complexes to regulate oncogene and tumor suppressor pathways, as well as their contribution as nononcogenes, makes them potentially a desirable therapeutic target. Targeting chromatin remodeling subunits, such as SMARCA2 and SMARCA4, has proven favorable in reducing cancer cell growth *in-vitro*. Additionally, many remodelers' subunits, such as BPTF, SMARCD1, SMARCA2, SMARCA4, CHD1, CHD4, and CHD7, have been associated with chemosensitivity [254]. To overcome chemosensitivity, we must first understand the pathway by which remodelers overcome the resistance. Taken together, a further challenge is to characterize genes that are wrongly regulated because of remodeling mutations and to show how they participate in carcinogenesis.

EPIGENETICALLY SILENCED GENES: THE MOLECULAR ANATOMY

Identifying silenced genes in cancerous cells is crucial to understanding how cancer develops. Additionally, finding silenced loci within tumor-related genes considers a crucial point to get insight into the mechanism behind gene silencing in malignant cells. Generally, epigenetic transcriptional suppressing requires a complex interplay between different epigenetic levels to drive epigenetic inactivation and cancer development.

Epigenetic modifications interact with each other. CpG methylation can be induced *via* nucleosome remodeling. For instance, nucleosome remodeler DDM1 is required to establish DNA methylation, thereby enabling DNA methyltransferases to methylate nucleosome core DNA. Any disruption in remodeler genes leads to the loss of cytosine methylation [255]. Mutation in the DDM1 gene causes defects in the global chromatin structure through partial inhibition in γ-H2AX [256].

The development of many different types of malignancies can be caused by activating mutations within key genes. Nevertheless, there is limited knowledge of how this could occur. As an example, non-receptor tyrosine kinase JAK2 catalyzes the phosphorylation of many functional proteins to drive several cellular processes either by activation or repression of some genes [257, 258]. It has been found that JAK2V617F mutation is implicated in JAK2 activation in oncogenic transformation in many myeloproliferative disorders [259 - 261]. From an epigenetic point of view, histone modification is directly affected by aberrant JAK2 activation. For instance, histone H3 at tyrosine residue 41 (Y41) is a major JAK2-responsive target protein [262]. The phosphorylation of histone H3Y41 by activated JAK2 prevents heterochromatin protein 1α (HP1α) from binding to the H3-specific region. It thereby releases the transcriptional repressor HP1α from chromatin, resulting in the gene transcription of genes suppressed by HP1α, such as lmo2 [262 - 264]. Advanced in-depth analyses of DNA methylation give a clear idea of the makeup of epigenomic alterations across cancer genomes.

The DNA promoter region of normal cells consists of open chromatin, depleted nucleosomes, and histone post-translational modifications that indicate the gene is actively being expressed [265, 266]. Compared to normal cells, cancer cells have hypermethylated cytosines in the promoter region that disrupt histone modification patterns and change the chromatin structure, leading to the repression of transcription. Several studies have shown that histone marks can be affected by dysregulated DNA methylation [267 - 270]. Mainly, promoter CpG-island hypermethylation correlates with higher levels of H3K27me3 and deacetylation of the histones. Several primary tumors exhibit a reduction in the acetylation of H4K16 resulting from the hypomethylation of DNA [271]. H4K16ac is a distinctive regulator for chromatin folding by influencing the functional interaction between the chromatin fiber and histones [272, 273]. Loss of the H4K16ac mark results in a more relaxed, unfolded chromatin structure, which contributes to genome instability and increases sensitivity to chemotherapy [274, 275]; it is also related to tumor progression [271]. Hypomethylation of the repetitive sequence containing regions of DNA is associated with reduced H4K20me3 levels. As a result of low H4K20me3 levels, many neoplastic tissues show abnormal expression of the Suv4-20h2 enzyme and DNA methyltransferase 1 [276, 277].

ONCOGENIC PRODUCTS DISRUPT THE EPIGENETIC MACHINERY

Chromosomal rearrangements are common abnormalities occurring in hematological malignancies that are usually implicated in the formation of oncogenic fused genes. Epigenetic machinery is distorted *via* oncogenic translocation products, especially when genes linked with epigenetic modifications are involved.

As we mentioned previously, histone acetylation promotes a normal gene's function by freeing the chromatin conformation. The mistargeted histone deacetylase enzymes can interrupt such a mechanism, causing aberrant gene suppression and preventing cellular differentiation. For example, the PML-RARA gene fusion induces the recruitment of histone deacetylase enzymes and increases DNA methylation activity through the PML moiety of the fusion receptor. Consequently, it inhibits the normal function of RARs. This ultimately promotes a granulocytic differentiation block [278], resulting in the lethal accumulation of immature promyelocytes [279].

Another oncogenic phenotype is chromosomal translocations at 11q23 that affect the normal function of the MLL gene [280]. The MLL-fused proteins promote chromatin activation by activating the DOT1L enzyme, which catalyzes H3K79 methylation. Fusion MLL proteins can also drive DNA hypermethylation in some promoter regions [281].

EPIGENETIC THERAPY

Epigenetic therapy emerged as one of the forefronts of cancer research in the last decade as a potential therapy for cancer treatment. Such treatment is likely to have fewer side effects than standard anti-cancer therapies because they specifically target chromatin-mediated mechanisms. Among the benefits of such targeted therapies are their reversibility [282]. We are still learning to target epigenetic dysregulation as a therapeutic strategy. Although, many ongoing clinical trials test several epigenetic therapies, a limited number have received approval for medical use.

Unfortunately, not all patients obtain a clinical benefit from epigenetic therapy, and it might take several months after the initiation of treatment before clinical responses are seen. Thus, the identification of good pretreatment biomarkers predicting response would be of great value. However, the results have been miscellaneous until now, leaving substantial room for improvement. The use of DNA methyltransferase inhibitors for treating leukemia has already been approved, as have some markers that can be used as a predictor for response [283, 284].

Epigenetic therapies are available in a variety of forms. The first epigenetic agents that have proven to be used in the clinic are those that inhibit DNMT, such as 5-azacytidine and its derivatives [285]. Myelodysplastic syndromes and malignant lymphoma are the most common diseases treated by azacytidine. The underlying mechanism of the therapeutic impact arises from the ability of such an agent to disrupt DNA methylation at specific tumor suppressor genes' promoters. These epigenetic drugs foster the body's ability to fight cancer on its own by stimulating an anti-tumor response [286].

A common form of epigenetic therapy is to inhibit histone-modifying enzymes, including HDACs and HMTs inhibitors [287]. For instance, patients with cutaneous T-cell lymphoma can receive vorinostat as a treatment since it is an inhibitor of HDAC [288]. Moreover, there are currently multiple myeloma-specific inhibitors in clinical trials, such as HDAC6 inhibitors [289]. There is a trial in non-Hodgkin lymphoma testing EZH2 inhibitors to deactivate H3K27 methylation [290]. Clinical tests are also conducted on inhibitor DOT1L, the enzyme responsible for H3K79 methylation, for leukemias malignant [291]. One of the latest types of epigenetic therapies is BET bromodomain inhibitors. Such inhibitors compete for binding with acetyl-lysine for the expulsion of BET-containing proteins from the chromatin. Various clinical studies have confirmed favorable data for using BET bromodomain inhibitors in treating a range of malignancies [292].

There are many challenges to epigenetic therapy in cancer therapy, including starting treatment at the earliest stages of tumor development. It is also challenging to get the drug to infiltrate deeper into a tumor site. There are also additional challenges related to the specificity of therapy. Therefore, overcoming these challenges will require much effort. There is a necessity for more research to find treatments that are more durable, manageable, and with minimal side effects.

SUMMARY

Advances in mapping technologies have demonstrated the significance of abnormal epigenetic pathways in carcinogenesis. Thus, targeting the epigenome offers a great approach to cancer treatment. Although epigenetic-targeted therapy has been effective against hematological neoplastic, many limitations need to be overcome to make it more effective against solid tumors. For example, recent DNMT and HDAC inhibitors seem to be ineffective against solid tumor cells proliferating under hypoxic conditions. Therefore, analyzing epigenetic patterns in hypoxic cancer cells may help identify specific predictors of early cancer recognition, diagnosis, survival and treatment response. Genetic and epigenetic alterations drive cancer's development. In this sense, genetic modification of epigenomic modifiers can alter DNA methylation profile, histone modification status, chromatin remodeling, and microRNA levels.

CONCLUSION

A comprehensive understanding of epigenome–genome interactions poses opportunities for effective epigenetic-targeted therapy for cancers. However, extensive work must be conducted to optimize treatment options and discover the safest combinations of multiple drugs.

CONSENT FOR PUBLICATION

Not applicable.

CONFLICT OF INTEREST

The authors declare that there are no conflicts of interest.

ACKNOWLEDGEMENTS

The authors would like to thank King Abdullah International Medical Research Center (KAIMRC) and King Fahad Specialist Hospital, Saudi Arabia. The authors would also like to thank both Prof. Faris and their families for their continued support.

REFERENCES

[1] Holliday R. The inheritance of epigenetic defects. Science 1987; 238(4824): 163-70. [http://dx.doi.org/10.1126/science.3310230] [PMID: 3310230]

[2] Golbabapour S, Abdulla MA, Hajrezaei M. A concise review on epigenetic regulation: insight into molecular mechanisms. Int J Mol Sci 2011; 12(12): 8661-94. [http://dx.doi.org/10.3390/ijms12128661] [PMID: 22272098]

[3] Jones PA, Baylin SB. The fundamental role of epigenetic events in cancer. Nat Rev Genet 2002; 3(6): 415-28. [http://dx.doi.org/10.1038/nrg816] [PMID: 12042769]

[4] Herman JG, Baylin SB. Gene silencing in cancer in association with promoter hypermethylation. N Engl J Med 2003; 349(21): 2042-54. [http://dx.doi.org/10.1056/NEJMra023075] [PMID: 14627790]

[5] Bernstein BE, Meissner A, Lander ES. The mammalian epigenome. Cell 2007; 128(4): 669-81. [http://dx.doi.org/10.1016/j.cell.2007.01.033] [PMID: 17320505]

[6] Jaenisch R, Bird A. Epigenetic regulation of gene expression: how the genome integrates intrinsic and environmental signals. Nat Genet 2003; 33(S3) (Suppl.): 245-54. [http://dx.doi.org/10.1038/ng1089] [PMID: 12610534]

[7] Esteller M. Cancer epigenomics: DNA methylomes and histone-modification maps. Nat Rev Genet 2007; 8(4): 286-98. [http://dx.doi.org/10.1038/nrg2005] [PMID: 17339880]

[8] Jones PA, Baylin SB. The epigenomics of cancer. Cell 2007; 128(4): 683-92. [http://dx.doi.org/10.1016/j.cell.2007.01.029] [PMID: 17320506]

[9] Valente S, Liu Y, Schnekenburger M, *et al.* Selective non-nucleoside inhibitors of human DNA methyltransferases active in cancer including in cancer stem cells. J Med Chem 2014; 57(3): 701-13. [http://dx.doi.org/10.1021/jm4012627] [PMID: 24387159]

[10] Bestor TH. Activation of mammalian DNA methyltransferase by cleavage of a Zn binding regulatory domain. EMBO J 1992; 11(7): 2611-7. [http://dx.doi.org/10.1002/j.1460-2075.1992.tb05326.x] [PMID: 1628623]

[11] Kaneda M, Okano M, Hata K, *et al.* Essential role for *de novo* DNA methyltransferase Dnmt3a in paternal and maternal imprinting. Nature 2004; 429(6994): 900-3. [http://dx.doi.org/10.1038/nature02633] [PMID: 15215868]

[12] Kohli RM, Zhang Y. TET enzymes, TDG and the dynamics of DNA demethylation. Nature 2013; 502(7472): 472-9. [http://dx.doi.org/10.1038/nature12750] [PMID: 24153300]

[13] Yang J, Bashkenova N, Zang R, Huang X, Wang J. The roles of TET family proteins in development and stem cells. Development 2020; 147(2): dev183129. [http://dx.doi.org/10.1242/dev.183129] [PMID: 31941705]

[14] Fan J, Baeẓa J, Denu JM. Investigating Histone Acetylation Stoichiometry and Turnover Rate. Methods Enzymol 2016; 574: 125-48.

[http://dx.doi.org/10.1016/bs.mie.2016.01.007] [PMID: 27423860]

[15] Bannister AJ, Kouzarides T. Regulation of chromatin by histone modifications. Cell Res 2011; 21(3): 381-95.
[http://dx.doi.org/10.1038/cr.2011.22] [PMID: 21321607]

[16] Cheng Y, He C, Wang M, *et al.* Targeting epigenetic regulators for cancer therapy: mechanisms and advances in clinical trials. Signal Transduct Target Ther 2019; 4(1): 62.
[http://dx.doi.org/10.1038/s41392-019-0095-0] [PMID: 31871779]

[17] Hodawadekar SC, Marmorstein R. Chemistry of acetyl transfer by histone modifying enzymes: structure, mechanism and implications for effector design. Oncogene 2007; 26(37): 5528-40.
[http://dx.doi.org/10.1038/sj.onc.1210619] [PMID: 17694092]

[18] Heery DM, Fischer PM. Pharmacological targeting of lysine acetyltransferases in human disease: a progress report. Drug Discov Today 2007; 12(1-2): 88-99.
[http://dx.doi.org/10.1016/j.drudis.2006.11.012] [PMID: 17198977]

[19] Singh BN, Zhang G, Hwa YL, Li J, Dowdy SC, Jiang SW. Nonhistone protein acetylation as cancer therapy targets. Expert Rev Anticancer Ther 2010; 10(6): 935-54.
[http://dx.doi.org/10.1586/era.10.62] [PMID: 20553216]

[20] Yang X-J, Seto E. HATs and HDACs: from structure, function and regulation to novel strategies for therapy and prevention. Oncogene 2007; 26(37): 5310-8.
[http://dx.doi.org/10.1038/sj.onc.1210599] [PMID: 17694074]

[21] Choudhary C, Kumar C, Gnad F, *et al.* Lysine acetylation targets protein complexes and co-regulates major cellular functions. Science 2009; 325(5942): 834-40.
[http://dx.doi.org/10.1126/science.1175371] [PMID: 19608861]

[22] Ayer DE. Histone deacetylases: transcriptional repression with SINers and NuRDs. Trends Cell Biol 1999; 9(5): 193-8.
[http://dx.doi.org/10.1016/S0962-8924(99)01536-6] [PMID: 10322454]

[23] Yoon HG, Chan DW, Huang ZQ, *et al.* Purification and functional characterization of the human N-CoR complex: the roles of HDAC3, TBL1 and TBLR1. EMBO J 2003; 22(6): 1336-46.
[http://dx.doi.org/10.1093/emboj/cdg120] [PMID: 12628926]

[24] Imai S, Armstrong CM, Kaeberlein M, Guarente L. Transcriptional silencing and longevity protein Sir2 is an NAD-dependent histone deacetylase. Nature 2000; 403(6771): 795-800.
[http://dx.doi.org/10.1038/35001622] [PMID: 10693811]

[25] Yang XJ, Seto E. The Rpd3/Hda1 family of lysine deacetylases: from bacteria and yeast to mice and men. Nat Rev Mol Cell Biol 2008; 9(3): 206-18.
[http://dx.doi.org/10.1038/nrm2346] [PMID: 18292778]

[26] Wu G, Broniscer A, McEachron TA, *et al.* Somatic histone H3 alterations in pediatric diffuse intrinsic pontine gliomas and non-brainstem glioblastomas. Nat Genet 2012; 44(3): 251-3.
[http://dx.doi.org/10.1038/ng.1102] [PMID: 22286216]

[27] Frederiks F, Stulemeijer IJE, Ovaa H, van Leeuwen F. A modified epigenetics toolbox to study histone modifications on the nucleosome core. ChemBioChem 2011; 12(2): 308-13.
[http://dx.doi.org/10.1002/cbic.201000617] [PMID: 21243718]

[28] Cheng X, Collins RE, Zhang X. Structural and sequence motifs of protein (histone) methylation enzymes. Annu Rev Biophys Biomol Struct 2005; 34(1): 267-94.
[http://dx.doi.org/10.1146/annurev.biophys.34.040204.144452] [PMID: 15869391]

[29] Zhang X, Yang Z, Khan SI, *et al.* Structural basis for the product specificity of histone lysine methyltransferases. Mol Cell 2003; 12(1): 177-85.
[http://dx.doi.org/10.1016/S1097-2765(03)00224-7] [PMID: 12887903]

[30] Bedford MT, Clarke SG. Protein arginine methylation in mammals: who, what, and why. Mol Cell

2009; 33(1): 1-13.
[http://dx.doi.org/10.1016/j.molcel.2008.12.013] [PMID: 19150423]

[31] Tewary SK, Zheng YG, Ho MC. Protein arginine methyltransferases: insights into the enzyme structure and mechanism at the atomic level. Cell Mol Life Sci 2019; 76(15): 2917-32.
[http://dx.doi.org/10.1007/s00018-019-03145-x] [PMID: 31123777]

[32] Zurita-Lopez CI, Sandberg T, Kelly R, Clarke SG. Human protein arginine methyltransferase 7 (PRMT7) is a type III enzyme forming ω-NG-monomethylated arginine residues. J Biol Chem 2012; 287(11): 7859-70.
[http://dx.doi.org/10.1074/jbc.M111.336271] [PMID: 22241471]

[33] Meyer R, Wolf SS, Obendorf M. PRMT2, a member of the protein arginine methyltransferase family, is a coactivator of the androgen receptor. J Steroid Biochem Mol Biol 2007; 107(1-2): 1-14.
[http://dx.doi.org/10.1016/j.jsbmb.2007.05.006] [PMID: 17587566]

[34] Qi C, Chang J, Zhu Y, Yeldandi AV, Rao SM, Zhu YJ. Identification of protein arginine methyltransferase 2 as a coactivator for estrogen receptor alpha. J Biol Chem 2002; 277(32): 28624-30.
[http://dx.doi.org/10.1074/jbc.M201053200] [PMID: 12039952]

[35] Copeland RA, Solomon ME, Richon VM. Protein methyltransferases as a target class for drug discovery. Nat Rev Drug Discov 2009; 8(9): 724-32.
[http://dx.doi.org/10.1038/nrd2974] [PMID: 19721445]

[36] Zhang J, Jing L, Li M, He L, Guo Z. Regulation of histone arginine methylation/demethylation by methylase and demethylase (Review). Mol Med Rep 2019; 19(5): 3963-71.
[http://dx.doi.org/10.3892/mmr.2019.10111] [PMID: 30942418]

[37] Metzger E, Wissmann M, Yin N, *et al.* LSD1 demethylates repressive histone marks to promote androgen-receptor-dependent transcription. Nature 2005; 437(7057): 436-9.
[http://dx.doi.org/10.1038/nature04020] [PMID: 16079795]

[38] Shi Y, Lan F, Matson C, *et al.* Histone demethylation mediated by the nuclear amine oxidase homolog LSD1. Cell 2004; 119(7): 941-53.
[http://dx.doi.org/10.1016/j.cell.2004.12.012] [PMID: 15620353]

[39] Klose RJ, Zhang Y. Regulation of histone methylation by demethylimination and demethylation. Nat Rev Mol Cell Biol 2007; 8(4): 307-18.
[http://dx.doi.org/10.1038/nrm2143] [PMID: 17342184]

[40] Whetstine JR, Nottke A, Lan F, *et al.* Reversal of histone lysine trimethylation by the JMJD2 family of histone demethylases. Cell 2006; 125(3): 467-81.
[http://dx.doi.org/10.1016/j.cell.2006.03.028] [PMID: 16603238]

[41] Chang B, Chen Y, Zhao Y, Bruick RK. JMJD6 is a histone arginine demethylase. Science 2007; 318(5849): 444-7.
[http://dx.doi.org/10.1126/science.1145801] [PMID: 17947579]

[42] Cuthbert GL, Daujat S, Snowden AW, *et al.* Histone deimination antagonizes arginine methylation. Cell 2004; 118(5): 545-53.
[http://dx.doi.org/10.1016/j.cell.2004.08.020] [PMID: 15339660]

[43] Rossetto D, Avvakumov N, Côté J. Histone phosphorylation. Epigenetics 2012; 7(10): 1098-108.
[http://dx.doi.org/10.4161/epi.21975] [PMID: 22948226]

[44] Oki M, Aihara H, Ito T. Role of histone phosphorylation in chromatin dynamics and its implications in diseases. Subcell Biochem 2007; 41: 323-40.
[http://dx.doi.org/10.1007/1-4020-5466-1_14] [PMID: 17484134]

[45] Wei Y, Mizzen CA, Cook RG, Gorovsky MA, Allis CD. Phosphorylation of histone H3 at serine 10 is correlated with chromosome condensation during mitosis and meiosis in Tetrahymena. Proc Natl Acad Sci USA 1998; 95(13): 7480-4.

[http://dx.doi.org/10.1073/pnas.95.13.7480]

[46] Cheung P, Tanner KG, Cheung WL, Sassone-Corsi P, Denu JM, Allis CD. Synergistic coupling of histone H3 phosphorylation and acetylation in response to epidermal growth factor stimulation. Mol Cell 2000; 5(6): 905-15.
[http://dx.doi.org/10.1016/S1097-2765(00)80256-7] [PMID: 10911985]

[47] Clayton AL, Rose S, Barratt MJ, Mahadevan LC. Phosphoacetylation of histone H3 on c-*fos* - and c-*jun* -associated nucleosomes upon gene activation. EMBO J 2000; 19(14): 3714-26.
[http://dx.doi.org/10.1093/emboj/19.14.3714] [PMID: 10899125]

[48] Rogakou EP, Pilch DR, Orr AH, Ivanova VS, Bonner WM. DNA double-stranded breaks induce histone H2AX phosphorylation on serine 139. J Biol Chem 1998; 273(10): 5858-68.
[http://dx.doi.org/10.1074/jbc.273.10.5858] [PMID: 9488723]

[49] Wang H, Wang L, Erdjument-Bromage H, *et al.* Role of histone H2A ubiquitination in Polycomb silencing. Nature 2004; 431(7010): 873-8.
[http://dx.doi.org/10.1038/nature02985] [PMID: 15386022]

[50] Brown JS, Jackson SP. Ubiquitylation, neddylation and the DNA damage response. Open Biol 2015; 5(4): 150018.
[http://dx.doi.org/10.1098/rsob.150018] [PMID: 25833379]

[51] Shiio Y, Eisenman RN. Histone sumoylation is associated with transcriptional repression. Proc Natl Acad Sci USA 2003; 100(23): 13225-30.
[http://dx.doi.org/10.1073/pnas.1735528100] [PMID: 14578449]

[52] Sakabe K, Wang Z, Hart GW. -*N* -acetylglucosamine (O-GlcNAc) is part of the histone code. Proc Natl Acad Sci USA 2010; 107(46): 19915-20.
[http://dx.doi.org/10.1073/pnas.1009023107] [PMID: 21045127]

[53] Chen Y, Sprung R, Tang Y, *et al.* Lysine propionylation and butyrylation are novel post-translational modifications in histones. Mol Cell Proteomics 2007; 6(5): 812-9.
[http://dx.doi.org/10.1074/mcp.M700021-MCP200] [PMID: 17267393]

[54] Hassa PO, Haenni SS, Elser M, Hottiger MO. Nuclear ADP-ribosylation reactions in mammalian cells: where are we today and where are we going? Microbiol Mol Biol Rev 2006; 70(3): 789-829.
[http://dx.doi.org/10.1128/MMBR.00040-05] [PMID: 16959969]

[55] Nelson CJ, Santos-Rosa H, Kouzarides T. Proline isomerization of histone H3 regulates lysine methylation and gene expression. Cell 2006; 126(5): 905-16.
[http://dx.doi.org/10.1016/j.cell.2006.07.026] [PMID: 16959570]

[56] Tan M, Luo H, Lee S, *et al.* Identification of 67 histone marks and histone lysine crotonylation as a new type of histone modification. Cell 2011; 146(6): 1016-28.
[http://dx.doi.org/10.1016/j.cell.2011.08.008] [PMID: 21925322]

[57] Kuroishi T, Rios-Avila L, Pestinger V, Wijeratne SSK, Zempleni J. Biotinylation is a natural, albeit rare, modification of human histones. Mol Genet Metab 2011; 104(4): 537-45.
[http://dx.doi.org/10.1016/j.ymgme.2011.08.030] [PMID: 21930408]

[58] Muers M. A haul of new histone modifications. Nat Rev Genet 2011; 12(11): 744.
[http://dx.doi.org/10.1038/nrg3086] [PMID: 21946920]

[59] Jiang T, Zhou X, Taghizadeh K, Dong M, Dedon PC. N-formylation of lysine in histone proteins as a secondary modification arising from oxidative DNA damage. Proc Natl Acad Sci USA 2007; 104(1): 60-5.
[http://dx.doi.org/10.1073/pnas.0606775103] [PMID: 17190813]

[60] Kouzarides T. Chromatin modifications and their function. Cell 2007; 128(4): 693-705.
[http://dx.doi.org/10.1016/j.cell.2007.02.005] [PMID: 17320507]

[61] Rajagopal N, Ernst J, Ray P, *et al.* Distinct and predictive histone lysine acetylation patterns at

promoters, enhancers, and gene bodies. G3 (Bethesda) 2014; 4(11): 2051-63. [http://dx.doi.org/10.1534/g3.114.013565] [PMID: 25122670]

[62] Li X, Corsa CAS, Pan PW, *et al.* MOF and H4 K16 acetylation play important roles in DNA damage repair by modulating recruitment of DNA damage repair protein Mdc1. Mol Cell Biol 2010; 30(22): 5335-47. [http://dx.doi.org/10.1128/MCB.00350-10] [PMID: 20837706]

[63] Swatek KN, Komander D. Ubiquitin modifications. Cell Res 2016; 26(4): 399-422. [http://dx.doi.org/10.1038/cr.2016.39] [PMID: 27012465]

[64] Azad GK, Swagatika S, Kumawat M, Kumawat R, Tomar RS. Modifying Chromatin by Histone Tail Clipping. J Mol Biol 2018; 430 (18 Pt B): 3051-67. [http://dx.doi.org/10.1016/j.jmb.2018.07.013] [PMID: 30009770]

[65] Wysocka J, Swigut T, Xiao H, *et al.* A PHD finger of NURF couples histone H3 lysine 4 trimethylation with chromatin remodelling. Nature 2006; 442(7098): 86-90. [http://dx.doi.org/10.1038/nature04815] [PMID: 16728976]

[66] Shi X, Hong T, Walter KL, *et al.* ING2 PHD domain links histone H3 lysine 4 methylation to active gene repression. Nature 2006; 442(7098): 96-9. [http://dx.doi.org/10.1038/nature04835] [PMID: 16728974]

[67] Peña PV, Davrazou F, Shi X, *et al.* Molecular mechanism of histone H3K4me3 recognition by plant homeodomain of ING2. Nature 2006; 442(7098): 100-3. [http://dx.doi.org/10.1038/nature04814] [PMID: 16728977]

[68] Sims RJ III, Chen CF, Santos-Rosa H, Kouzarides T, Patel SS, Reinberg D. Human but not yeast CHD1 binds directly and selectively to histone H3 methylated at lysine 4 *via* its tandem chromodomains. J Biol Chem 2005; 280(51): 41789-92. [http://dx.doi.org/10.1074/jbc.C500395200] [PMID: 16263726]

[69] Huang Y, Fang J, Bedford MT, Zhang Y, Xu RM. Recognition of histone H3 lysine-4 methylation by the double tudor domain of JMJD2A. Science 2006; 312(5774): 748-51. [http://dx.doi.org/10.1126/science.1125162] [PMID: 16601153]

[70] Bannister AJ, Zegerman P, Partridge JF, *et al.* Selective recognition of methylated lysine 9 on histone H3 by the HP1 chromo domain. Nature 2001; 410(6824): 120-4. [http://dx.doi.org/10.1038/35065138] [PMID: 11242054]

[71] Mishima Y, Watanabe M, Kawakami T, *et al.* Hinge and chromoshadow of HP1α participate in recognition of K9 methylated histone H3 in nucleosomes. J Mol Biol 2013; 425(1): 54-70. [http://dx.doi.org/10.1016/j.jmb.2012.10.018] [PMID: 23142645]

[72] Mujtaba S, Zeng L, Zhou M-M. Structure and acetyl-lysine recognition of the bromodomain. Oncogene 2007; 26(37): 5521-7. [http://dx.doi.org/10.1038/sj.onc.1210618] [PMID: 17694091]

[73] Hassan AH, Prochasson P, Neely KE, *et al.* Function and selectivity of bromodomains in anchoring chromatin-modifying complexes to promoter nucleosomes. Cell 2002; 111(3): 369-79. [http://dx.doi.org/10.1016/S0092-8674(02)01005-X] [PMID: 12419247]

[74] Li W, Zhao A, Tempel W, Loppnau P, Liu Y. Crystal structure of DPF3b in complex with an acetylated histone peptide. J Struct Biol 2016; 195(3): 365-72. [http://dx.doi.org/10.1016/j.jsb.2016.07.001] [PMID: 27402533]

[75] Fischle W, Tseng BS, Dormann HL, *et al.* Regulation of HP1-chromatin binding by histone H3 methylation and phosphorylation. Nature 2005; 438(7071): 1116-22. [http://dx.doi.org/10.1038/nature04219] [PMID: 16222246]

[76] Xhemalce B, Kouzarides T. A chromodomain switch mediated by histone H3 Lys 4 acetylation regulates heterochromatin assembly. Genes Dev 2010; 24(7): 647-52. [http://dx.doi.org/10.1101/gad.1881710] [PMID: 20299449]

[77] Clements A, Poux AN, Lo WS, Pillus L, Berger SL, Marmorstein R. Structural basis for histone and phosphohistone binding by the GCN5 histone acetyltransferase. Mol Cell 2003; 12(2): 461-73. [http://dx.doi.org/10.1016/S1097-2765(03)00288-0] [PMID: 14536085]

[78] Khorasanizadeh S. The Nucleosome. Cell 2004; 116(2): 259-72. [http://dx.doi.org/10.1016/S0092-8674(04)00044-3] [PMID: 14744436]

[79] Clapier CR, Cairns BR. The biology of chromatin remodeling complexes. Annu Rev Biochem 2009; 78(1): 273-304. [http://dx.doi.org/10.1146/annurev.biochem.77.062706.153223] [PMID: 19355820]

[80] Vignali M, Hassan AH, Neely KE, Workman JL. ATP-dependent chromatin-remodeling complexes. Mol Cell Biol 2000; 20(6): 1899-910. [http://dx.doi.org/10.1128/MCB.20.6.1899-1910.2000] [PMID: 10688638]

[81] Côté J, Peterson CL, Workman JL. Perturbation of nucleosome core structure by the SWI/SNF complex persists after its detachment, enhancing subsequent transcription factor binding. Proc Natl Acad Sci USA 1998; 95(9): 4947-52. [http://dx.doi.org/10.1073/pnas.95.9.4947]

[82] Gurard-Levin ZA, Quivy JP, Almouzni G. Histone chaperones: assisting histone traffic and nucleosome dynamics. Annu Rev Biochem 2014; 83(1): 487-517. [http://dx.doi.org/10.1146/annurev-biochem-060713-035536] [PMID: 24905786]

[83] Fei J, Torigoe SE, Brown CR, *et al.* The prenucleosome, a stable conformational isomer of the nucleosome. Genes Dev 2015; 29(24): 2563-75. [http://dx.doi.org/10.1101/gad.272633.115] [PMID: 26680301]

[84] Torigoe SE, Urwin DL, Ishii H, Smith DE, Kadonaga JT. Identification of a rapidly formed nonnucleosomal histone-DNA intermediate that is converted into chromatin by ACF. Mol Cell 2011; 43(4): 638-48. [http://dx.doi.org/10.1016/j.molcel.2011.07.017] [PMID: 21855802]

[85] Corona DFV, Längst G, Clapier CR, *et al.* ISWI is an ATP-dependent nucleosome remodeling factor. Mol Cell 1999; 3(2): 239-45. [http://dx.doi.org/10.1016/S1097-2765(00)80314-7] [PMID: 10078206]

[86] Ito T, Bulger M, Pazin MJ, Kobayashi R, Kadonaga JT. ACF, an ISWI-containing and ATP-utilizing chromatin assembly and remodeling factor. Cell 1997; 90(1): 145-55. [http://dx.doi.org/10.1016/S0092-8674(00)80321-9] [PMID: 9230310]

[87] Brown CR, Mao C, Falkovskaia E, Law JK, Boeger H. *In vivo* role for the chromatin-remodeling enzyme SWI/SNF in the removal of promoter nucleosomes by disassembly rather than sliding. J Biol Chem 2011; 286(47): 40556-65. [http://dx.doi.org/10.1074/jbc.M111.289918] [PMID: 21979950]

[88] Boeger H, Griesenbeck J, Strattan JS, Kornberg RD. Removal of promoter nucleosomes by disassembly rather than sliding *in vivo*. Mol Cell 2004; 14(5): 667-73. [http://dx.doi.org/10.1016/j.molcel.2004.05.013] [PMID: 15175161]

[89] Papamichos-Chronakis M, Watanabe S, Rando OJ, Peterson CL. Global regulation of H2A.Z localization by the INO80 chromatin-remodeling enzyme is essential for genome integrity. Cell 2011; 144(2): 200-13. [http://dx.doi.org/10.1016/j.cell.2010.12.021] [PMID: 21241891]

[90] Clapier CR, Iwasa J, Cairns BR, Peterson CL. Mechanisms of action and regulation of ATP-dependent chromatin-remodelling complexes. Nat Rev Mol Cell Biol 2017; 18(7): 407-22. [http://dx.doi.org/10.1038/nrm.2017.26] [PMID: 28512350]

[91] Bultman S, Gebuhr T, Yee D, *et al.* A Brg1 null mutation in the mouse reveals functional differences among mammalian SWI/SNF complexes. Mol Cell 2000; 6(6): 1287-95. [http://dx.doi.org/10.1016/S1097-2765(00)00127-1] [PMID: 11163203]

[92] Reyes JC, Barra J, Muchardt C, Camus A, Babinet C, Yaniv M. Altered control of cellular proliferation in the absence of mammalian brahma (SNF2α). EMBO J 1998; 17(23): 6979-91. [http://dx.doi.org/10.1093/emboj/17.23.6979] [PMID: 9843504]

[93] Yip DJ, Corcoran CP, Alvarez-Saavedra M, *et al.* Snf2l regulates Foxg1-dependent progenitor cell expansion in the developing brain. Dev Cell 2012; 22(4): 871-8. [http://dx.doi.org/10.1016/j.devcel.2012.01.020] [PMID: 22516202]

[94] Yang W, Lee DY, Ben-David Y. The roles of microRNAs in tumorigenesis and angiogenesis. Int J Physiol Pathophysiol Pharmacol 2011; 3(2): 140-55. [PMID: 21760972]

[95] Peng Y, Croce CM. The role of MicroRNAs in human cancer. Signal Transduct Target Ther 2016; 1(1): 15004. [http://dx.doi.org/10.1038/sigtrans.2015.4] [PMID: 29263891]

[96] Vasudevan S, Tong Y, Steitz JA. Switching from repression to activation: microRNAs can up-regulate translation. Science 2007; 318(5858): 1931-4. [http://dx.doi.org/10.1126/science.1149460] [PMID: 18048652]

[97] Fabbri M, Paone A, Calore F, *et al.* MicroRNAs bind to Toll-like receptors to induce prometastatic inflammatory response. Proc Natl Acad Sci USA 2012; 109(31): E2110-6. [http://dx.doi.org/10.1073/pnas.1209414109] [PMID: 22753494]

[98] Cao YL, Zhuang T, Xing BH, Li N, Li Q. Exosomal DNMT1 mediates cisplatin resistance in ovarian cancer. Cell Biochem Funct 2017; 35(6): 296-303. [http://dx.doi.org/10.1002/cbf.3276] [PMID: 28791708]

[99] Rajendran G, Shanmuganandam K, Bendre A, Mujumdar D, Goel A, Shiras A. Epigenetic regulation of DNA methyltransferases: DNMT1 and DNMT3B in gliomas. J Neurooncol 2011; 104(2): 483-94. [http://dx.doi.org/10.1007/s11060-010-0520-2] [PMID: 21229291]

[100] Peng DF, Kanai Y, Sawada M, *et al.* DNA methylation of multiple tumor-related genes in association with overexpression of DNA methyltransferase 1 (DNMT1) during multistage carcinogenesis of the pancreas. Carcinogenesis 2006; 27(6): 1160-8. [http://dx.doi.org/10.1093/carcin/bgi361] [PMID: 16537562]

[101] Hong L, Sun G, Peng L, *et al.* The interaction between miR-148a and DNMT1 suppresses cell migration and invasion by reactivating tumor suppressor genes in pancreatic cancer. Oncol Rep 2018; 40(5): 2916-25. [http://dx.doi.org/10.3892/or.2018.6700] [PMID: 30226601]

[102] Wang Y, Hu Y, Guo J, Wang L. miR-148a-3p Suppresses the Proliferation and Invasion of Esophageal Cancer by Targeting DNMT1. Genet Test Mol Biomarkers 2019; 23(2): 98-104. [http://dx.doi.org/10.1089/gtmb.2018.0285] [PMID: 30735457]

[103] Feinberg AP, Vogelstein B. Hypomethylation distinguishes genes of some human cancers from their normal counterparts. Nature 1983; 301(5895): 89-92. [http://dx.doi.org/10.1038/301089a0] [PMID: 6185846]

[104] Gama-Sosa MA, Slagel VA, Trewyn RW, *et al.* The 5-methylcytosine content of DNA from human tumors. Nucleic Acids Res 1983; 11(19): 6883-94. [http://dx.doi.org/10.1093/nar/11.19.6883] [PMID: 6314264]

[105] de Capoa A, Musolino A, Della Rosa S, *et al.* DNA demethylation is directly related to tumour progression: evidence in normal, pre-malignant and malignant cells from uterine cervix samples. Oncol Rep 2003; 10(3): 545-9. [PMID: 12684621]

[106] Brothman AR, Swanson G, Maxwell TM, *et al.* Global hypomethylation is common in prostate cancer cells: a quantitative predictor for clinical outcome? Cancer Genet Cytogenet 2005; 156(1): 31-6. [http://dx.doi.org/10.1016/j.cancergencyto.2004.04.004] [PMID: 15588853]

[107] Kankava K, Kvaratskhelia E, Burkadze G, *et al.* Assessment of the value of methylation features in different tissues for preoperative identification of high-risk breast tumors. Georgian Med News 2019; (289): 143-51.
[PMID: 31215897]

[108] Widschwendter M, Jiang G, Woods C, *et al.* DNA hypomethylation and ovarian cancer biology. Cancer Res 2004; 64(13): 4472-80.
[http://dx.doi.org/10.1158/0008-5472.CAN-04-0238] [PMID: 15231656]

[109] Zhang W, Klinkebiel D, Barger CJ, *et al.* Global DNA Hypomethylation in Epithelial Ovarian Cancer: Passive Demethylation and Association with Genomic Instability. Cancers (Basel) 2020; 12(3): 764.
[http://dx.doi.org/10.3390/cancers12030764] [PMID: 32213861]

[110] Anwar S, Wulaningsih W, Lehmann U. Transposable Elements in Human Cancer: Causes and Consequences of Deregulation. Int J Mol Sci 2017; 18(5): 974.
[http://dx.doi.org/10.3390/ijms18050974] [PMID: 28471386]

[111] Van Tongelen A, Loriot A, De Smet C. Oncogenic roles of DNA hypomethylation through the activation of cancer-germline genes. Cancer Lett 2017; 396: 130-7.
[http://dx.doi.org/10.1016/j.canlet.2017.03.029] [PMID: 28342986]

[112] Alberge JB, Magrangeas F, Wagner M, *et al.* DNA hydroxymethylation is associated with disease severity and persists at enhancers of oncogenic regions in multiple myeloma. Clin Epigenetics 2020; 12(1): 163.
[http://dx.doi.org/10.1186/s13148-020-00953-y] [PMID: 33138842]

[113] Ehrlich M. DNA hypomethylation in cancer cells. Epigenomics 2009; 1(2): 239-59.
[http://dx.doi.org/10.2217/epi.09.33] [PMID: 20495664]

[114] Jeong S, Lee K, Wen X, *et al.* Tumoral LINE-1 hypomethylation is associated with poor survival of patients with intrahepatic cholangiocarcinoma. BMC Cancer 2017; 17(1): 588.
[http://dx.doi.org/10.1186/s12885-017-3595-8] [PMID: 28851390]

[115] Ross JP, Rand KN, Molloy PL. Hypomethylation of repeated DNA sequences in cancer. Epigenomics 2010; 2(2): 245-69.
[http://dx.doi.org/10.2217/epi.10.2] [PMID: 22121873]

[116] Vera E, Canela A, Fraga MF, Esteller M, Blasco MA. Epigenetic regulation of telomeres in human cancer. Oncogene 2008; 27(54): 6817-33.
[http://dx.doi.org/10.1038/onc.2008.289] [PMID: 18762811]

[117] Ehrlich M, Hopkins NE, Jiang G, *et al.* Satellite DNA hypomethylation in karyotyped Wilms tumors. Cancer Genet Cytogenet 2003; 141(2): 97-105.
[http://dx.doi.org/10.1016/S0165-4608(02)00668-4] [PMID: 12606126]

[118] Kalkat M, De Melo J, Hickman K, *et al.* MYC Deregulation in Primary Human Cancers. Genes (Basel) 2017; 8(6): 151.
[http://dx.doi.org/10.3390/genes8060151] [PMID: 28587062]

[119] Destefanis F, Manara V, Bellosta P. Myc as a Regulator of Ribosome Biogenesis and Cell Competition: A Link to Cancer. Int J Mol Sci 2020; 21(11): 4037.
[http://dx.doi.org/10.3390/ijms21114037] [PMID: 32516899]

[120] He S, Liu Z, Oh DY, Thiele CJ. MYCN and the epigenome. Front Oncol 2013; 3: 1.
[http://dx.doi.org/10.3389/fonc.2013.00001] [PMID: 23373009]

[121] Shen L, Qui D, Fang J. Correlation between hypomethylation of c-myc and c-N-ras oncogenes and pathological changes in human hepatocellular carcinoma. Zhonghua Zhong Liu Za Zhi 1997; 19(3): 173-6.
[PMID: 10920889]

[122] de Souza CRT, Leal MF, Calcagno DQ, *et al.* MYC deregulation in gastric cancer and its

clinicopathological implications. PLoS One 2013; 8(5): e64420. [http://dx.doi.org/10.1371/journal.pone.0064420] [PMID: 23717612]

[123] Cui H. Loss of imprinting of IGF2 as an epigenetic marker for the risk of human cancer. Dis Markers 2007; 23(1-2): 105-12. [http://dx.doi.org/10.1155/2007/363464] [PMID: 17325430]

[124] Kasprzak A, Adamek A. Insulin-Like Growth Factor 2 (IGF2) Signaling in Colorectal Cancer—from Basic Research to Potential Clinical Applications. Int J Mol Sci 2019; 20(19): 4915. [http://dx.doi.org/10.3390/ijms20194915] [PMID: 31623387]

[125] Cruz-Correa M, Cui H, Giardiello FM, *et al.* Loss of imprinting of insulin growth factor II gene: a potential heritable biomarker for colon neoplasia predisposition. Gastroenterology 2004; 126(4): 964-70. [http://dx.doi.org/10.1053/j.gastro.2003.12.051] [PMID: 15057734]

[126] Murata A, Baba Y, Watanabe M, *et al.* IGF2 DMR0 methylation, loss of imprinting, and patient prognosis in esophageal squamous cell carcinoma. Ann Surg Oncol 2014; 21(4): 1166-74. [http://dx.doi.org/10.1245/s10434-013-3414-7] [PMID: 24318096]

[127] Tsai KW, Hu LY, Wu CW, *et al.* Epigenetic regulation of miR-196b expression in gastric cancer. Genes Chromosomes Cancer 2010; 49(11): 969-80. [http://dx.doi.org/10.1002/gcc.20804] [PMID: 20662076]

[128] Li A, Omura N, Hong SM, *et al.* Pancreatic cancers epigenetically silence SIP1 and hypomethylate and overexpress miR-200a/200b in association with elevated circulating miR-200a and miR-200b levels. Cancer Res 2010; 70(13): 5226-37. [http://dx.doi.org/10.1158/0008-5472.CAN-09-4227] [PMID: 20551052]

[129] Robertson KD, Ait-Si-Ali S, Yokochi T, Wade PA, Jones PL, Wolffe AP. DNMT1 forms a complex with Rb, E2F1 and HDAC1 and represses transcription from E2F-responsive promoters. Nat Genet 2000; 25(3): 338-42. [http://dx.doi.org/10.1038/77124] [PMID: 10888886]

[130] Reis RS, Santos JA, Abreu PM, *et al.* Hypermethylation status of DAPK, MGMT and RUNX3 in HPV negative oral and oropharyngeal squamous cell carcinoma. Genet Mol Biol 2020; 43(3): e20190334. [http://dx.doi.org/10.1590/1678-4685-gmb-2019-0334] [PMID: 32870234]

[131] Qiao X, Yang X, Zhou Y, *et al.* Characterization of DAPK1 as a novel transcriptional target of BRMS1. Int J Oncol 2017; 50(5): 1760-6. [http://dx.doi.org/10.3892/ijo.2017.3930] [PMID: 28339067]

[132] Yadav P, Masroor M, Nandi K, *et al.* Promoter Methylation of BRCA1, DAPK1 and RASSF1A is Associated with Increased Mortality among Indian Women with Breast Cancer. Asian Pac J Cancer Prev 2018; 19(2): 443-8. [http://dx.doi.org/10.22034/APJCP.2018.19.2.443] [PMID: 29480000]

[133] Wang X, Cui N, Liu X, *et al.* Identification of. Front Genet 2018; 9: 258. [http://dx.doi.org/10.3389/fgene.2018.00258] [PMID: 30065752]

[134] Chan A, Chan M, Lee TL, *et al.* Promoter hypermethylation of Death-associated protein-kinase gene associated with advance stage gastric cancer. Oncol Rep 2005; 13(5): 937-41. [http://dx.doi.org/10.3892/or.13.5.937] [PMID: 15809761]

[135] Shivakumar L, Minna J, Sakamaki T, Pestell R, White MA. The RASSF1A tumor suppressor blocks cell cycle progression and inhibits cyclin D1 accumulation. Mol Cell Biol 2002; 22(12): 4309-18. [http://dx.doi.org/10.1128/MCB.22.12.4309-4318.2002] [PMID: 12024041]

[136] Hasegawa M, Nelson HH, Peters E, Ringstrom E, Posner M, Kelsey KT. Patterns of gene promoter methylation in squamous cell cancer of the head and neck. Oncogene 2002; 21(27): 4231-6. [http://dx.doi.org/10.1038/sj.onc.1205528] [PMID: 12082610]

[137] Ye M, Huang T, Ni C, Yang P, Chen S. Diagnostic Capacity of RASSF1A Promoter Methylation as a

Biomarker in Tissue, Brushing, and Blood Samples of Nasopharyngeal Carcinoma. EBioMedicine 2017; 18: 32-40.
[http://dx.doi.org/10.1016/j.ebiom.2017.03.038] [PMID: 28396012]

[138] Meng RW, Li YC, Chen X, *et al.* Aberrant Methylation of RASSF1A Closely Associated with HNSCC, a Meta-Analysis. Sci Rep 2016; 6(1): 20756.
[http://dx.doi.org/10.1038/srep20756] [PMID: 26857374]

[139] Cohen Y, Singer G, Lavie O, Dong SM, Beller U, Sidransky D. The RASSF1A tumor suppressor gene is commonly inactivated in adenocarcinoma of the uterine cervix. Clin Cancer Res 2003; 9(8): 2981-4.
[PMID: 12912945]

[140] Regel I, Eichenmüller M, Mahajan UM, *et al.* Downregulation of SFRP1 is a protumorigenic event in hepatoblastoma and correlates with beta-catenin mutations. J Cancer Res Clin Oncol 2020; 146(5): 1153-67.
[http://dx.doi.org/10.1007/s00432-020-03182-1] [PMID: 32189106]

[141] Vincent KM, Postovit LM. A pan-cancer analysis of secreted Frizzled-related proteins: re-examining their proposed tumour suppressive function. Sci Rep 2017; 7(1): 42719.
[http://dx.doi.org/10.1038/srep42719] [PMID: 28218291]

[142] Kumar A, Gosipatala SB, Pandey A, Singh P. Prognostic Relevance of SFRP1 Gene Promoter Methylation in Colorectal Carcinoma. Asian Pac J Cancer Prev 2019; 20(5): 1571-7.
[http://dx.doi.org/10.31557/APJCP.2019.20.5.1571] [PMID: 31128064]

[143] Alsofyani AA, Alsiary RA, Samkari A, *et al.* Prognostic potential of KLOTHO and SFRP1 promoter methylation in head and neck squamous cell carcinoma. J Appl Genet 2017; 58(4): 459-65.
[http://dx.doi.org/10.1007/s13353-017-0404-7] [PMID: 28812223]

[144] Chen H, Xu Z, Yang B, Zhou X, Kong H. RASGRF1 Hypermethylation, a Putative Biomarker of Colorectal Cancer. Ann Clin Lab Sci 2018; 48(1): 3-10.
[PMID: 29530990]

[145] Romero-Garcia S, Prado-Garcia H, Carlos-Reyes A. Role of DNA Methylation in the Resistance to Therapy in Solid Tumors. Front Oncol 2020; 10: 1152.
[http://dx.doi.org/10.3389/fonc.2020.01152] [PMID: 32850327]

[146] Zhang J, Stevens MFG, Laughton CA, Madhusudan S, Bradshaw TD. Acquired resistance to temozolomide in glioma cell lines: molecular mechanisms and potential translational applications. Oncology 2010; 78(2): 103-14.
[http://dx.doi.org/10.1159/000306139] [PMID: 20357518]

[147] Esteller M, Garcia-Foncillas J, Andion E, *et al.* Inactivation of the DNA-repair gene MGMT and the clinical response of gliomas to alkylating agents. N Engl J Med 2000; 343(19): 1350-4.
[http://dx.doi.org/10.1056/NEJM200011093431901] [PMID: 11070098]

[148] Esteller M, Gaidano G, Goodman SN, *et al.* Hypermethylation of the DNA repair gene O(6)-methylguanine DNA methyltransferase and survival of patients with diffuse large B-cell lymphoma. J Natl Cancer Inst 2002; 94(1): 26-32.
[http://dx.doi.org/10.1093/jnci/94.1.26] [PMID: 11773279]

[149] Palomeras S, Diaz-Lagares Á, Viñas G, *et al.* Epigenetic silencing of TGFBI confers resistance to trastuzumab in human breast cancer. Breast Cancer Res 2019; 21(1): 79.
[http://dx.doi.org/10.1186/s13058-019-1160-x] [PMID: 31277676]

[150] Chang SY, Kuo CC, Wu CC, *et al.* *NKX6.1* hypermethylation predicts the outcome of stage II colorectal cancer patients undergoing chemotherapy. Genes Chromosomes Cancer 2018; 57(5): 268-77.
[http://dx.doi.org/10.1002/gcc.22529] [PMID: 29363224]

[151] Baharudin R, Ab Mutalib NS, Othman SN, *et al.* Identification of Predictive DNA Methylation Biomarkers for Chemotherapy Response in Colorectal Cancer. Front Pharmacol 2017; 8: 47.

[http://dx.doi.org/10.3389/fphar.2017.00047] [PMID: 28243201]

[152] Sun J, Du N, Li J, *et al.* Transcription Factor AP2ε. Technol Cancer Res Treat 2016; 15(2): 285-95. [http://dx.doi.org/10.1177/1533034615577028] [PMID: 25810491]

[153] Guo R, Wu G, Li H, *et al.* Promoter methylation profiles between human lung adenocarcinoma multidrug resistant A549/cisplatin (A549/DDP) cells and its progenitor A549 cells. Biol Pharm Bull 2013; 36(8): 1310-6. [http://dx.doi.org/10.1248/bpb.b13-00153] [PMID: 23902976]

[154] Tian FM, Zhong CY, Wang XN, Meng Y. PDE3A is hypermethylated in cisplatin resistant non-small cell lung cancer cells and is a modulator of chemotherapy response. Eur Rev Med Pharmacol Sci 2017; 21(11): 2635-41. [PMID: 28678321]

[155] Fan H, Zhang M, Liu W. Hypermethylated KCNQ1 acts as a tumor suppressor in hepatocellular carcinoma. Biochem Biophys Res Commun 2018; 503(4): 3100-7. [http://dx.doi.org/10.1016/j.bbrc.2018.08.099] [PMID: 30144972]

[156] Fujiyoshi S, Honda S, Minato M, *et al.* Hypermethylation of *CSF3R* is a novel cisplatin resistance marker and predictor of response to postoperative chemotherapy in hepatoblastoma. Hepatol Res 2020; 50(5): 598-606. [http://dx.doi.org/10.1111/hepr.13479] [PMID: 31894653]

[157] Zhang N, Wang AY, Wang XK, Sun XM, Xue HZ. GAS5 is downregulated in gastric cancer cells by promoter hypermethylation and regulates adriamycin sensitivity. Eur Rev Med Pharmacol Sci 2016; 20(15): 3199-205. [PMID: 27466992]

[158] Tang X, Wu W, Sun SY, Wistuba II, Hong WK, Mao L. Hypermethylation of the death-associated protein kinase promoter attenuates the sensitivity to TRAIL-induced apoptosis in human non-small cell lung cancer cells. Mol Cancer Res 2004; 2(12): 685-91. [http://dx.doi.org/10.1158/1541-7786.685.2.12] [PMID: 15634757]

[159] Han N, Shi L, Guo Q, *et al.* HAT1 induces lung cancer cell apoptosis *via* up regulating Fas. Oncotarget 2017; 8(52): 89970-7. [http://dx.doi.org/10.18632/oncotarget.21205] [PMID: 29163803]

[160] Jin X, Tian S, Li P. Histone Acetyltransferase 1 Promotes Cell Proliferation and Induces Cisplatin Resistance in Hepatocellular Carcinoma. Oncol Res 2017; 25(6): 939-46. [http://dx.doi.org/10.3727/096504016X14809827856524] [PMID: 27938492]

[161] Miao BP, Zhang RS, Yang G, *et al.* Histone acetyltransferase 1 up regulates Bcl2L12 expression in nasopharyngeal cancer cells. Arch Biochem Biophys 2018; 646: 72-9. [http://dx.doi.org/10.1016/j.abb.2018.03.040] [PMID: 29621521]

[162] Fan P, Zhao J, Meng Z, *et al.* Overexpressed histone acetyltransferase 1 regulates cancer immunity by increasing programmed death-ligand 1 expression in pancreatic cancer. J Exp Clin Cancer Res 2019; 38(1): 47. [http://dx.doi.org/10.1186/s13046-019-1044-z] [PMID: 30709380]

[163] Yin YW, Jin HJ, Zhao W, *et al.* The Histone Acetyltransferase GCN5 Expression Is Elevated and Regulated by c-Myc and E2F1 Transcription Factors in Human Colon Cancer. Gene Expr 2015; 16(4): 187-96. [http://dx.doi.org/10.3727/105221615X14399878166230] [PMID: 26637399]

[164] Zhao C, Li Y, Qiu W, *et al.* C5a induces A549 cell proliferation of non-small cell lung cancer *via* GDF15 gene activation mediated by GCN5-dependent KLF5 acetylation. Oncogene 2018; 37(35): 4821-37. [http://dx.doi.org/10.1038/s41388-018-0298-9] [PMID: 29773900]

[165] Zhao L, Pang A, Li Y. Function of GCN5 in the TGF-β1-induced epithelial-to-mesenchymal transition

in breast cancer. Oncol Lett 2018; 16(3): 3955-63.
[http://dx.doi.org/10.3892/ol.2018.9134] [PMID: 30128014]

[166] Shao G, Liu Y, Ma T, Zhang L, Yuan M, Zhao S. GCN5 inhibition prevents IL-6-induced prostate cancer metastases through PI3K/PTEN/Akt signaling by inactivating Egr-1. Biosci Rep 2018; 38(6): BSR20180816.
[http://dx.doi.org/10.1042/BSR20180816] [PMID: 30333255]

[167] Fei HJ, Zu LD, Wu J, *et al.* PCAF acts as a gastric cancer suppressor through a novel PCAF-p16-CDK4 axis. Am J Cancer Res 2016; 6(12): 2772-86.
[PMID: 28042499]

[168] Watts GS, Oshiro MM, Junk DJ, *et al.* The acetyltransferase p300/CBP-associated factor is a p53 target gene in breast tumor cells. Neoplasia 2004; 6(3): 187-94.
[http://dx.doi.org/10.1593/neo.03292] [PMID: 15153330]

[169] Yu C, Gong AY, Chen D, Solelo Leon D, Young CYF, Chen XM. Phenethyl isothiocyanate inhibits androgen receptor-regulated transcriptional activity in prostate cancer cells through suppressing PCAF. Mol Nutr Food Res 2013; 57(10): 1825-33.
[http://dx.doi.org/10.1002/mnfr.201200810] [PMID: 23661605]

[170] Liu T, Wang X, Hu W, *et al.* Epigenetically Down-Regulated Acetyltransferase PCAF Increases the Resistance of Colorectal Cancer to 5-Fluorouracil. Neoplasia 2019; 21(6): 557-70.
[http://dx.doi.org/10.1016/j.neo.2019.03.011] [PMID: 31042625]

[171] Okada Y, Jiang Q, Lemieux M, Jeannotte L, Su L, Zhang Y. Leukaemic transformation by CALM-AF10 involves upregulation of Hoxa5 by hDOT1L. Nat Cell Biol 2006; 8(9): 1017-24.
[http://dx.doi.org/10.1038/ncb1464] [PMID: 16921363]

[172] Hayashi Y, Harada Y, Kagiyama Y, *et al.* NUP98-HBO1-fusion generates phenotypically and genetically relevant chronic myelomonocytic leukemia pathogenesis. Blood Adv 2019; 3(7): 1047-60.
[http://dx.doi.org/10.1182/bloodadvances.2018025007] [PMID: 30944097]

[173] Imamura T, Kakazu N, Hibi S, *et al.* Rearrangement of theMOZ gene in pediatric therapy-related myelodysplastic syndrome with a novel chromosomal translocation t(2;8)(p23;p11). Genes Chromosomes Cancer 2003; 36(4): 413-9.
[http://dx.doi.org/10.1002/gcc.10172] [PMID: 12619166]

[174] Pelletier N, Champagne N, Stifani S, Yang XJ. MOZ and MORF histone acetyltransferases interact with the Runt-domain transcription factor Runx2. Oncogene 2002; 21(17): 2729-40.
[http://dx.doi.org/10.1038/sj.onc.1205367] [PMID: 11965546]

[175] Murati A, Adélaïde J, Mozziconacci MJ, *et al.* Variant *MYST4-CBP* gene fusion in a t(10;16) acute myeloid leukaemia. Br J Haematol 2004; 125(5): 601-4.
[http://dx.doi.org/10.1111/j.1365-2141.2004.04960.x] [PMID: 15147375]

[176] Francis NJ, Kingston RE, Woodcock CL. Chromatin compaction by a polycomb group protein complex. Science 2004; 306(5701): 1574-7.
[http://dx.doi.org/10.1126/science.1100576] [PMID: 15567868]

[177] He LR, Liu MZ, Li BK, *et al.* Prognostic impact of H3K27me3 expression on locoregional progression after chemoradiotherapy in esophageal squamous cell carcinoma. BMC Cancer 2009; 9(1): 461.
[http://dx.doi.org/10.1186/1471-2407-9-461] [PMID: 20028503]

[178] Wei Y, Xia W, Zhang Z, *et al.* Loss of trimethylation at lysine 27 of histone H3 is a predictor of poor outcome in breast, ovarian, and pancreatic cancers. Mol Carcinog 2008; 47(9): 701-6.
[http://dx.doi.org/10.1002/mc.20413] [PMID: 18176935]

[179] Yoo KH, Hennighausen L. EZH2 methyltransferase and H3K27 methylation in breast cancer. Int J Biol Sci 2012; 8(1): 59-65.
[http://dx.doi.org/10.7150/ijbs.8.59] [PMID: 22211105]

[180] Hansen KH, Bracken AP, Pasini D, *et al.* A model for transmission of the H3K27me3 epigenetic mark. Nat Cell Biol 2008; 10(11): 1291-300.
[http://dx.doi.org/10.1038/ncb1787] [PMID: 18931660]

[181] Guan X, Deng H, Choi UL, *et al.* EZH2 overexpression dampens tumor-suppressive signals *via* an EGR1 silencer to drive breast tumorigenesis. Oncogene 2020; 39(48): 7127-41.
[http://dx.doi.org/10.1038/s41388-020-01484-9] [PMID: 33009487]

[182] Koh CM, Iwata T, Zheng Q, Bethel C, Yegnasubramanian S, De Marzo AM. Myc enforces overexpression of EZH2 in early prostatic neoplasia *via* transcriptional and post-transcriptional mechanisms. Oncotarget 2011; 2(9): 669-83.
[http://dx.doi.org/10.18632/oncotarget.327] [PMID: 21941025]

[183] Eichenauer T, Simmendinger L, Fraune C, *et al.* High level of EZH2 expression is linked to high density of CD8-positive T-lymphocytes and an aggressive phenotype in renal cell carcinoma. World J Urol 2021; 39(2): 481-90.
[http://dx.doi.org/10.1007/s00345-020-03200-4] [PMID: 32303902]

[184] Wang H, Albadine R, Magheli A, *et al.* Increased EZH2 protein expression is associated with invasive urothelial carcinoma of the bladder. Urol Oncol 2012; 30(4): 428-33.
[http://dx.doi.org/10.1016/j.urolonc.2010.09.005] [PMID: 21396836]

[185] Lund K, Adams PD, Copland M. EZH2 in normal and malignant hematopoiesis. Leukemia 2014; 28(1): 44-9.
[http://dx.doi.org/10.1038/leu.2013.288] [PMID: 24097338]

[186] Yu J, Yu J, Rhodes DR, *et al.* A polycomb repression signature in metastatic prostate cancer predicts cancer outcome. Cancer Res 2007; 67(22): 10657-63.
[http://dx.doi.org/10.1158/0008-5472.CAN-07-2498] [PMID: 18006806]

[187] van Haaften G, Dalgliesh GL, Davies H, *et al.* Somatic mutations of the histone H3K27 demethylase gene UTX in human cancer. Nat Genet 2009; 41(5): 521-3.
[http://dx.doi.org/10.1038/ng.349] [PMID: 19330029]

[188] Kim JH, Sharma A, Dhar SS, *et al.* UTX and MLL4 coordinately regulate transcriptional programs for cell proliferation and invasiveness in breast cancer cells. Cancer Res 2014; 74(6): 1705-17.
[http://dx.doi.org/10.1158/0008-5472.CAN-13-1896] [PMID: 24491801]

[189] Seligson DB, Horvath S, Shi T, *et al.* Global histone modification patterns predict risk of prostate cancer recurrence. Nature 2005; 435(7046): 1262-6.
[http://dx.doi.org/10.1038/nature03672] [PMID: 15988529]

[190] Barlési F, Giaccone G, Gallegos-Ruiz MI, *et al.* Global histone modifications predict prognosis of resected non small-cell lung cancer. J Clin Oncol 2007; 25(28): 4358-64.
[http://dx.doi.org/10.1200/JCO.2007.11.2599] [PMID: 17906200]

[191] Manuyakorn A, Paulus R, Farrell J, *et al.* Cellular histone modification patterns predict prognosis and treatment response in resectable pancreatic adenocarcinoma: results from RTOG 9704. J Clin Oncol 2010; 28(8): 1358-65.
[http://dx.doi.org/10.1200/JCO.2009.24.5639] [PMID: 20142597]

[192] Wagner KW, Alam H, Dhar SS, *et al.* KDM2A promotes lung tumorigenesis by epigenetically enhancing ERK1/2 signaling. J Clin Invest 2013; 123(12): 5231-46.
[http://dx.doi.org/10.1172/JCI68642] [PMID: 24200691]

[193] Tzatsos A, Paskaleva P, Ferrari F, *et al.* KDM2B promotes pancreatic cancer *via* Polycomb-dependent and -independent transcriptional programs. J Clin Invest 2013; 123(2): 727-39.
[http://dx.doi.org/10.1172/JCI64535] [PMID: 23321669]

[194] Xiong W, Deng Z, Tang Y, Deng Z, Li M. Downregulation of KMT2D suppresses proliferation and induces apoptosis of gastric cancer. Biochem Biophys Res Commun 2018; 504(1): 129-36.
[http://dx.doi.org/10.1016/j.bbrc.2018.08.143] [PMID: 30177394]

[195] Fenizia C, Bottino C, Corbetta S, *et al.* SMYD3 promotes the epithelial-mesenchymal transition in breast cancer. Nucleic Acids Res 2019; 47(3): 1278-93. [http://dx.doi.org/10.1093/nar/gky1221] [PMID: 30544196]

[196] Sarris ME, Moulos P, Haroniti A, Giakountis A, Talianidis I. Smyd3 Is a Transcriptional Potentiator of Multiple Cancer-Promoting Genes and Required for Liver and Colon Cancer Development. Cancer Cell 2016; 29(3): 354-66. [http://dx.doi.org/10.1016/j.ccell.2016.01.013] [PMID: 26908355]

[197] Lv T, Yuan D, Miao X, *et al.* Over-expression of LSD1 promotes proliferation, migration and invasion in non-small cell lung cancer. PLoS One 2012; 7(4): e35065. [http://dx.doi.org/10.1371/journal.pone.0035065] [PMID: 22493729]

[198] Lim S, Janzer A, Becker A, *et al.* Lysine-specific demethylase 1 (LSD1) is highly expressed in ER-negative breast cancers and a biomarker predicting aggressive biology. Carcinogenesis 2010; 31(3): 512-20. [http://dx.doi.org/10.1093/carcin/bgp324] [PMID: 20042638]

[199] Li X, Li T, Chen D, *et al.* Overexpression of lysine-specific demethylase 1 promotes androgen-independent transition of human prostate cancer LNCaP cells through activation of the AR signaling pathway and suppression of the p53 signaling pathway. Oncol Rep 2016; 35(1): 584-92. [http://dx.doi.org/10.3892/or.2015.4362] [PMID: 26534764]

[200] Qin Y, Zhu W, Xu W, *et al.* LSD1 sustains pancreatic cancer growth *via* maintaining HIF1α-dependent glycolytic process. Cancer Lett 2014; 347(2): 225-32. [http://dx.doi.org/10.1016/j.canlet.2014.02.013] [PMID: 24561118]

[201] Zhang J, Zhao D, Li Q, *et al.* Upregulation of LSD1 promotes migration and invasion in gastric cancer through facilitating EMT. Cancer Manag Res 2019; 11: 4481-91. [http://dx.doi.org/10.2147/CMAR.S186649] [PMID: 31191010]

[202] Huang D, Xiao F, Hao H, *et al.* JARID1B promotes colorectal cancer proliferation and Wnt/-catenin signaling *via* decreasing CDX2 level. Cell Commun Signal 2020; 18(1): 169. [http://dx.doi.org/10.1186/s12964-020-00660-4] [PMID: 33109187]

[203] Yamamoto S, Wu Z, Russnes HG, *et al.* JARID1B is a luminal lineage-driving oncogene in breast cancer. Cancer Cell 2014; 25(6): 762-77. [http://dx.doi.org/10.1016/j.ccr.2014.04.024] [PMID: 24937458]

[204] Zhang J, An X, Han Y, *et al.* Overexpression of JARID1B promotes differentiation *via* SHIP1/AKT signaling in human hypopharyngeal squamous cell carcinoma. Cell Death Dis 2016; 7(9): e2358. [http://dx.doi.org/10.1038/cddis.2016.262] [PMID: 27584795]

[205] Calin GA, Croce CM. MicroRNAs and chromosomal abnormalities in cancer cells. Oncogene 2006; 25(46): 6202-10. [http://dx.doi.org/10.1038/sj.onc.1209910] [PMID: 17028600]

[206] Tagawa H, Seto M. A microRNA cluster as a target of genomic amplification in malignant lymphoma. Leukemia 2005; 19(11): 2013-6. [http://dx.doi.org/10.1038/sj.leu.2403942] [PMID: 16167061]

[207] Mavrakis KJ, Wolfe AL, Oricchio E, *et al.* Genome-wide RNA-mediated interference screen identifies miR-19 targets in Notch-induced T-cell acute lymphoblastic leukaemia. Nat Cell Biol 2010; 12(4): 372-9. [http://dx.doi.org/10.1038/ncb2037] [PMID: 20190740]

[208] Calin GA, Sevignani C, Dumitru CD, *et al.* Human microRNA genes are frequently located at fragile sites and genomic regions involved in cancers. Proc Natl Acad Sci USA 2004; 101(9): 2999-3004. [http://dx.doi.org/10.1073/pnas.0307323101] [PMID: 14973191]

[209] O'Donnell KA, Wentzel EA, Zeller KI, Dang CV, Mendell JT. c-Myc-regulated microRNAs modulate E2F1 expression. Nature 2005; 435(7043): 839-43.

[http://dx.doi.org/10.1038/nature03677] [PMID: 15944709]

[210] Chang TC, Yu D, Lee YS, *et al.* Widespread microRNA repression by Myc contributes to tumorigenesis. Nat Genet 2008; 40(1): 43-50.
[http://dx.doi.org/10.1038/ng.2007.30] [PMID: 18066065]

[211] Hermeking H. The miR-34 family in cancer and apoptosis. Cell Death Differ 2010; 17(2): 193-9.
[http://dx.doi.org/10.1038/cdd.2009.56] [PMID: 19461653]

[212] Han L, Witmer PDW, Casey E, Valle D, Sukumar S. DNA methylation regulates microRNA expression. Cancer Biol Ther 2007; 6(8): 1290-4.
[http://dx.doi.org/10.4161/cbt.6.8.4486] [PMID: 17660710]

[213] Saito Y, Jones PM. Epigenetic activation of tumor suppressor microRNAs in human cancer cells. Cell Cycle 2006; 5(19): 2220-2.
[http://dx.doi.org/10.4161/cc.5.19.3340] [PMID: 17012846]

[214] Hanahan D, Weinberg RA. Hallmarks of cancer: the next generation. Cell 2011; 144(5): 646-74.
[http://dx.doi.org/10.1016/j.cell.2011.02.013] [PMID: 21376230]

[215] Hatley ME, Patrick DM, Garcia MR, *et al.* Modulation of K-Ras-dependent lung tumorigenesis by MicroRNA-21. Cancer Cell 2010; 18(3): 282-93.
[http://dx.doi.org/10.1016/j.ccr.2010.08.013] [PMID: 20832755]

[216] Kalluri R, Weinberg RA. The basics of epithelial-mesenchymal transition. J Clin Invest 2009; 119(6): 1420-8.
[http://dx.doi.org/10.1172/JCI39104] [PMID: 19487818]

[217] Ferrara N. VEGF and the quest for tumour angiogenesis factors. Nat Rev Cancer 2002; 2(10): 795-803.
[http://dx.doi.org/10.1038/nrc909] [PMID: 12360282]

[218] Nallamshetty S, Chan SY, Loscalzo J. Hypoxia: a master regulator of microRNA biogenesis and activity. Free Radic Biol Med 2013; 64: 20-30.
[http://dx.doi.org/10.1016/j.freeradbiomed.2013.05.022]

[219] Luo J, Solimini NL, Elledge SJ. Principles of cancer therapy: oncogene and non-oncogene addiction. Cell 2009; 136(5): 823-37.
[http://dx.doi.org/10.1016/j.cell.2009.02.024] [PMID: 19269363]

[220] Mayes K, Qiu Z, Alhazmi A, Landry JW. ATP-dependent chromatin remodeling complexes as novel targets for cancer therapy. Adv Cancer Res 2014; 121: 183-233.
[http://dx.doi.org/10.1016/B978-0-12-800249-0.00005-6] [PMID: 24889532]

[221] Lai AY, Wade PA. Cancer biology and NuRD: a multifaceted chromatin remodelling complex. Nat Rev Cancer 2011; 11(8): 588-96.
[http://dx.doi.org/10.1038/nrc3091] [PMID: 21734722]

[222] Magdinier F, Wolffe AP. Selective association of the methyl-CpG binding protein MBD2 with the silent p14/p16 locus in human neoplasia. Proc Natl Acad Sci USA 2001; 98(9): 4990-5.
[http://dx.doi.org/10.1073/pnas.101617298]

[223] Stirzaker C, Song JZ, Ng W, *et al.* Methyl-CpG-binding protein MBD2 plays a key role in maintenance and spread of DNA methylation at CpG islands and shores in cancer. Oncogene 2017; 36(10): 1328-38.
[http://dx.doi.org/10.1038/onc.2016.297] [PMID: 27593931]

[224] Cai Y, Geutjes E-J, de Lint K, *et al.* The NuRD complex cooperates with DNMTs to maintain silencing of key colorectal tumor suppressor genes. Oncogene 2014; 33(17): 2157-68.
[http://dx.doi.org/10.1038/onc.2013.178] [PMID: 23708667]

[225] Bracken AP, Brien GL, Verrijzer CP. Dangerous liaisons: interplay between SWI/SNF, NuRD, and Polycomb in chromatin regulation and cancer. Genes Dev 2019; 33(15-16): 936-59.

[http://dx.doi.org/10.1101/gad.326066.119] [PMID: 31123059]

[226] Basta J, Rauchman M. The nucleosome remodeling and deacetylase complex in development and disease. Transl Res 2015; 165(1): 36-47.
[http://dx.doi.org/10.1016/j.trsl.2014.05.003] [PMID: 24880148]

[227] Denslow SA, Wade PA. The human Mi-2/NuRD complex and gene regulation. Oncogene 2007; 26(37): 5433-8.
[http://dx.doi.org/10.1038/sj.onc.1210611] [PMID: 17694084]

[228] McKenzie LD, LeClair JW, Miller KN, *et al.* CHD4 regulates the DNA damage response and RAD51 expression in glioblastoma. Sci Rep 2019; 9(1): 4444.
[http://dx.doi.org/10.1038/s41598-019-40327-w] [PMID: 30872624]

[229] Srinivasan R, Mager GM, Ward RM, Mayer J, Svaren J. NAB2 represses transcription by interacting with the CHD4 subunit of the nucleosome remodeling and deacetylase (NuRD) complex. J Biol Chem 2006; 281(22): 15129-37.
[http://dx.doi.org/10.1074/jbc.M600775200] [PMID: 16574654]

[230] Xia L, Huang W, Bellani M, *et al.* CHD4 Has Oncogenic Functions in Initiating and Maintaining Epigenetic Suppression of Multiple Tumor Suppressor Genes. Cancer Cell 2017; 31(5): 653-668.e7.
[http://dx.doi.org/10.1016/j.ccell.2017.04.005] [PMID: 28486105]

[231] Li R, Zhang H, Yu W, *et al.* ZIP: a novel transcription repressor, represses EGFR oncogene and suppresses breast carcinogenesis. EMBO J 2009; 28(18): 2763-76.
[http://dx.doi.org/10.1038/emboj.2009.211] [PMID: 19644445]

[232] Wang HC, Chou CL, Yang CC, *et al.* Over-Expression of CHD4 Is an Independent Biomarker of Poor Prognosis in Patients with Rectal Cancers Receiving Concurrent Chemoradiotherapy. Int J Mol Sci 2019; 20(17): 4087.
[http://dx.doi.org/10.3390/ijms20174087] [PMID: 31438571]

[233] Mills AA. The Chromodomain Helicase DNA-Binding Chromatin Remodelers: Family Traits that Protect from and Promote Cancer. Cold Spring Harb Perspect Med 2017; 7(4): a026450.
[http://dx.doi.org/10.1101/cshperspect.a026450] [PMID: 28096241]

[234] Quan J, Adelmant G, Marto JA, Look AT, Yusufzai T. The chromatin remodeling factor CHD5 is a transcriptional repressor of WEE1. PLoS One 2014; 9(9): e108066.
[http://dx.doi.org/10.1371/journal.pone.0108066] [PMID: 25247294]

[235] Wang L, He S, Tu Y, *et al.* Downregulation of chromatin remodeling factor CHD5 is associated with a poor prognosis in human glioma. J Clin Neurosci 2013; 20(7): 958-63.
[http://dx.doi.org/10.1016/j.jocn.2012.07.021] [PMID: 23707602]

[236] Wong RRY, Chan LKY, Tsang TPT, *et al.* CHD5 Downregulation Associated with Poor Prognosis in Epithelial Ovarian Cancer. Gynecol Obstet Invest 2011; 72(3): 203-7.
[http://dx.doi.org/10.1159/000323883] [PMID: 21860208]

[237] Wu X, Zhu Z, Li W, *et al.* Chromodomain helicase DNA binding protein 5 plays a tumor suppressor role in human breast cancer. Breast Cancer Res 2012; 14(3): R73.
[http://dx.doi.org/10.1186/bcr3182] [PMID: 22569290]

[238] Du X, Wu T, Lu J, *et al.* Decreased expression of chromodomain helicase DNA-binding protein 5 is an unfavorable prognostic marker in patients with primary gallbladder carcinoma. Clin Transl Oncol 2013; 15(3): 198-204.
[http://dx.doi.org/10.1007/s12094-012-0903-2] [PMID: 22855185]

[239] Fatemi M, Paul TA, Brodeur GM, Shokrani B, Brim H, Ashktorab H. Epigenetic silencing of *CHD5*, a novel tumor-suppressor gene, occurs in early colorectal cancer stages. Cancer 2014; 120(2): 172-80.
[http://dx.doi.org/10.1002/cncr.28316] [PMID: 24243398]

[240] Du Z, Li L, Huang X, *et al.* The epigenetic modifier CHD5 functions as a novel tumor suppressor for renal cell carcinoma and is predominantly inactivated by promoter CpG methylation. Oncotarget 2016;

7(16): 21618-30.
[http://dx.doi.org/10.18632/oncotarget.7822] [PMID: 26943038]

[241] Tsukiyama T, Wu C. Purification and properties of an ATP-dependent nucleosome remodeling factor. Cell 1995; 83(6): 1011-20.
[http://dx.doi.org/10.1016/0092-8674(95)90216-3] [PMID: 8521501]

[242] Li H, Ilin S, Wang W, *et al.* Molecular basis for site-specific read-out of histone H3K4me3 by the BPTF PHD finger of NURF. Nature 2006; 442(7098): 91-5.
[http://dx.doi.org/10.1038/nature04802] [PMID: 16728978]

[243] Pan Y, Yuan F, Li Y, Wang G, Lin Z, Chen L. Bromodomain PHD-finger transcription factor promotes glioma progression and indicates poor prognosis. Oncol Rep 2018; 41(1): 246-56.
[http://dx.doi.org/10.3892/or.2018.6832] [PMID: 30542695]

[244] Dar AA, Nosrati M, Bezrookove V, *et al.* The role of BPTF in melanoma progression and in response to BRAF-targeted therapy. J Natl Cancer Inst 2015; 107(5): djv034.
[http://dx.doi.org/10.1093/jnci/djv034] [PMID: 25713167]

[245] Xiao S, Liu L, Lu X, Long J, Zhou X, Fang M. The prognostic significance of bromodomain PHD-finger transcription factor in colorectal carcinoma and association with vimentin and E-cadherin. J Cancer Res Clin Oncol 2015; 141(8): 1465-74.
[http://dx.doi.org/10.1007/s00432-015-1937-y] [PMID: 25716692]

[246] Zhao X, Zheng F, Li Y, *et al.* BPTF promotes hepatocellular carcinoma growth by modulating hTERT signaling and cancer stem cell traits. Redox Biol 2019; 20: 427-41.
[http://dx.doi.org/10.1016/j.redox.2018.10.018] [PMID: 30419422]

[247] Badenhorst P, Voas M, Rebay I, Wu C. Biological functions of the ISWI chromatin remodeling complex NURF. Genes Dev 2002; 16(24): 3186-98.
[http://dx.doi.org/10.1101/gad.1032202] [PMID: 12502740]

[248] Song H, Spichiger-Haeusermann C, Basler K. The ISWI-containing NURF complex regulates the output of the canonical Wingless pathway. EMBO Rep 2009; 10(10): 1140-6.
[http://dx.doi.org/10.1038/embor.2009.157] [PMID: 19713963]

[249] Kwon SY, Xiao H, Glover BP, Tjian R, Wu C, Badenhorst P. The nucleosome remodeling factor (NURF) regulates genes involved in Drosophila innate immunity. Dev Biol 2008; 316(2): 538-47.
[http://dx.doi.org/10.1016/j.ydbio.2008.01.033] [PMID: 18334252]

[250] Witkiewicz AK, McMillan EA, Balaji U, *et al.* Whole-exome sequencing of pancreatic cancer defines genetic diversity and therapeutic targets. Nat Commun 2015; 6(1): 6744.
[http://dx.doi.org/10.1038/ncomms7744] [PMID: 25855536]

[251] Chandler RL, Brennan J, Schisler JC, Serber D, Patterson C, Magnuson T. ARID1a-DNA interactions are required for promoter occupancy by SWI/SNF. Mol Cell Biol 2013; 33(2): 265-80.
[http://dx.doi.org/10.1128/MCB.01008-12] [PMID: 23129809]

[252] Wang W, Friedland SC, Guo B, *et al.* ARID1A, a SWI/SNF subunit, is critical to acinar cell homeostasis and regeneration and is a barrier to transformation and epithelial-mesenchymal transition in the pancreas. Gut 2019; 68(7): 1245-58.
[http://dx.doi.org/10.1136/gutjnl-2017-315541] [PMID: 30228219]

[253] Guan B, Wang TL, Shih IM. ARID1A, a factor that promotes formation of SWI/SNF-mediated chromatin remodeling, is a tumor suppressor in gynecologic cancers. Cancer Res 2011; 71(21): 6718-27.
[http://dx.doi.org/10.1158/0008-5472.CAN-11-1562] [PMID: 21900401]

[254] Hasan N, Ahuja N. The Emerging Roles of ATP-Dependent Chromatin Remodeling Complexes in Pancreatic Cancer. Cancers (Basel) 2019; 11(12): 1859.
[http://dx.doi.org/10.3390/cancers11121859] [PMID: 31769422]

[255] Jeddeloh JA, Stokes TL, Richards EJ. Maintenance of genomic methylation requires a SWI2/SNF2-

like protein. Nat Genet 1999; 22(1): 94-7.
[http://dx.doi.org/10.1038/8803] [PMID: 10319870]

[256] Choi SH, Ryu TH, Kim JI, Lee S, Lee SS, Kim JH. Mutation in DDM1 inhibits the homology directed repair of double strand breaks. PLoS One 2019; 14(2): e0211878.
[http://dx.doi.org/10.1371/journal.pone.0211878] [PMID: 30742642]

[257] Campbell PJ, Green AR. The myeloproliferative disorders. N Engl J Med 2006; 355(23): 2452-66.
[http://dx.doi.org/10.1056/NEJMra063728] [PMID: 17151367]

[258] Levine RL, Pardanani A, Tefferi A, Gilliland DG. Role of JAK2 in the pathogenesis and therapy of myeloproliferative disorders. Nat Rev Cancer 2007; 7(9): 673-83.
[http://dx.doi.org/10.1038/nrc2210] [PMID: 17721432]

[259] James C, Ugo V, Le Couédic JP, *et al.* A unique clonal JAK2 mutation leading to constitutive signalling causes polycythaemia vera. Nature 2005; 434(7037): 1144-8.
[http://dx.doi.org/10.1038/nature03546] [PMID: 15793561]

[260] Levine RL, Loriaux M, Huntly BJ, *et al.* The JAK2V617F activating mutation occurs in chronic myelomonocytic leukemia and acute myeloid leukemia, but not in acute lymphoblastic leukemia or chronic lymphocytic leukemia. Blood 2005; 106(10): 3377-9.
[http://dx.doi.org/10.1182/blood-2005-05-1898] [PMID: 16081687]

[261] Kralovics R, Passamonti F, Buser AS, *et al.* A gain-of-function mutation of JAK2 in myeloproliferative disorders. N Engl J Med 2005; 352(17): 1779-90.
[http://dx.doi.org/10.1056/NEJMoa051113] [PMID: 15858187]

[262] Dawson MA, Bannister AJ, Göttgens B, *et al.* JAK2 phosphorylates histone H3Y41 and excludes HP1α from chromatin. Nature 2009; 461(7265): 819-22.
[http://dx.doi.org/10.1038/nature08448] [PMID: 19783980]

[263] Yamada Y, Warren AJ, Dobson C, Forster A, Pannell R, Rabbitts TH. The T cell leukemia LIM protein Lmo2 is necessary for adult mouse hematopoiesis. Proc Natl Acad Sci USA 1998; 95(7): 3890-5.
[http://dx.doi.org/10.1073/pnas.95.7.3890]

[264] McCormack MP, Rabbitts TH. Activation of the T-cell oncogene LMO2 after gene therapy for X-linked severe combined immunodeficiency. N Engl J Med 2004; 350(9): 913-22.
[http://dx.doi.org/10.1056/NEJMra032207] [PMID: 14985489]

[265] Kelly TK, Liu Y, Lay FD, Liang G, Berman BP, Jones PA. Genome-wide mapping of nucleosome positioning and DNA methylation within individual DNA molecules. Genome Res 2012; 22(12): 2497-506.
[http://dx.doi.org/10.1101/gr.143008.112] [PMID: 22960375]

[266] Yang X, Noushmehr H, Han H, Andreu-Vieyra C, Liang G, Jones PA. Gene reactivation by 5-aza- 2′-deoxycytidine-induced demethylation requires SRCAP-mediated H2A.Z insertion to establish nucleosome depleted regions. PLoS Genet 2012; 8(3): e1002604.
[http://dx.doi.org/10.1371/journal.pgen.1002604] [PMID: 22479200]

[267] Nguyen CT, Gonzales FA, Jones PA. Altered chromatin structure associated with methylation-induced gene silencing in cancer cells: correlation of accessibility, methylation, MeCP2 binding and acetylation. Nucleic Acids Res 2001; 29(22): 4598-606.
[http://dx.doi.org/10.1093/nar/29.22.4598]

[268] Fahrner JA, Eguchi S, Herman JG, Baylin SB. Dependence of histone modifications and gene expression on DNA hypermethylation in cancer. Cancer Res 2002; 62(24): 7213-8.
[PMID: 12499261]

[269] Baylin SB, Jones PA. A decade of exploring the cancer epigenome — biological and translational implications. Nat Rev Cancer 2011; 11(10): 726-34.
[http://dx.doi.org/10.1038/nrc3130] [PMID: 21941284]

[270] Shen H, Laird PW. Interplay between the cancer genome and epigenome. Cell 2013; 153(1): 38-55. [http://dx.doi.org/10.1016/j.cell.2013.03.008] [PMID: 23540689]

[271] Fraga MF, Ballestar E, Villar-Garea A, *et al.* Loss of acetylation at Lys16 and trimethylation at Lys20 of histone H4 is a common hallmark of human cancer. Nat Genet 2005; 37(4): 391-400. [http://dx.doi.org/10.1038/ng1531] [PMID: 15765097]

[272] Shogren-Knaak M, Ishii H, Sun JM, Pazin MJ, Davie JR, Peterson CL. Histone H4-K16 acetylation controls chromatin structure and protein interactions. Science 2006; 311(5762): 844-7. [http://dx.doi.org/10.1126/science.1124000] [PMID: 16469925]

[273] Shogren-Knaak M, Peterson CL. Switching on chromatin: mechanistic role of histone H4-K16 acetylation. Cell Cycle 2006; 5(13): 1361-5. [http://dx.doi.org/10.4161/cc.5.13.2891] [PMID: 16855380]

[274] Elsheikh SE, Green AR, Rakha EA, *et al.* Global histone modifications in breast cancer correlate with tumor phenotypes, prognostic factors, and patient outcome. Cancer Res 2009; 69(9): 3802-9. [http://dx.doi.org/10.1158/0008-5472.CAN-08-3907] [PMID: 19366799]

[275] Hajji N, Wallenborg K, Vlachos P, Füllgrabe J, Hermanson O, Joseph B. Opposing effects of hMOF and SIRT1 on H4K16 acetylation and the sensitivity to the topoisomerase II inhibitor etoposide. Oncogene 2010; 29(15): 2192-204. [http://dx.doi.org/10.1038/onc.2009.505] [PMID: 20118981]

[276] Pogribny IP, Ross SA, Tryndyak VP, Pogribna M, Poirier LA, Karpinets TV. Histone H3 lysine 9 and H4 lysine 20 trimethylation and the expression of Suv4-20h2 and Suv-39h1 histone methyltransferases in hepatocarcinogenesis induced by methyl deficiency in rats. Carcinogenesis 2006; 27(6): 1180-6. [http://dx.doi.org/10.1093/carcin/bgi364] [PMID: 16497704]

[277] Tryndyak VP, Kovalchuk O, Pogribny IP. Loss of DNA methylation and histone H4 lysine 20 trimethylation in human breast cancer cells is associated with aberrant expression of DNA methyltransferase 1, Suv4-20h2 histone methyltransferase and methyl-binding proteins. Cancer Biol Ther 2006; 5(1): 65-70. [http://dx.doi.org/10.4161/cbt.5.1.2288] [PMID: 16322686]

[278] Di Croce L, Raker VA, Corsaro M, *et al.* Methyltransferase recruitment and DNA hypermethylation of target promoters by an oncogenic transcription factor. Science 2002; 295(5557): 1079-82. [http://dx.doi.org/10.1126/science.1065173] [PMID: 11834837]

[279] Collins SJ. The role of retinoids and retinoic acid receptors in normal hematopoiesis. Leukemia 2002; 16(10): 1896-905. [http://dx.doi.org/10.1038/sj.leu.2402718] [PMID: 12357341]

[280] Popovic R, Licht JD. Emerging epigenetic targets and therapies in cancer medicine. Cancer Discov 2012; 2(5): 405-13. [http://dx.doi.org/10.1158/2159-8290.CD-12-0076] [PMID: 22588878]

[281] Slany RK. The molecular biology of mixed lineage leukemia. Haematologica 2009; 94(7): 984-93. [http://dx.doi.org/10.3324/haematol.2008.002436] [PMID: 19535349]

[282] Azad N, Zahnow CA, Rudin CM, Baylin SB. The future of epigenetic therapy in solid tumours—lessons from the past. Nat Rev Clin Oncol 2013; 10(5): 256-66. [http://dx.doi.org/10.1038/nrclinonc.2013.42] [PMID: 23546521]

[283] Peters I, Dubrowinskaja N, Abbas M, *et al.* DNA methylation biomarkers predict progression-free and overall survival of metastatic renal cell cancer (mRCC) treated with antiangiogenic therapies. PLoS One 2014; 9(3): e91440. [http://dx.doi.org/10.1371/journal.pone.0091440] [PMID: 24633192]

[284] Treppendahl MB, Kristensen LS, Grønbæk K. Predicting response to epigenetic therapy. J Clin Invest 2014; 124(1): 47-55. [http://dx.doi.org/10.1172/JCI69737] [PMID: 24382389]

[285] Christman JK. 5-Azacytidine and 5-aza-2′-deoxycytidine as inhibitors of DNA methylation: mechanistic studies and their implications for cancer therapy. Oncogene 2002; 21(35): 5483-95. [http://dx.doi.org/10.1038/sj.onc.1205699] [PMID: 12154409]

[286] Li H, Chiappinelli KB, Guzzetta AA, *et al.* Immune regulation by low doses of the DNA methyltransferase inhibitor 5-azacitidine in common human epithelial cancers. Oncotarget 2014; 5(3): 587-98.
[http://dx.doi.org/10.18632/oncotarget.1782] [PMID: 24583822]

[287] Ropero S, Esteller M. The role of histone deacetylases (HDACs) in human cancer. Mol Oncol 2007; 1(1): 19-25.
[http://dx.doi.org/10.1016/j.molonc.2007.01.001] [PMID: 19383284]

[288] Zhang Q, Wang S, Chen J, Yu Z. Histone Deacetylases (HDACs) Guided Novel Therapies for T-cell lymphomas. Int J Med Sci 2019; 16(3): 424-42.
[http://dx.doi.org/10.7150/ijms.30154] [PMID: 30911277]

[289] Cea M, Cagnetta A, Gobbi M, *et al.* New insights into the treatment of multiple myeloma with histone deacetylase inhibitors. Curr Pharm Des 2013; 19(4): 734-44.
[http://dx.doi.org/10.2174/138161213804581945] [PMID: 23016853]

[290] Ribeiro ML, Reyes-Garau D, Armengol M, Fernández-Serrano M, Roué G. Recent Advances in the Targeting of Epigenetic Regulators in B-Cell Non-Hodgkin Lymphoma. Front Genet 2019; 10: 986. [http://dx.doi.org/10.3389/fgene.2019.00986] [PMID: 31681423]

[291] Stein EM, Garcia-Manero G, Rizzieri DA, *et al.* The DOT1L inhibitor pinometostat reduces H3K79 methylation and has modest clinical activity in adult acute leukemia. Blood 2018; 131(24): 2661-9. [http://dx.doi.org/10.1182/blood-2017-12-818948] [PMID: 29724899]

[292] Xu Y, Vakoc CR. Targeting Cancer Cells with BET Bromodomain Inhibitors. Cold Spring Harb Perspect Med 2017; 7(7): a026674.
[http://dx.doi.org/10.1101/cshperspect.a026674]

SUBJECT INDEX

A

B

C

D

E

M

N

O

P

R

S

T